COPING WITH LIFE CRISES

LIFE CRISES

An Integrated Approach

The Plenum Series on Stress and Coping

Series Editor:
Donald Meichenbaum, *University of Waterloo, Waterloo, Ontario, Canada*

COPING WITH LIFE CRISIS
An Integrated Approach
Edited by Rudolf H. Moos

Forthcoming
DYNAMICS OF STRESS
Physiological, Psychological, and Social Perspectives
Edited by Mortimer H. Appley and Richard A. Trumbull

A Continuation Order Plan is available for this series. A continuation order will bring delivery of each new volume immediately upon publication. Volumes are billed only upon actual shipment. For further information please contact the publisher.

COPING WITH LIFE CRISES

An Integrated Approach

Edited by
Rudolf H. Moos

Stanford University and
Veterans Administration Medical Center
Palo Alto, California

In collaboration with
Jeanne A. Schaefer

PLENUM PRESS • NEW YORK AND LONDON

Library of Congress Cataloging in Publication Data

Main entry under title:

Coping with life crises.

Includes bibliographical references and index.
1. Adjustment (Psychology). 2. Life change events. 3. Stress (Psychology). 4. Developmental psychology. I. Moos, Rudolf H., 1934–   . II. Schaefer, Jeanne A.
BF335.C59   1986   155   85-28149
ISBN 0-306-42133-X
ISBN 0-306-42144-5 (pbk.)

© 1986 Plenum Press, New York
A Division of Plenum Publishing Corporation
233 Spring Street, New York, N.Y. 10013

Printed in the United States of America

Contributors

David Balk, Ph.D., Director of Program Evaluation, La Frontera Center, Tucson, Arizona

Allan Beigel, M.D., Director, Southern Arizona Mental Health Center, Tucson, Arizona

Michael R. Berren, Ph.D., Director of Research and Evaluation, Southern Arizona Mental Health Center, Tucson, Arizona

Lesley Bradbury, Repatriation General Hospital, Sydney, Australia

Leland P. Bradford, deceased, a founder and former director of the National Training Laboratory, Arlington, Virginia

Kathleen B. Bryer, M.F.T., West End Medical Center, Lancaster, Pennsylvania

Ann Wolbert Burgess, R.N., D.N.Sc., Boston City Hospital, Boston, Massachusetts

Paul Chodoff, M.D., Department of Psychiatry, George Washington University, Washington, D.C.

Eve K. Brown Crandall, R.N., M.S., M.N., School of Nursing, Washburn University, Topeka, Kansas

Andre P. Derdeyn, M.D., Division of Child and Adolescent Psychiatry, University of Virginia Medical Center, Charlottesville, Virginia

Esther Elizur, Ph.D., Senior Research Associate, Kibbutz Child and Family Clinic, Derech Haifa 147, Tel Aviv, Israel

Arthur B. Elster, M.D., College of Medicine, University of Utah, Salt Lake City, Utah

Stuart Ghertner, Ph.D., Director of Treatment Support Services, Southern Arizona Mental Health Center, Tucson, Arizona

Lynda Lytle Holmstrom, Ph.D., Department of Sociology, Boston College, Chestnut Hill, Massachusetts

David R. Jones, Colonel, USAFSAM/NGN, Brooks Air Force Base, San Antonio, Texas

Mordecai Kaffman, M.D., Medical Director, Kibbutz Child and Family Clinic, Derech Haifa 147, Tel Aviv, Israel

Kenneth Kressel, Ph.D., University College, Rutgers University, Newark, New Jersey

Robert Jay Lifton, M.D., City University of New York, John Jay College, New York, New York

Katharyn Antle May, D.N.S., R.N., School of Nursing, Department of Family Health Care Nursing, University of California, San Francisco, California

Margaret Shandor Miles, R.N., Ph.D., F.A.A.N., School of Nursing, University of North Carolina, Chapel Hill, North Carolina

Brent C. Miller, Ph.D., Department of Family and Human Development, Utah State University, Logan, Utah

Jean Baker Miller, M.D., Stone Center, Wellesley College, Wellesley, Massachusetts

Rudolf H. Moos, Ph.D., Department of Psychiatry and Behavioral Sciences, Stanford University and Veterans Administration Medical Center, Palo Alto, California

Frank Ochberg, M.D., 4383 Maumee, Okemos, Michigan

Eric Olson, Sven Rinmansgaten, 3 TR/S-11237, Stockholm, Sweden

Susan Panzarine, R.N., Ph.D., School of Nursing, University of Maryland, Baltimore, Maryland

Dorothy Paulay, L.C.S.W., 10401 Wilshire Boulevard, Los Angeles, California

Jane W. Ransom, M.S.W., The Department of Social Services, Charlottesville, Virginia

Beverly Raphael, M.D., Faculty of Medicine, University of Newcastle, New South Wales, Australia

Betsy Robinson, Ph.D., Division of Family and Community Medicine, University of California, San Francisco, California

Jeanne A. Schaefer, R.N., Ph.D., Department of Psychiatry and Behavioral Sciences, Stanford University and Veterans Administration Medical Center, Palo Alto, California

Stephen Schlesinger, M.D., Division of Child and Adolescent Psychiatry, University of Virginia Medical Center, Charlottesville, Virginia

Bruce Singh, Faculty of Medicine, University of Newcastle, New South Wales, Australia

Denise A. Skinner, Ph.D., Department of Human Development, Family Relations, and Community Educational Services, University of Wisconsin-Stout, Menomonie, Wisconsin

Carlos E. Sluzki, M.D., Department of Psychiatry, Berkshire Medical Center, Pittsfield, Massachusetts

Donna L. Sollie, Department of Home and Family Life, Texas Tech University, Lubbock, Texas

Lois M. Tamir, Ph.D., Department of Psychology, University of Texas Health Sciences Center, Dallas, Texas

Lenore C. Terr, M.D., 450 Sutter Street, San Francisco, California

Majda Thurnher, Ph.D., Human Development and Aging Program, University of California, San Francisco, California

Judith S. Wallerstein, Ph.D., Center for the Family in Transition, Corte Madera, California

Robert S. Weiss, Ph.D., Department of Sociology, University of Massachusetts, Boston, Massachusetts

Cindy Cook Williams, R.N., M.S.W., Survey Research Center, Institute for Social Research, Social Environment and Health Program, University of Michigan, Ann Arbor, Michigan

Jacqueline P. Wiseman, Ph.D., Department of Sociology, University of California-San Diego, La Jolla, California

Preface

This book examines new developments in the area of human competence and coping behavior. It sets forth a conceptual framework that considers the interplay between environmental contexts and personal resources and their impact on how individuals cope with life transitions and crises. The selections cover the tasks confronted in varied life crises and describe the coping strategies employed in managing them. The material identifies the long-term effects of such life events as divorce and bereavement as well as the way in which these stressors can promote personal growth and maturity. The book contains a broad selection of recent literature on coping and adaptation, integrative commentaries that provide the background for each of the areas as well as conceptual linkages among them, and an introductory overview that presents a general perspective on human competence and coping. Illustrative case examples are included.

The first part of the book is organized chronologically according to developmental life transitions confronted by many people—from the childhood years through adolescence, career choice and parenthood, divorce and remarriage, middle age and retirement, and death and bereavement. The second part covers unusual life crises and other hazards that typically involve extreme stress such as man-made and natural disasters and terrorism.

The book highlights effective coping behavior among healthy individuals rather than psychological breakdown and psychiatric symptoms. The emphasis is on successful adaptation, the ability to cope with life transitions and crises, and the process by which such crises can promote personal maturity. The selections are drawn from a wide range of disciplines including psychology, psychiatry, gerontology, sociology, political science, and social work. The material reviews recent developments in these areas; most of the articles were published in the 1980s. Thus, the selections cover newly emerging patterns of life transitions, such as dual-career families and the process of remarriage and stepfamily formation after divorce. Other timely topics involve the course of adaptation to terrorism and rape and patterns of long-term adjustment among Vietnam veterans and prisoners of war.

Coping with Life Crises: An Integrated Approach is broadly conceived to meet the needs of a diverse audience. There is a wealth of knowledge about how individuals manage diverse life events, but the information is scattered widely throughout the literature. The selections included here were identified after a search of well over 100 journals and periodicals. The developmental life-cycle focus will make the book useful for undergraduate courses on the psychology of adjustment, personality theory and assessment, abnormal psychology, and life-span psychology. The selections are also appropriate for courses in the health sciences, such as community health, family medicine, psychiatry, and epidemiology, and they should be of interest to students in schools of nursing, social work, and public health.

The concepts and practical ideas are of special value to social workers, family and marital counselors, individual and group therapists, and other counselors who work in mental health care settings. They will also be useful in training programs for school psychologists, vocational counselors, and paraprofessionals who work with individuals who are experiencing varied life crises.

The book has 11 parts. Part I provides an overview of the broad perspectives that have shaped current approaches to the study of life crises: evolutionary theory and an emphasis on behavioral adaptation, psychoanalysis and ideas about personal fulfillment and growth, a life-cycle focus on human development, and observations on the process of coping with extreme life crises. The overview describes the formulation of crisis theory and presents a conceptual approach to understand the development of life crises and transitions and the forces that affect their outcome.

Parts II through VII provide information on developmental

life transitions. Part II covers childhood and the early years and emphasizes the psychological tasks faced by children of divorce and children's bereavement reactions following the death of a parent. Part III considers adolescence and the high school years. The articles address the experience of adolescents in single-parent households, adolescents' grief reactions and changes in self-concept following the death of a sibling, and the coping strategies of adolescent expectant fathers.

Part IV highlights issues of career choice and parenthood. The selections cover dual-career family life-styles and coping behavior, the changing reactions of first-time fathers during their partner's pregnancy, and the issues couples face in managing the first year of parenthood. Part V describes the increasingly common life transitions of divorce and remarriage. The selections highlight the stages of a couple's decision making and coping with divorce, the patterns of psychological recovery after divorce among low-income single parents, and the tasks involved in remarriage and the formation of effective and satisfying step-families.

Part VI considers middle age and retirement. The articles emphasize the tasks and transitions faced by men at midlife, the issues confronted by middle-aged persons (mostly women) who become caregivers for their infirm and elderly parents, and the problems that may arise when individuals retire from active, productive careers and the ways in which these problems can be overcome. Part VII, the last section on life transitions, focuses on death and bereavement. The first selection is a poignant personal account of how a dedicated woman coped with the slow decline and eventual death of her husband after a critical injury sustained in a sudden accident. The other articles cover how bereaved parents search for meaning to help them come to terms with their child's death, and the way in which Amish beliefs and rituals about death and their family and community support systems help survivors adapt.

Parts VIII through XI consider the process of coping with unusual life crises. Part VIII describes special family stressors and emphasizes how women try to adapt to an alcoholic husband and the relative effectiveness of some of their coping styles. We also focus on how relocation and migration create complex problems and conflicts and on how families cope with these issues and adapt to their new home.

Part IX concentrates on man-made and natural disasters. The articles present a typology by which to classify disasters, describe the experiences of residents of a small West Virginia mining town in the aftermath of a devastating flood, and consider how emergency rescue workers and other helpers in a disaster manage the special stressors they experience.

Part X turns to the growing prevalence of violence and terrorism. The selections consider the psychic trauma and process of adaptation among children involved in a school-bus kidnapping, the adaptive strategies employed by rape victims and how they foreshadow eventual patterns of recovery, and the short- and long-term coping styles that lead to adjustment among the survivors of terrorism.

The concluding Part XI considers war and imprisonment. The material describes how Vietnam veterans often are haunted by painful memories and search for a meaningful way to comprehend them, how repatriated prisoners of war conceptualize and try to come to terms with their experience, and the ways in which some individuals managed to survive the Nazi Holocaust.

This book can be used together with a companion volume: *Coping with Physical Illness: New Perspectives* (Plenum, 1984). The companion volume covers coping with selected health crises, such as birth defects and perinatal death, childhood and adult cancer, and chronic physical disability. It also considers the "crisis of treatment" and the coping tasks evoked by the hospital environment and radical new medical procedures as well as the stressors faced by health-care staff and issues elicited by death and the fear of dying. Both books highlight the idea that a life crisis is a critical juncture—a key turning point—during which individuals and their families are uniquely open to the positive influence of professional caregivers.

Jeanne Schaefer helped me compile and organize this book. She searched through an extensive amount of information, assisted in selecting the articles, and co-authored the overview chapter and the commentaries. The work was supported in part by Grant MH28177 from the National Institute of Mental Health, Grants AA02863 and AA06699 from the National Institute on

Alcohol Abuse and Alcoholism, and Veterans Administration Medical and Health Services Research and Development Service research funds. I wish to thank Adrienne Juliano and Pauline Burton who performed word-processing and secretarial tasks involved in the preparation of the book.

This book is for Karen. Fortunately, she has experienced only minor life crises thus far, though she might dispute this judgment. I hope she manages any future problems at least as well as she coped with the "Big C." l like to think that the events and changes she experiences will help her grow and make her life more vital and fulfilling.

RUDOLF H. MOOS

Contents

I

Overview and Perspective

Life Transitions and Crises

A Conceptual Overview

RUDOLF H. MOOS and JEANNE A. SCHAEFER

While awaiting an ambulance after sustaining a grave injury in a sudden, terrifying automobile accident, Jon Krapfl mentally prepared for death. The ambulance attendants wanted him to remain hopeful and hesitated to tell him that his neck was broken. By sharing his intense fear of imminent death, Jon managed to obtain the information he sought. During his lengthy rehabilitation, Jon experienced sharp, insistent pain, felt he was losing his mind due to intrusive hallucinations, found it hard to accept his injury and physical limitations, and ruminated about how his wife and children would confront his disability. Jon faced these issues effectively and eventually returned to his job as a professor of psychology at the University of West Virginia. He later construed the forced review of his life as a "freeing experience" and came to see his ordeal as having "enriched my life."[12]

A middle-aged man who became a quadriplegic after an accident found that his relationship with his wife matured in the ensuing months. He later evaluated the accident as "the best thing that ever happened to me. For the first time in my life, I think I

RUDOLF H. MOOS and JEANNE A. SCHAEFER • Social Ecology Laboratory, Department of Psychiatry and Behavioral Sciences, Stanford University and Veterans Administration Medical Centers, Palo Alto, California 94305.

really know what love means" (p. 13).[5] Even more remarkable is the reaction of a young girl who experienced unthinkable personal horror in a Nazi concentration camp, where she was confronted with abject chaos and the constant threat of imminent death. After liberation, when her captors and torturers themselves were imprisoned, she "felt sorry for the SS men behind the wire. I know what pain and hunger can be, so I used to slip them extra bread through the wire" (p. 409).[7]

How can individuals such as these transcend the most profound life crises, whereas others break down after experiencing seemingly minor stressors? Why do some people seek change and thrive on challenge, whereas others shy away from novel experiences? What are the major adaptive tasks encountered in managing varied life transitions? Are there common phases or stages through which individuals progress as they negotiate a life crisis? Finally, how do personal and environmental resources affect the ultimate psychosocial outcome of a life crisis? We deal with these issues here by considering a range of life transitions and crises and describing how individuals cope with them and their consequences.

Historical Overview

Several broad perspectives have shaped current approaches to understanding life crises: evolutionary theory and an emphasis on behavioral adaptation, psychoanalytic concepts and ideas about personal fulfillment and growth, a focus on human development through the life cycle, and information on the process of coping with severe crises.

Evolutionary Theory and Behavioral Adaptation

Charles Darwin's theory of evolution examined the adaptation of animals (and humans) to their environment. The two central elements in Darwinian theory are variation in the reproduction and inheritance of living organisms and natural selection for the survival of the fittest. The internal factor of variation is seen as positive and creative; it produces the diversity needed for progress. The external factor of natural selection eliminates the harmful or less useful variations and enables those that are beneficial to develop and reproduce. Living organisms exist in the "web of life" in which they "struggle for existence" in a specific environment.

Darwin's ideas shaped the formation of ecology, which is the study of the links between organisms or groups of organisms and their environments. Evolutionary thought and human ecology have focused primarily on communal adaptation. Human beings cannot adapt to their environment alone; they are interdependent and must make collective efforts to survive. Human ecology posits that the formation of social bonds is an essential aspect of humankind's effective transaction with the environment. Communal adaptation is an outgrowth of individual adaptation and of specific coping strategies that serve to contribute to group survival and promote human community.

This orientation led to an emphasis on behavioral problem-solving activities that enhance individual and species survival. The behaviorist tradition initially considered the functional aspects of goal-directed behavior, but more recent approaches have highlighted the role of cognition in effective adaptation. Cognitive behaviorism is concerned with an individual's appraisal of the self and the meaning of an event as well as with behavioral problem-solving skills. A sense of self-efficacy is thought to be an essential coping resource. Successful coping promotes expectations of self-efficacy, which lead to more vigorous and persistent efforts to master new tasks.[1]

Psychoanalytic Concepts and Human Growth Approaches

Sigmund Freud's psychoanalytic perspective set the stage for an intrapsychic and cognitive counterpoint to the evolutionary emphasis on behavioral factors. Freud attributed behavior to the drive to reduce tension by satisfying sexual and aggressive instincts. He believed that ego processes served to resolve conflicts between an individual's impulses and the constraints of external reality. In essence, their function is to reduce tension by enabling the individual to express sexual and aggressive impulses indirectly without recognizing their "true" intent. These ego processes are cognitive mechanisms (though their expression may involve behavioral components) whose main functions are defensive (reality distorting) and emotion focused (oriented toward tension reduction).

The neo-Freudian ego psychologists objected to these ideas. They posited a "conflict-free ego sphere" with "autonomous" energy that fueled reality-oriented processes such as attention and perception. Moreover, the exercise of ego functions such as cognition and memory is rewarding in its own right. Although there is a strong drive to reduce excessive tension, most individuals search for novelty and excitement and try to master their environment. They possess such aspects of competence motivation as curiosity and an exploratory drive, a need for new and varied stimulation ("stimulus hunger"), and a sense of agency and of being in control of their life.

These ideas formed the basis for a new set of growth or fulfillment theories of human development. For example, Carl Rogers believes that individuals try to actualize or develop their capacities in ways that serve to maintain life and promote growth. Abraham Maslow has distinguished between *deficiency* and *growth motivation*. Deficiency motivation reflects a drive to survive and aims to decrease tension arising from such needs as hunger and thirst. In contrast, growth motivation reflects an orientation toward self-actualization and entails the urge to enrich one's experience and expand one's horizons. According to Maslow, mature, healthy persons perceive reality accurately, are solution-centered and spontaneous in behavior, and have a strong social interest, a genuine desire to help others, and a broad perspective on life.

Developmental Life-Cycle Approaches

Psychoanalytic theorists posited that life events in infancy strongly affect or even determine adult personality. But information about the growth of ego functions and normal patterns of maturation shows that early life events do not necessarily foreshadow an individual's character or pattern of reaction to crises and transitions. In addition to highlighting the processes of defense and coping, psychoanalysis and ego psychology thus provided the basis for developmental approaches that consider the gradual acquisition of personal resources over the life span.

Erik Erikson[8] described eight life stages, each of which encompasses a new challenge or "crisis" that must be negotiated successfully in order for an individual to cope adequately with the next stage. Personal coping resources (such as the formation of trust and ego integrity) "accrued" during the adolescent and young-adult years are integrated into the self-concept and shape the process of coping in adulthood and old age. Adequate resolution of the issues that occur at one stage in the life cycle leave a legacy of coping resources that can help to resolve subsequent crises.

Stage models such as Erikson's often are depicted as a spiral staircase; failure to attain one landing implies failure to attain the next. According to Neugarten,[21] however, adulthood is not usually composed of an invariant sequence of stages that occur at specific chronological ages. Most people do expect certain life events to occur at particular times, and they develop a mental clock stipulating whether they are "on time" or "off time." Events that occur on time can be anticipated, rehearsed, and managed without taxing individuals' coping capacity or shattering their sense of continuity. But our idea of social timing has changed dramatically over the past two decades. The rhythm of the life cycle is much more fluid as more men and women are divorcing and remarrying, children are reared in different households, and more middle-aged persons go back to college or begin a new family. The increasing flexibility of adulthood has highlighted the transitions of middle and old age and how individuals cope with them.[14]

Coping with Extreme Crises

In-depth studies of adaptation under extreme conditions have sparked renewed interest in human competence and coping. The most compelling accounts are of the harrowing conditions in the Nazi concentration camps of World War II. The camps reflected a situation of degradation comparable to the most hellish circumstances ever endured by humankind. But even under these conditions, many inmates managed to salvage some control over their fate (see Part XI). For example, an extensive underground organization in Camp Buchenwald was able to monitor inmates' work assignments and hide and protect valuable members of the underground. The inmates of Camp Treblinka staged a revolution against overwhelming odds. Such feats raise a compelling question: How can anyone face such suffering and the ever-present threat of painful death and yet survive psychologically to "bear witness" about the experience in objective and even creative terms?

Other work in this vein has considered such crises as parental and sibling death (see Parts II and III), disasters such as a flood or tornado (Part IX), being the victim of rape or kidnapping (Part X), and long-term internment in a prisoner of war camp (Part XI). Similar studies have examined how individuals adapt to serious illness or injury and face life-threatening surgery and other painful medical treatment.[19] In general, such studies highlight the adaptive aspects of individual and group coping instead of the formation of "neurotic" symptoms and psychopathology. The surprising fact is that many persons cope effectively with crises of such magnitude.

Another empirical trend grew from an emphasis on life changes as predictors of health and illness. A well-known psychiatrist, Adolph Meyer, noted the importance of such events as school entrance, graduation, job changes or failures, family births and deaths, migration, and the like. These life events were thought to foreshadow the development of symptoms and disease. Subsequently, Holmes and his colleagues used the Meyerian perspective to study life events and their connections to the onset and progression of illness. They constructed an assessment procedure that consists of different life events scaled according to the amount of "readjustment" they presumably require; for instance, death of a spouse (100 life-change units), divorce (73 units), and retirement (45 units).

Holmes and his associates found that life changes of greater magnitude (or life crises) carried a higher chance of an associated illness or disease. But the link between life stressors and illness actually is quite modest, because most persons who experience life crises remain healthy. This fact has fueled the search for "resistance resources" (such as coping skills and social support) that enable an individual to prevent stress or to manage it effectively (for an overview of this area, see Lazarus & Folkman[13]).

Crisis Theory

The historical trends we have described shaped the formation of crisis theory, which is concerned with how individuals manage major life transitions and crises. The theory provides a conceptual framework for preventive mental health care and for understanding severe life crises. The fundamental ideas were developed by Erich Lindemann who described the process of grief and mourning and the role of community caretakers in helping bereaved family members cope with the loss of their loved ones.[16] Combined with Erikson's formulation of "developmental crises" at transition points in the life cycle, these ideas paved the way for the outgrowth of crisis theory.[4]

Crisis theory deals with the impact of disruptions on established patterns of personal and social identity. Similar to the requirement for physiological homeostasis, individuals have a need for social and psychological equilibrium. When people encounter an event that upsets their characteristic patterns of thought and behavior, they employ habitual problem-solving strategies until a balance is restored. A crisis is a situation that is so novel or major that habitual responses are insufficient; it leads to a state of turbulence typically accompanied by heightened fear, anger, or guilt. Because a person cannot remain in a state of disequilibrium, a crisis is necessarily self-limited. Even though it may be temporary, some resolution must be found. The new balance may be a healthy adaptation that promotes personal growth or a maladaptive response that foreshadows psychological problems. Thus, a crisis is a transition or turning point that has profound implications for an individual's adaptation and ability to meet future crises.

Crisis theory has focused more heavily on the harmful or catabolic than on the positive or anabolic influence of life events. In fact, life transitions and crises often provide an essential condition for psychological development. Stressful life episodes may enrich a person's beliefs and values by making it necessary to assimilate new experiences. This process can promote cognitive integration and stimulate personal growth that helps to manage the problematic aspects of the new situation. In this view, life crises impel the development of new cognitive and personal skills primarily because such skills are needed for effective adaptation.[18]

A Guiding Conceptual Framework

We have evolved a framework to help understand the development and outcome of normative transitions and life crises. Through a cognitive appraisal of its significance, a crisis sets forth basic adaptive tasks to which varied coping skills can be applied. The individual's appraisal, task definition, and selection and effectiveness of coping skills are influenced by three sets of factors: demographic and personal characteristics, aspects of the transition or the crisis itself, and features of the physical and social environments. These sets of factors jointly affect the resolution of the initial phase of the crisis; this resolution can alter all three sets and change the ultimate outcome. It is important to recognize that family members and friends are directly or indirectly affected by an event, encounter many of the same or closely related adaptive tasks, and use the same kinds of coping skills (for an application of the framework to the crisis of physical illness, see Moos[19]).

Major Adaptive Tasks

Five major sets of tasks are encountered in managing a life transition or crisis (see Table 1).

The first set of tasks is to *establish the meaning and understand the personal significance of the situation*. This is an ongoing issue to which the individual will return again and again. After a crisis, there typically is an initial reaction of shock and confusion and then a slow dawning awareness of the reality of the event. An individual then tries to assimilate the meaning of each aspect of a crisis as it and its aftermath unfold. In a divorce, for example, a child must acknowledge the reality of the marital rupture and try

Table 1. Major Sets of Adaptive Tasks

1. Establish the meaning and understand the personal significance of the situation
2. Confront reality and respond to the requirements of the external situation
3. Sustain relationships with family members and friends as well as with other individuals who may be helpful in resolving the crisis and its aftermath
4. Maintain a reasonable emotional balance by managing upsetting feelings aroused by the situation
5. Preserve a satisfactory self-image and maintain a sense of competence and mastery

to understand its immediate consequences. At a later point, the child needs to accept the loss of the predivorce family and the permanence of the divorce (see Chapter 2). When a death occurs, the loss must be accepted intellectually and be somehow explained. Victims of a disaster must appraise their personal losses and try to imbue their experience and the catastrophe itself with an acceptable meaning (see Chapter 22).

The second set of tasks entails *confronting reality and responding to the requirements of the external situation.* During a separation or divorce, for example, there are such tasks as restructuring family roles, accommodating to less income, finding a job or developing new skills to make one more employable, and coping with the overload of being a single parent. After a death, the survivor faces the task of planning a funeral or memorial service and making decisions about the disposition of the body by burial or cremation; longer term tasks may entail managing a household by oneself and learning to handle financial and other matters that usually were taken care of by a spouse. Survivors of a disaster must face the immediate danger, see to the security of their families, find temporary shelter, and then begin to rebuild their lives by tackling such tasks as applying for low-cost loans and dealing with the government bureaucracy.

The third set of tasks is to *sustain relationships with family members and friends as well as with other individuals who may be helpful in resolving the crisis and its aftermath.* Experiencing a life crisis can make it hard to keep communication lines open and to accept comfort and support at the very time when these are most essential. Close personal relationships can help individuals obtain information necessary to make wise decisions, find emotional support for them, and secure reassurance about the problems they face. These tasks are especially difficult for children of divorce because they must maintain their ability to form trusting relationships even though they have experienced the anger and grief that often follow the dissolution of such relationships. A divorced adult must be able to develop new social attachments and, when considering remarriage, invest in new family members as primary sources of emotional support (see Part V).

In many crisis situations, this set of tasks also entails forming adequate relationships with "community caretakers" such as medical and other health-care staff (after a physical illness or injury), police and law enforcement officials (in the case of an assault or violent crime), and counselors and mental health professionals (in the case of bereavement or family violence). As noted earlier, Jon Krapfl's self-disclosure enabled him to establish a bond with his ambulance attendants that prompted them to explain honestly the extent of his injury and probable prognosis.[12] When a hostage can form such a bond, it may cause terrorists to refrain from killing him or her (see Chapter 26).

The fourth category of tasks entails *preserving a reasonable emotional balance by managing upsetting feelings aroused by the situation.* Life crises arouse many powerful emotions, such as a sense of failure and self-blame for a divorce or an accidental death, tension and fear that are linked to the uncertainty of an outcome, alienation that may arise from being the victim of an assault, and anger and grief in the face of a sudden, unexpected death. An important aspect of this set of tasks is for the individual to maintain some hope even when its scope is sharply limited by circumstances. The ability to sustain hope can be a matter of survival because prisoners of war and those in concentration camps who hold out no chance of eventual escape or release are likely to become depressed and apathetic and to die in captivity (see Part XI).

The fifth and closely linked set of tasks consists of *preserving a satisfactory self-image and maintaining a sense of competence and mastery.* For instance, individuals who have experienced a divorce may face a lack of self-confidence about their ability to sustain relationships and establish an independent life-style. Moreover, changes in an individual's life circumstances must be blended into a revised self-image. This "identity crisis" may require a shift in personal values and behavior as, for example, when a divorced or widowed homemaker resumes her education and obtains a full-time job. Some persons who have surmounted a crisis develop a new sense of purpose by helping others adjust to similar crises, as when a rape victim volunteers at a rape crisis center. Overall, it is important to find a balance between accepting help and taking an active and responsible part in controlling the direction of one's life.

These five groups of tasks generally are encountered in each life transition or crisis, but their relative importance varies depending on the personal characteristics of the individual, the nature of the stressor, and the unique set of circumstances. Thus, for example, it is harder to establish the meaning of a sudden, untimely death of a child than of the expected death of an older person. It may be virtually impossible for a father to preserve his emotional balance after he has accidentally killed his son in a "preventable" automobile mishap. The special trauma experienced by childhood victims of incest, in which a protective parental relationship is subverted into an exploitive one, makes the formation of new intimate social bonds especially hard. Because problems that affect one member of a family also touch the others, these five sets of tasks will be encountered by family members and friends as well as individuals who themselves are in a crisis.

Major Types of Coping Skills

We now offer an overview of the major sets of coping skills that are employed to deal with the adaptive tasks just described. These skills may be used individually, consecutively, or more likely in various combinations. Specific coping strategies are not inherently adaptive or maladaptive. Skills that are effective in one situation may not be in another. Skills that may be beneficial, given moderate or temporary use, may be harmful if relied upon exclusively. The word *skill* underscores the positive aspects of coping and depicts coping as an ability that can be taught and used flexibly as the situation requires.

Coping skills can be organized into three domains according to their primary focus.[20] *Appraisal-focused coping* entails attempts to understand and find a pattern of meaning in a crisis. The process of appraisal and reappraisal is a form of coping in that it serves to modify the meaning and comprehend the threat aroused by a situation. *Problem-focused coping* seeks to confront the reality of a crisis and its aftermath by dealing with the tangible consequences and trying to construct a more satisfying situation. *Emotion-focused coping* aims to manage the feelings provoked by a crisis and to maintain affective equilibrium. Thus, coping skills can focus on the meaning, the practical aspects, or the emotions linked to a crisis. We use these ideas to categorize coping responses into nine types (see Table 2).

1. *Logical analysis and mental preparation.* This set of skills covers paying attention to one aspect of the crisis at a time, breaking a seemingly overwhelming problem into small, potentially manageable bits, drawing on past experiences, and mentally rehearsing alternative actions and their probable consequences. Such skills are commonly used to prepare for unfamiliar experiences such as testifying in court or visiting a morgue to identify a dead person. Trying to bolster one's confidence by reminding oneself of prior successes in facing difficult problems fits into this category. On a broader scale, it also encompasses the anticipatory mourning process in which an expected death or other loss is acknowledged

Table 2. Major Types of Coping Skills

Appraisal-focused coping
   Logical analysis and mental preparation
   Cognitive redefinition
   Cognitive avoidance or denial
Problem-focused coping
   Seeking information and support
   Taking problem-solving action
   Identifying alternative rewards
Emotion-focused coping
   Affective regulation
   Emotional discharge
   Resigned acceptance

beforehand as well as the review of one's prior relationship and experiences with an individual who has died.

When life's happenings seem capricious and uncontrollable, as with a sudden death or a serious disaster, it often is easier to manage if one can find a general purpose or pattern of meaning in the course of events. Efforts in this direction constitute a related type of coping skill. Belief in a divine purpose or in the general goodness of a divine spirit may serve as consolation or as encouragement to do one's best to deal with the difficulties one encounters. Putting an experience into a long-term perspective (with or without religious orientation) often makes individual events more tolerable.

2. *Cognitive redefinition.* This category covers cognitive strategies by which an individual accepts the basic reality of a situation but restructures it to find something favorable. Such strategies include reminding oneself that things could be worse, thinking of oneself as well off in comparison to other people, altering values and priorities in line with changing reality, and concentrating on something good that might grow out of a crisis. For instance, individuals who have experienced a natural disaster may compare themselves to others who have more serious problems, whereas some parents come to see the experience of raising a handicapped child as being of positive value in that the suffering brought them closer together and helped them redirect their life.

Taylor and her colleagues[27] have described five ways in which individuals may selectively enhance themselves and their crisis situation. Individuals can compare themselves with others who are less fortunate, focus on personal attributes that make them appear advantaged, create hypothetical situations that are worse than those they experienced (such as when a rape victim feels that she might have been killed), identify normative standards of adjustment that make their own adjustment appear exceptional, and construe benefits from the victimizing event (such as believing that it fostered self-esteem or personal maturity). Such selective perceptions can minimize the aversive aspects of stressful events and help promote adjustment.

3. *Cognitive avoidance or denial.* This category encompasses an array of skills aimed at denying or minimizing the seriousness of a

crisis. These may be directed at the crisis itself, as when a widow initially maintains that her husband "cannot be dead and will return," or when adolescent fathers-to-be refuse to acknowledge that the baby will change their life. They also can involve the immediate consequences of an event, such as the denial and bland affect that often occur right after a natural disaster. Once the event is accepted, they may be aimed at its long-term significance, as when the survivors of a disaster believe that their lives will return to normal quickly. Another example entails conscious suppression, as when a woman tries to put the memory of being raped or abused out of her mind. These skills tend to be described as "defensive mechanisms" because they are self-protective responses to stress. This term does not convey their constructive value; they can temporarily rescue an individual from being overwhelmed or provide the time needed to garner other personal coping resources.

4. *Seeking information and support.* This set of skills covers obtaining information about the crisis and alternate courses of action and their probable outcome. Women who have been assaulted seek information about their responsibility (initially blaming themselves, for example, for not having attended to early warning signs or not following usual "safety rules"), about hospital and police procedures, and about ways of coming to terms with their experience. Learning about the causes of family violence can mitigate a sense of guilt or failure felt by the victim of spouse or child abuse. These skills often are used in combination with logical analysis as individuals try to restore a sense of control by learning about the demands that might be made on them and mentally preparing themselves to overcome expected problems by thinking through the steps involved.

A related group of coping skills concerns the ability to seek support and reassurance from family, friends, and other helpful persons in the community. Such help can be a valuable source of strength in facing difficult times, but individuals must deal with the tension between seeking comfort and wanting to remain self-reliant. Persons who keep their feelings "bottled up" or who withdraw from social interaction cut themselves off from help of this type. Many persons obtain support by joining special groups such as national self-help organizations or smaller ad hoc groups for individuals undergoing specific crises. These groups can provide a type of aid that is less available from alternate sources, such as information about how persons in a similar situation handle their predicament.

5. *Taking problem-solving action.* This array of skills involves taking concrete action to deal directly with a crisis or its aftermath. In family and parental transitions, for example, individuals may make tentative plans on a day-to-day basis, structure and share household tasks, learn how to bargain or compromise with their spouse, try to obtain flexible jobs and job-sharing arrangements, and cope with overload by establishing priorities and compartmentalizing their work and family roles (see Part IV). Survivors of a disaster use such active behavioral strategies as repairing or rebuilding their homes, helping to reinstitute essential local services, cleaning and restoring the community, and perhaps (when the disaster is man-made) seeking redress by participating in legal action (see Part IX). Such accomplishments can recreate a sense of competence and self-esteem at a time when opportunities for effective action may be scarce. Individuals take pride in assertive coping strategies; friends and relatives find relief in offering concrete help.

6. *Pursuing alternate rewards.* These skills encompass attempts to replace the losses involved in certain transitions and crises by changing one's activities and creating new sources of satisfaction. Such coping responses entail making short-range plans to deal with reality issues and setting concrete limited goals. Many ongoing stressors, such as the enforced separation that occurs when a husband is a prisoner of war, cannot be dealt with directly. Nevertheless, most of the coping strategies adopted by wives in this situation (such as trying to maintain family integrity and establishing independence by obtaining a job or participating in community activities) are problem-focused in that they involve changing the self or the environment to meet the demands of the crisis situation.

Other examples include the decision to redirect one's energy toward work or school after the sudden death of a child, or to actively help fellow "sufferers" by sharing information or raising funds. One effective way to come to terms with an unalterable situation is to assist other individuals to negotiate a similar crisis or transition. In this way, individuals who have experienced an event leave a legacy of knowledge and bolster their self-esteem. Some persons pursue this line of coping energetically and give lectures, write books, or take legal and political action in an effort to change public attitudes (such as by developing crisis services for rape victims or special educational programs for handicapped children).

7. *Affective regulation*. These skills cover efforts to maintain hope and control one's emotions when dealing with a distressing situation. This occurs when an individual reacts to a disaster or hostage situation calmly rather than showing terror or dismay, or when bereaved individuals discuss their situation with an air of detachment. Other ways to regulate affect are tolerating ambiguity and withholding immediate action, experiencing and working through one's feelings, and maintaining a sense of pride and keeping a "stiff upper lip." The strategy of "progressive desensitization," whereby individuals gradually "expose" themselves to aspects of the stressor and dull their sensitivity to their own and others' reactions, falls within this category. For instance, a widow may progress from avoiding contact with anything that reminds her of her deceased husband to being able to glance at his picture, and, eventually, to being able to sort out his clothes and other personal effects.

8. *Emotional discharge*. This diverse array of responses includes openly venting one's feelings of anger and despair, crying or screaming in protest at news of a fateful prognosis or the sudden death of a loved one, and using jokes and gallows humor to help allay constant strain. It also includes "acting out" by not complying with social norms as well as behavior that may temporarily reduce tension, such as when an adolescent girl goes on eating binges or engages in promiscuous sexual activity after the death of her father. Other examples of tension-reduction strategies include drinking and smoking more, taking tranquilizers and other medications, and directing severe anger or criticism at individuals who are trying to be helpful, such as police investigating an assault or a friend assisting with practical tasks after a spouse's death. Such behaviors may involve a temporary failure of affective regulation, but we categorize them separately because

many individuals alternate between emotional control and emotional discharge.

9. *Resigned acceptance.* This category covers coming to terms with a situation and accepting it as it is, deciding that the basic circumstances cannot be altered, and submitting to "certain" fate. For instance, when the death of an individual seems inevitable, a conscious decision to accept the situation helps to promote disengagement and mitigate distress. Strategies that fall into this category include concluding that nothing can be done to change things (in regard to a natural disaster or enforced migration, for example), trying to avoid the situation (staying away from an alcoholic husband and keeping the children out of his way), and behavioral withdrawal (such as a death row inmate remaining in his cell even at exercise and mealtimes). In the face of seemingly overwhelming demands, some individuals develop a fatalistic belief in which life is seen as unpredictable and disaster as inevitable. Such a resigned acceptance of fate does not necessarily preclude problem-solving activities; it simply helps individuals accept tragedy when it occurs.

These nine categories cover the most common types of coping skills employed to deal with life change. Such skills are seldom used singly or exclusively. An individual may deny or minimize the seriousness of a crisis while talking to a family member, seek relevant information from a lawyer or other community helper, request reassurance or emotional support from a friend, and so on. A life crisis typically presents a set of related tasks and requires a combination or sequence of coping skills.

General Determinants of Outcome

Why does one person respond differently than another to a life crisis or transition? What factors influence the appraisal of an event, the nature of specific tasks, and the choice and progression of coping strategies? The relevant determinants fall into three categories: demographic and personal factors, event-related factors, and features of the physical and social environments (see Figure 1). For instance, the nature and difficulty of adaptive tasks are affected by aspects of the event (it is especially hard to fathom

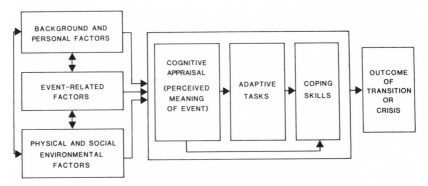

Figure 1. A conceptual model for understanding life crises and transitions.

the meaning of an untimely event such as the sudden death of a child), by personal factors (a divorced woman with little income faces the task of finding a suitable job), and by environmental factors (in a high-crime area a victim of assault may find it hard to protect himself or herself). In turn, the coping efforts stimulated by these tasks can change personal factors (a person may seek and obtain information that changes her or his attitudes), environmental factors (a burglary victim may place locks on windows and doors), and event-related factors (learning how to empathize with a spouse's point of view may change the likelihood that a separation will be followed by divorce).

Demographic and Personal Factors. Demographic and personal factors include age, gender, ethnicity, and socioeconomic status as well as cognitive and emotional maturity, ego strength and self-confidence, philosophical or religious commitments, and prior crisis and coping experiences. These factors help to define psychosocial crises as well as to resolve them. For instance, men may be especially threatened by the change of role that accompanies the death of a spouse because, in comparison to women, they are less likely to be competent at household tasks. Conversely, men may cope better with a disaster, especially when they can employ active coping behavior such as cleaning and restoring a flooded home.

There also are strong age-related variations in how events are appraised and managed. In reaction to a separation or divorce, for example, preschool and kindergarten children are likely to feel bewildered and to engage in fantasy denial, whereas young school-age children tend to feel responsible and try to reconcile their parents. Older school-age children actively try to understand the situation and master their upsetting feelings by courage and bravado, reaching out to others for support or defensively engaging in constant activity. Adolescents are most likely to experience a loss of family stability and to suffer from the need to achieve self-direction and maturity too quickly.[31]

More generally, life events are imbued with meaning by relatively stable features of personality and by an individual's unique set of obligations and beliefs. Patterns of commitment help to define which events are stressful, whereas beliefs about personal control, religion, and the role of fate or chance in human affairs alter the appraisal of an event and the choice of coping strategies. Personal strength and resiliency typically predict positive outcomes of stress, but individuals who feel invulnerable may have a hard time when their illusions are shattered due to a natural disaster or an assault.[22]

Event-Related Factors. These factors encompass the characteristics of life transitions and crises such as the type and context of an event. Rees and Smyer[24] have identified four types of events: biological (such as illness and death), personal/psychological (such as getting married), physical/environmental (such as being exposed to a disaster), and social/cultural (such as adopting a child). Other aspects of life events include their focus (self or other), suddenness of onset or predictability, controllability, likelihood of occurrence, and extent or pervasiveness (the diversity of life areas that may be affected).

In regard to the type of stressor, the characteristics of divorce and bereavement are quite different. The reality of death is easier to acknowledge because death usually has an identifiable calendar date and because the loss is final and the lost person irretrievable. By contrast, divorce often is preceded by several separations and thus appears (especially to a child) to be modifiable or reversible. The fact that divorce is always a voluntary decision for one of the partners, however, may heighten the plight for the other partner and the children. Moreover, the spouse and child of divorce often travel a lonely road and must actively seek out help. In contrast, death is a universal experience and typically elicits considerable support.[30]

Such variations among stressors define the nature of the tasks individuals and their family members face and, consequently, their adaptive responses. Events over which individuals have some control are more likely to elicit problem-solving coping strategies, whereas those that are essentially uncontrollable tend to evoke cognitive and emotion-focused responses. In comparison to natural disasters, for instance, technological mishaps may elicit more focused anger and action because a specific individual or group seems to be responsible (see Part IX). When an event or its aftermath cannot be changed, individuals will try to alter the meaning of the situation and their feelings about it. Thus, endemic intractable stressors, such as unemployment, noise, and air pollution, are likely to lead to passive adaptation and gradual retrenchment and resignation.

Social and Physical Environmental Factors. Aspects of the social and physical environments affect the adaptive tasks individuals and their families face and the choice and outcome of the coping skills they use. The human environment encompasses the relationships of individuals and their families and the support and expectations of the wider community. Social cohesion is linked to better adaptation to such life transitions as becoming a parent, retirement, and aging as well as to more positive outcomes of crises such as bereavement, rape, and imprisonment (see Parts VII, X, and XI). Conversely, close social bonds sometimes make it more difficult to transcend a life crisis. In adjusting to the death of a child, for instance, more cohesive families may elicit stronger feelings of depression, because the death is seen as more of a loss. Threats to family stability are not distressing in families that lack cohesion because the family is not as important a source of security.

From a broader perspective, adaptation can be fostered by the cooperative efforts of the community. Such institutional resources as the provision of child-care centers provide valuable help for working parents with young children. Community self-help organizations serve as a focus for people who share a common concern and can furnish information, guidance, and hope in dealing with a community disaster. Conversely, macrosocial or contextual factors may make adaptation more difficult. Refugees who settle in communities in which unemployment is high are more likely to have to compete for jobs and to be unemployed or underemployed. The lack of an established ethnic community on which to draw for guidance and support makes the plight of a refugee more severe. Overall, such contextual factors can alter the appraisal of threat as well as the choice, sequence, and relative effectiveness of coping skills.

Preventive Intervention and Treatment

Life transitions and crises confront a person with a critical juncture or turning point. Personal growth and an expanded repertoire of coping skills often follow the successful resolution of a crisis. But failure to manage a situation effectively may foreshadow impaired adjustment and problems in handling future transitions and crises.

According to crisis theory, an individual is especially receptive to outside influence in a time of flux. Such accessibility offers family and friends as well as counselors and psychotherapists a special opportunity to exert a constructive impact. Caregivers who are mindful of the typical issues that arise in normative transitions and prevalent crises can prepare individuals and their families for the experiences they are likely to encounter and help them to expand their coping resources and repertoires. More generally, prevention programs can teach individuals to recognize and reduce sources of stress and help them to strengthen their personal competence, coping skills, and social resources.[6] (For an overview of prevention programs, see Heller and associates.[11])

Our conceptual framework emphasizes that individuals' cognitive appraisal, definition of adaptive tasks, and selection of coping skills are influenced by the person, by aspects of the transition or crisis, and by the environment (see Figure 1). This framework is useful for identifying foci for prevention programs. Interventions can be directed at one or more of these sets of factors. For example, programs may focus on lessening the prevalence of a stressor, helping individuals avoid conditions that lead to stress, changing the appraisal of a transition or crisis, or providing information to alert individuals to the tasks they will confront and to potential coping strategies for managing them.

For the most part, preventive interventions have focused on enhancing high-risk individuals' coping skills and social resources. Adolescents who are parents are an especially vulnerable group. They must manage the demands of parenting while struggling with the normal developmental tasks of adolescence (see Chapter 6). The Parent-to-Parent Program[10] in rural Vermont is an example of a community-based intervention for this high-risk group. Trained community volunteers make home visits on a long-term basis and work with the young parents to enhance their child-rearing, interpersonal, and financial skills. Group meetings with other adolescent parents provide social contact and an opportunity to share experiences. The program has a positive impact on the adolescents' parenting skills in that they learn more about their children's needs and abilities. Simultaneously, many parents make progress themselves by returning to high school, getting vocational training, working, and making new friends.

The divorcing family provides another fertile area for preventive interventions. Emotional upheavals, losses, and painful role changes reverberate through the family, touching children as well as adults (Chapters 2 and 10). Bloom and his associates[2,3] initiated a preventive intervention program for newly separated adults. This program provided support and augmented competencies via study groups on socialization, parenting, employment and career planning, legal and financial matters, and housing. Follow-up revealed that program participants adjusted better psychologically and reported fewer problems than members of a control group. Even 4 years later, the positive effects of the intervention continued to be evident. Another primary prevention program, the Divorce Adjustment Project, is composed of school-based children's support groups that teach interpersonal skills and provide emotional support and community-based support groups that help single parents improve their parenting skills, learn how to deal with their feelings, and become more assertive. The program improved parental adjustment and increased children's positive self-concept and adaptive social skills.[26]

Growing numbers of self-help groups and lay helper programs are key resources that serve a preventive function for those who are divorced, have become stepparents, or are bereaved or victimized. For example, Mary Vachon and her associates[28] established a program in which recent widows were contacted by widows who had resolved their grief and who had been trained as supportive counselors. The widow contacts arranged group meetings and made themselves available for one-to-one support for as long as the new widows needed it. Compared to a control group, widows who received this self-help intervention progressed more rapidly toward good adaptation.

In many instances, persons experiencing a crisis find that their own coping is facilitated by acting as a lay helper or a counselor in self-help groups (for an overview of self-help groups, see Lieberman, Borman, & associates[15]). Helping others provides a sense of purpose and is a way for the bereaved and victimized to find meaning in their suffering. Self-help groups also may be vehicles for emotion- and problem-focused coping on an individual or a community level. A Homeowner's Association[9] provided victims of the toxic chemical disaster at Love Canal with a way to address community concerns, diffuse angry feelings, and provide residents a community power base. Association members engaged in problem-solving actions such as conducting a health survey that provided evidence of health risks outside the original evacuation area. As a result, members were able to persuade the authorities to evacuate additional residents.

The suddenness of massive disasters requires that caregivers be prepared to mobilize teams of professionals to serve large numbers of people in a stricken community. The primary prevention program established by Beverly Raphael[23] in the wake of a major rail disaster is one example of such an effort. Immediately after the accident, counselors were available to provide support to distraught relatives waiting at the morgue to identify the bodies of their loved ones. Special counseling programs were established for high-risk families who were identified as having inadequate support networks, multiple crises, or preexisting relationship problems with the victim, or whose loved one's death involved traumatic circumstances. A team of consultants provided services to those who worked with the families of the victims, and debriefing sessions were held for the rescue teams. Finally, the mass media were used to educate people in the community about bereavement reactions and ways to handle them. Those who received bereavement counseling tended to do better than those who did not.[25]

Despite the dire need of people facing certain devastating

crises, caregivers must understand that their help may be declined. In an attempt to cope with a disaster, survivors may minimize its impact and try to put painful experiences behind them. They reject help from professionals because the thoughts and memories they are trying valiantly to suppress surface when they discuss their experiences. In other instances, caregivers may find that access to survivors of a disaster is limited by family, friends, or other professionals who form a "trauma membrane" to protect survivors from further stress.[17] Caregivers may also be the unwitting target of anger aroused by the victims' plight. For example, victims of devastating bushfires in Australia expressed ambivalence toward outside helpers. Although they were grateful for offers of food and shelter, they resented their forced dependence and loss of status. Victims' directed their pent-up anger at the helpers, and blamed them for not being able to meet all of their needs.[29]

The success of prevention programs is closely linked to the caregivers' ability to be responsive to the needs of those in crisis. The individuals who worked with victims of the Australian bushfires displayed the sensitivity that is essential for effective intervention. Outreach workers used the media and pamphlets to provide information about the range of reactions to disaster. This helped reassure victims who were engulfed in powerful emotions that made them wonder if they were crazy. Victims needed to talk about their experiences. The helpers listened and encouraged the expression of troubling feelings, as when a woman talked of her guilt for having a good time in town while, unknown to her, neighbors rescued her children from the sweeping fire. Victims stayed away from centers offering mental health services because seeking help was an admission of their failure to cope and evidence of their lack of control. Outreach workers were sensitive to this reaction and responded by contacting everyone in the community, thereby avoiding the problem of singling out certain people who were experiencing special problems.[29]

Caregivers need to be conversant with knowledge of coping tasks and skills and to be sensitive to people's emotional reactions and needs. Coupled with their own empathy and understanding of crisis situations, this information can help them diffuse the negative impact of life's crises and nurture the potential for growth intrinsic in such situations.

References

1. Bandura, A. Self-efficacy mechanism in human agency. *American Psychologist*, 1982, *37*, 122–147.
2. Bloom, B. L., Hodges, W. F., & Caldwell, R. A. A preventive intervention program for the newly separated: Initial evaluations. *American Journal of Community Psychology*, 1982, *10*, 251–264.
3. Bloom, B. L., Hodges, W. F., Kern, M. B., & McFaddin, S. C. A preventive intervention program for the newly separated: Final evaluations. *American Journal of Orthopsychiatry*, 1985, *55*, 9–26.
4. Caplan, G. *Principles of preventive psychiatry*. New York: Basic Books, 1964.
5. Cassem, N. Bereavement as indispensable for growth. In N. B. Schoenberg & Others (Eds.), *Bereavement: Its psychosocial aspects*. New York: Columbia University Press, 1975.
6. Cowen, E. L. Primary prevention in mental health: Past, present, and future. In R. D. Felner, L. A. Jason, J. N. Moritsugu, & S. S. Farber (Eds.), *Preventive psychology: Theory, research and practice*. New York: Pergamon Press, 1983.
7. Dimsdale, J. Coping—every man's war. *American Journal of Psychotherapy*, 1978, *32*, 402–413.
8. Erikson, E. H. *Childhood and society* (2nd ed.). New York: Norton, 1963.
9. Gibbs, L. M. Community response to an emergency situation: Psychological destruction and the Love Canal. *American Journal of Community Psychology*, 1983, *11*, 116–125.
10. Halpern, R., & Covey, L. Community support for adolescent parents and their children: The Parent-to-Parent Program in Vermont. *Journal of Primary Prevention*, 1983, *3*, 160–173.
11. Heller, K., Price, R. H., Reinharz, S., Riger, S., & Wandersman, A. *Psychology and community change: Challenges of the future* (2nd ed.). Homewood, Il.: Dorsey, 1984.
12. Krapfl, J. Traumatic injury in mid-life. In E. Callahan & K. McCluskey (Eds.), *Life span developmental psychology: Non-normative life events*. New York: Academic Press, 1983.
13. Lazarus, R., & Folkman, S. *Stress, appraisal, and coping*. New York: Springer, 1984.
14. Levinson, D. The mid-life transition: A period in adult psychosocial development. *Psychiatry*, 1977, *40*, 99–112.
15. Lieberman, M. A., Borman, L. D., & Associates. *Self-help groups for coping with crisis: Origins, members, processes, and impact*. San Francisco: Jossey-Bass, 1979.
16. Lindemann, E., & Lindemann, E. *Beyond grief: Studies in crisis intervention*. New York: Aronson, 1979.
17. Lindy, J. D., Grace, M. C., & Green, B. L. Survivors: Outreach to a reluctant population. *American Journal of Orthopsychiatry*, 1981, *51*, 468–478.
18. Medinger, F., & Varghese, R. Psychological growth and the impact of stress in middle age. *International Journal of Aging and Human Development*, 1981, *13*, 247–263.

19. Moos, R. *Coping with physical illness: New perspectives.* New York: Plenum Press, 1984.
20. Moos, R., & Billings, A. Conceptualizing and measuring coping resources and processes. In L. Goldberger & S. Breznitz (Eds.), *Handbook of stress: Theoretical and clinical aspects.* New York: Macmillan, 1982.
21. Neugarten, B. Time, age, and the life cycle. *American Journal of Psychiatry,* 1979, *136,* 887–894.
22. Perloff, L. Perceptions of vulnerability to victimization. *Journal of Social Issues,* 1983, *39,* 41–61.
23. Raphael, B. A primary prevention action programme: Psychiatric involvement following a major rail disaster. *Omega,* 1979–1980, *10,* 211–226.
24. Rees, H., & Smyer, M. The dimensionalization of life events. In E. Callahan & K. McCluskey (Eds.), *Life span developmental psychology: Non-normative life events.* New York: Academic Press, 1983.
25. Singh, B., & Raphael, B. Postdisaster morbidity of the bereaved: A possible role for preventive psychiatry. *Journal of Nervous and Mental Disease,* 1981, *169,* 203–212.
26. Stolberg, A. L., & Garrison, K. M. Evaluating a primary prevention program for children of divorce. *American Journal of Community Psychology,* 1985, *13,* 111–124.
27. Taylor, S., Wood, J., & Lichtman, R. It could be worse: Selective evaluation as a response to victimization. *Journal of Social Issues,* 1983, *39,* 1–40.
28. Vachon, M. L. S., Lyall, W. A. L., Rogers, J., Freedman-Letofsky, K., & Freeman, S. J. J. A controlled study of self-help intervention for widows. *American Journal of Psychiatry,* 1980, *137,* 1380–1384.
29. Valent, P. The Ash Wednesday bushfires in Australia. *Medical Journal of Australia,* 1984, *141,* 291–300.
30. Wallerstein, J. Children of divorce: Stress and developmental tasks. In N. Garmezy & M. Rutter (Eds.), *Stress, coping and development in children.* New York: McGraw-Hill, 1983.
31. Wallerstein, J., & Kelly, J. *Surviving the breakup: How children and parents cope with divorce.* New York: Basic Books, 1980.

II

Developmental Life Transitions
Childhood and the Early Years

The coping skills we rely on as adults begin to emerge in childhood. One essential skill is the ability to deal with loss. Rupture of the family through separation and divorce is a commonplace crisis that confronts many children with their first significant loss. Children of divorce must cope with the loss of a parent and the frightening vulnerability that comes when their beliefs in the security of the family unit are shattered. Such children must make sense of the vagaries of adult love relationships and master intense emotions—sadness, loneliness, and fear of abandonment; anger at their parents for divorcing; and worry about who will care for them and for the departed parent.[9] The losses the child faces in divorce are similar to and perhaps even more difficult to master than those that arise from the death of a parent. The lack of finality in separation and divorce hinders acceptance of the loss and allows the child to cling to the lingering hope that the parents will reunite. Also, the child who loses a parent through divorce often receives less support than a child whose parent has died. No "funeral" or other ritual acknowledges the loss when there is a separation and one of the parents moves out of the home.

The years of parental conflict prior to divorce may be especially stressful for children. Deborah Luepnitz[5] found that children's coping strategies varied with age. Younger children sometimes withdraw from parental conflicts by blocking their ears, retreating to their rooms, and engaging in wish-fulfilling fantasies. Some older children cope by staying away from home as much as possible, whereas others take a more direct problem-focused approach and try to intervene in parental arguments. Some children are successful in managing stress at home by investing in schoolwork, joining scouts, engaging in sports or other extracurricular activities, or relying on social support from siblings and friends.

Following the divorce, children's psychological responses again reflect their age and developmental level.[9] Younger children's reactions are the most acute. They respond with anxiety and fear of abandonment. Adolescents act in ways that help them maintain distance from the pain of the divorce. They minimize the impact of the divorce, deny that it has any emotional effect on them, and use humor and sarcasm. They also keep busy with friends and develop interests away from their family.

In the first article, Judith Wallerstein describes six tasks confronting children of divorce. The initial task is to acknowledge the reality of the breakup of the marriage. Acknowledgment can be hindered by fears of parental abandonment or overwhelming feelings of sorrow, rejection, or anger. Even so, all of the children studied mastered this task by the end of the first year of separation. The second task involves disengagement from parental conflict and distress and a return to customary activities and relationships at school and play. Children who succeeded in negotiating this task mastered their anxiety and depression, established some psychological distance from their parents, and reestablished earlier levels of learning and participation in usual activities.

The third task, resolution of the loss, is one of the most difficult to master. Children must come to terms with multiple losses associated with the divorce and simultaneously overcome feelings of rejection and powerlessness. Regular visits with the departed parent may facilitate mastery of this task. Joint-custody arrangements in which parents have a cooperative relationship may also mitigate children's feelings that they have lost a parent and aid their adjustment to the divorce. Susan Steinman[7] found that children in joint-custody arrangements sometimes were burdened by switching between their parents' homes and by trying to be equally loyal to each parent. In general, however, these problems were outweighed by the benefits of access to both parents. Children in joint-custody arrangements did not experience the rejection and feelings of abandonment that plagued children who had little or no contact with their departed parent.

Children may blame themselves for their parents' divorce. The fourth task facing children is to resolve their self-blame and anger. Anger diminishes as children better understand their parents' relationship and the reasons for the divorce. Self-blame decreases as children acquire the ability to forgive themselves for failing to save their parents' marriage or for wanting the divorce to occur. The fifth task involves acceptance of the permanence of the divorce. It requires that children give up their tenacious hold on the idea that their family will be reunited. The sixth and final task is to achieve a realistic hope regarding future relationships. Young persons must be able to risk establishing a loving relationship in the hope that it will succeed and the realization that it may not. Mastery of this final task is a long-term process.

Judith Wallerstein's[8] 10-year follow-up study of children of divorce revealed signs of successful adaptation. Most children were performing adequately in school, had close relationships with their custodial mother, and looked forward to marrying and having children of their own. Although the youngest children were the most upset at the time of the divorce, 10 years later they were less troubled by the divorce than their older siblings. The younger children had few memories of their intact predivorce family and of their reactions to the divorce, whereas the older children recalled family conflicts and the pain they experienced at the time of the divorce.

Like divorce, death of a parent is a devastating loss that permanently alters the family. Young children who have lost a mother wonder who will feed and care for them, whereas those whose father has died may be frightened about where the money will come from for food. Surviving parents may be so absorbed in their own grief that the child's profound emotional needs are denied and go unmet.[6] The emotional pain of parental loss can reverberate through a lifetime. Even among adults who have coped with the loss of a parent in childhood, holidays or life-cycle milestones such as a graduation, marriage, or birth of a child may trigger surges of maturational grief. At these times, the adult reexperiences the loss of the parent. This type of grief is a normal response and differs from lingering unresolved grief—the prod-

uct of a failure in adaptation.[3] As with divorce, the aftermath of
parental death is a prolonged, painful period of adjustment.

The second article addresses the issue of long-term adaptation to childhood bereavement. Esther Elizur and Mordecai Kaffman describe a longitudinal study of young, kibbutz children's
bereavement reactions following the death of their father in the
Yom Kippur War. In the early months, the children's coping
reactions included crying, moodiness, longing for the lost father,
and attempts to remember the father by imitating him or talking
to his photograph. Anger and protest were also among the immediate reactions to the loss. In order to "gain distance and time"
from the disturbing reality of the parent's death, some children
tried to maintain the belief that their father was still present by
remembering past joint experiences and anticipating the father's
future return. The children also searched for a substitute father.
As time passed, the children began to discuss death and tried to
understand it and its meaning.

In the second year, denial and fantasy decreased, and the
children began to accept the reality of the loss. But this new understanding seemed to fuel their fears of being alone and of abandonment. The children coped with these emotions by being more
demanding, restless, and dependent and by openly expressing
their anger. By the third and fourth years, many of the children
had begun to adjust to the loss. Their fears and anger diminished.

More than two-thirds of the children experienced emotional
problems during the study. Even though many children improved, more than one-third still had significant problems $3\frac{1}{2}$
years after the death of their father. Clearly, the impact of a
parent's death is severe. When Kaffman and Elizur[4] compared
the bereavement reactions of these kibbutz children with nonkib-
butz children who had lost a father, they found that the kibbutz
children had fewer clinical symptoms. They attributed this
positive effect to the child-rearing methods, styles of family functioning, and other cultural factors in the supportive kibbutz
environment.

Unfortunately, the children in Elizur and Kaffman's study
had no opportunity to prepare for their devastating loss. "Death
preparation" may assuage some of the grief children experience
when a close family member dies. Exposing children to death

through the loss of a pet or through books that stimulate discussions about the meaning of death may help them to cope with the inevitable losses of close family members.[1] Surviving parents can enhance their children's long-term adjustment by telling them of the parent's death in a clear and direct way, encouraging them to vent longing and grief, providing the opportunity for them to participate in the funeral and visit the grave, offering reassurance that the grief-stricken surviving parent will still be able to care for them, and keeping their world as constant as possible by avoiding changes such as a move to a new home or school.[1,2]

If the crises of divorce and death of a parent are successfully negotiated, children may ultimately benefit from the growth-promoting aspects of these experiences. Such resilience is evident in findings that some children of divorce show increased maturity and independence, a greater willingness to help with household tasks, more mature views about finances, and a desire to avoid the mistakes of their parents.[9] Likewise, Elizur and Kaffman noted an "accelerated maturity" among children who had lost a parent. They took responsibility for the care of siblings, helped with household tasks, and identified with their father in a positive way by assuming some of his roles within the family.

References

1. Adams-Greenly, M., & Moynihan, R. T. Helping the children of fatally ill parents. *American Journal of Orthopsychiatry*, 1983, *53*, 219–229.
2. Brenner, A. *Helping children cope with stress.* Lexington, Mass: Lexington Books, 1984.
3. Johnson, P., & Rosenblatt, P. Grief following childhood loss of a parent. *American Journal of Psychotherapy*, 1981, *35*, 419–425.
4. Kaffman, M., & Elizur, E. Bereavement responses of kibbutz and non-kibbutz children following the death of the father. *Journal of Child Psychology and Psychiatry*, 1983, *24*, 435–442.
5. Luepnitz, D. A. Which aspects of divorce affect children? *The Family Coordinator*, 1979, *28*, 79–85.
6. Raphael, B. *The anatomy of bereavement.* New York: Basic Books, 1983.
7. Steinman, S. The experience of children in a joint-custody arrangement: A report of a study. *American Journal of Orthopsychiatry*, 1981, *51*, 403–414.
8. Wallerstein, J. S. Children of divorce: Preliminary report of a ten-year follow-up of young children. *American Journal of Orthopsychiatry*, 1984, *54*, 444–458.
9. Wallerstein, J. S., & Kelly, J. B. *Surviving the breakup: How children and parents cope with divorce.* New York: Basic Books, 1980.

2

Children of Divorce
The Psychological Tasks of the Child

JUDITH S. WALLERSTEIN

Divorce represents a special kind of stressful experience for the child who has been reared within a two-parent family. The child's experience in divorce is comparable in several ways to the experience of the child who loses a parent through death or to the child who loses his or her community following a natural disaster. Each of these experiences strikes at and disrupts close family relationships. Each weakens the protection that the nuclear family provides, leaving in its wake a diminished, more vulnerable family structure. Each traces a pattern of time that begins with an acute, time-limited crisis, and is followed by an extended period of disequilibrium which may last several years—or even longer—past the central event. And each introduces a chain of long-lasting changes that are not predictable at the outset and that reach into multiple domains of family life.

Thus, divorce, bereavement, and the loss of community pose powerful continuing demands for major psychological, social, and often economic reorganization. For the child, the readjustments

This chapter appears in abridged form from the *American Journal of Orthopsychiatry*, 1983, *53*, 230–243. Copyright 1983, the American Orthopsychiatric Association, Inc. Reprinted by permission.

JUDITH S. WALLERSTEIN • Center for the Family in Transition, Corte Madera, California 94925.

that are required are likely, in our observations, to stretch over the years of childhood and adolescence. We have conceptualized these required readjustments as a series of tasks to be addressed immediately as well as over the many years that follow. In accord with Erikson's architectural conception of the tasks that attend the successive stages of the life cycle,[3] and in accord with the formulations of Lindemann[7] and Caplan[2] regarding the succession of tasks imposed by bereavement, elaborated later and more complexly within crisis theory, this chapter will delineate a series of tasks that attend the child's experience in the divorcing family. These are the coping tasks that are shaped by the threats or perceived threats to psychic integrity and development which the divorce process poses to the child. They are conceptualized as hierarchical, as following a particular time sequence beginning with the critical events of parental separation and culminating at late adolescence and young adulthood.

The reorganization and readjustments that are required of the child of the divorcing family, namely the tasks that need to be addressed, represent a major addition to the expectable customary tasks of childhood and adolescence in our society. In this view, the child of divorce faces a special set of challenges and carries an added burden.

My colleagues and I have followed over many years the course of 60 divorcing families with children from the time of the decisive marital separation and the initial filing for dissolution through the first 5 years following divorce and, more recently, through the first 10-year period. The sample drawn in 1971 from a northern California population of primarily, but not entirely, white, middle-class families consisted at the outset of 60 divorcing families with 131 children aged 3 to 18 at the time of the decisive separation. The families were seen again a year later, or approximately 18 months after separation. By that time most were legally divorced. They were seen again at the 5-year mark by the same clinical team. At that time, 58 of the original 60 families were recontacted. Finally, during the year 1981–1982, at the 10-year mark, we have renewed contact with the same families using three members of the original five-person clinical team, and we have been successful thus far in reaching 86%, or 51 families and 98 children. The methods of the project and its findings at the decisive separation, at 18 months and at 5 years have been previously reported.[5,6,8-15]

Task 1: Acknowledging the Reality of the Marital Rupture

The first and simplest task for the child is to acknowledge the reality of the marital rupture and to understand the family and household changes that ensue separate from the frightening fantasies which have been evoked in the child's mind.

Overall, the child's perceptions and understanding of the family events are filtered through a prism that has been cut and shaped by the child's chronological age and developmentally related needs, conflicts, and wishes, as well as a great many factors, including individual differences. The major divorce-related obstacles to an accurate, age-appropriate acknowledgment are the child's vivid and terrifying fantasies of parental abandonment and disaster; these have been triggered by the parental conflict, by the troubled—sometimes wildly raging, bizarre, and unprecedented—behavior of one or both parents and by the departure of one parent from the home. And as so often happens, the macabre conclusions to which the child's fantasy constructions lead far exceed the unhappy reality. Additionally, the hapless child's fear of being overwhelmed by the intense feelings of sorrow, anger, rejection, and yearning further block the acknowledgment of the family rupture. Therefore, the child's powerful need to deny, to defer, and to avoid the terrifying thoughts and feelings is greatly strengthened and is joined with the comfort derived from fantasy and denial. Sometimes the power of fantasy is called upon additionally to undo and reverse the distressing reality. Indeed, fantasy can undo the child's feelings of powerlessness and enable the child heroically to mend the rift and reunite the parents or reunite the child with the departed parent. All of the preschool children in our study who played house placed the mother and father dolls in bed together, hugging each other. The complex ego-syntonic interweaving of denial through fantasy with the child's enfolding developmental agenda was so well reflected in the response of little girls at the oedipal stage of development in their response to the father's departure:

> *"My daddy sleeps in my bed every night," we were informed by a smiling child who had not seen her father for many weeks. "He will come back to me when he grows up," another bravely assured us and herself.*

We have elsewhere described the diminished parenting, the lessened supports from the parents and other adults, and the failure of so many parents to explain the family events to the children or to prepare them for what lay ahead.[13] Given the powerful fears generated by the family events, it is understandable that the falling away of parental support at this critical time would gravely burden the child, especially the young child, in this first task of coming to grips with reality.

All of the children whom we studied mastered this first task by the end of the first year of separation. A significant number achieved this recognition earlier. Older children and adolescents were helped in their understanding of the divorce because of the high incidence of divorce in their community which, while it did not reassure or comfort them, did promote realistic understanding.

The acknowledgment of the reality of the marital rupture presents a separate task from the more difficult task of acknowledging its permanence. Children address the issue of permanence with great reluctance and over a several-year period. We shall discuss this separately as Task 5.

Task 2: Disengaging from Parental Conflict and Distress and Resuming Customary Pursuits

The second task of the child is to return to customary activities and relationships at school and at play and to do so with the capacity for learning and for appropriate interests and pleasure unimpaired by the family crisis. This task poses a dual challenge. At a time of family disequilibrium, when one or both parents may be troubled, depressed, or very angry, when the household is likely to be in disarray,[4] the child needs to find, establish, and maintain some measure of psychological distance and separation from the adults. In order to achieve this distance, the child needs actively and very painfully to disengage from the parental distress or conflict despite what may be profound worry over a parent and despite what may be the intense need of one or both parents for nurturance and support from the child. In effect, with little or no expectable parental help, the child needs to take appropriate steps to safeguard his or her individual identity and separate life course.

The second part of this task requires that the child remove the family crisis from its commanding position in his or her inner world. The achievement of this task rests in turn on the mastery, or at least the diminution of anxiety, depression, and the many conflicting feelings that attend the marital rupture in order to gain or regain the perspective and composure sufficient to enable the child's return. Only by mastery of both aspects of this task, namely that which faces outward toward the family and involves relative disengagement from the parental orbit, and that which faces inward, namely toward the child's inner thoughts and feelings and involves relative mastery of anxiety and depression, can the child maintain his or her development unimpaired by the family crisis and make his or her way back to the world of children or adolescents.

A significant number of the latency-age and preadolescent youngsters whose parents were newly involved in sexual relationships with lovers reported that they had difficulty concentrating and that they were preoccupied with their parents' sexual activities. We have elsewhere[15] referred to Gwen, age 10:

> *Gwen complained to us that she had lost interest in her school, in her friends, and in her piano lessons, "in everything since Dad left." She reported that she thought all day that he was "making out with his girlfriend." She also thought constantly about her mother together with her boyfriend. "How," asked the child, "can I concentrate at school thinking about Mom and Dad kissing and making love with other people?"*

Unlike the first task, the mastery of this task of disengagement was not easier for the older children. It may, in fact, have been rendered more difficult by the fine shading between an all-too-realistic worry and phobic anxiety. How shall we assess the behavior of the many youngsters who paced the floor nervously when the parent was late in returning home? Or how shall we assess the behavior of the children who begged the custodial parent to quit smoking, asking, "What will happen to me if you get cancer?" Or how assess the despair of children to whom a parent had confided a suicidal preoccupation and who realized full well that their presence was needed by the parent in order to stave off the suicide attempt or the threat of ego disintegration?

Adolescent commitments to school and their usual round of extracurricular activities seemed particularly vulnerable to disruption at this time. Several adolescents became acutely depressed:

> *One 14-year-old youngster who had distinguished herself at school and competitive sports was truant for the remainder of the school year following the parental separation and was found to be riding the local buses 6 hours daily, preoccupied with suicidal thoughts.*

Some became newly involved at this time in sexual activity or delinquency, most notably stealing.

By the end of the first year or year and a half following the separation, most youngsters in our study were able to reestablish their earlier levels of learning and to reinvest in their other activities. They were able to regain relationships with friends whom they had driven away by their moodiness and their irritability during the period immediately following the marital separation. Children in families where the siblings formed a supportive subgroup appeared to have some advantage in addressing this difficult task. Nevertheless, it should be noted that a significant number of children at every age, but notably at adolescence, were not able to find their way back to an age-appropriate agenda after the derailment of the family crisis.

Task 3: Resolution of Loss

Divorce brings multiple losses in its wake, of which the most central is the partial or total loss of one parent from the family. But the losses of divorce may include, as well, the loss of the familiar daily routines, the loss of the symbols, traditions, and continuity of the intact family, and the loss of the protective physical presence of two parents who can spell and buffer each other as needed. Often, as well, the losses of divorce include the loss of the family home, school, and neighborhood, and sometimes the loss of a more privileged way of life, including private school and a wide range of pleasurable, exciting activities. While the departure of a parent who has been physically or psychologically brutal or demeaning to the child or parent provides great relief, by and large, children who have not been frightened on their own behalf or on behalf of a parent are likely to mourn the loss of one parent's departure even in the absence of a close relationship or frequent contact during the marriage.

This task of absorbing loss is perhaps the single most difficult task imposed by divorce. The child is required to mourn the multiple losses in order to come to terms with the constraints, limitations, and potentialities of the postdivorce or remarried family. At its core, this task demands that the child overcome his or her profound sense of rejection, of humiliation, of unlovability, and of powerlessness which the one parent's departure so often engenders. Children at all ages are likely to feel rejected. "He left me," they say and are likely secretly to conclude, "He left because I was not lovable." Our beginning findings regarding children who remain in the custody of their father suggest that these feelings of unlovability, unworthiness, and rejection are even stronger where the mother has relinquished or abandoned the child or is an inconsistent visitor.

This task is greatly facilitated by the establishment of a reliable visiting pattern which can enable father and child to restore a sense of psychic wholeness and rightness in their respective new roles of part-time parent and part-time child. The building of a good enough parent–child relationship within the visiting structure, which is governed realistically by the opportunities and the constraints of the visit, rests upon the working through of the yearning for the father within the intact family and an openness to the new relationship. It is reasonable that only if the loss of the full-time presence of the departed parent is accepted by both parent and child does the visiting relationship and its potential become fully realizable.[14] There is also the strong possibility that the child's relationship to the stepparent requires some modicum of resolution of this mourning process.

The resolution of this task often lasts many years. The voluntariness of both the divorce and the parent's departure burdens the child's coping efforts and increases the child's suffering, making this loss more difficult to assimilate than the involuntary loss associated with bereavement. This task is, of course, most easily accomplished when the loss of the relationship with the father (or the mother) is partial, and the outside parent and child are able to establish and maintain a loving relationship within an ongoing, reliable visiting pattern or under conditions of a good joint-custody plan. Even under ideal conditions this is no small achievement.

Task 4: Resolving Anger and Self-Blame

In order to understand this task it is important to note the importance of the social context of marital dissolution. Unlike bereavement or natural disaster, divorce is entirely man or woman made and represents a voluntary decision for at least one of the marital partners. The children are aware that divorce is not inevitable, that the immediate cause is the decision of one or both parents to separate and that its true cause is the unwillingness or failure to maintain the marriage. Moreover, the children, like the community, will have different responses when the divorce is sought to remedy a brutal or unhappy marriage, when the divorce is sought to pursue a postponed career, or when the divorce occurs because of one adult's impulsive decision to join a lover.

Our work indicates clearly that children and adolescents do not believe in no-fault divorce. They may blame one or both parents, or they may blame themselves. Divorce characteristically gives rise to anger at the one parent who sought the divorce or both parents for their perceived self-centeredness or unresponsiveness to the wishes of the child to maintain the intact family. The anger that these children experience is likely sometimes to be intense and long-lasting, especially among older children and adolescents who disapprove of the conduct of one or both parents.

We have earlier reported[13] the intense anger and sorrow expressed by one 14-year-old boy:

> *In a school composition written 5 years after the marital rupture, he wrote, "My father picked up his suitcases one day and walked out because, as he said, he wanted his freedom. We thought we were a close-knit family, and it was an unexpected shock. It was the death of our family."*

Our observations are that anger that has been generated within the context of divorce may well remain undiminished by the passage of time. Such anger not only keeps youngsters alienated from one parent but often, in our observation, correlates significantly with acting-out behavior at adolescence, including delinquency, school difficulty, and low achievement. Most of all, anger that does not subside seems to keep youngsters from achieving closure with regard to the divorce experience. The anger does seem to diminish within the context of greater understanding of the parents and their relationship with each other; this rests, in turn, on the achievement by the older child or the adolescent of some perspective regarding the reasons that prompted the divorce and a greater understanding of one or both parents.

Thus, the cooling of the anger and task of forgiveness go hand in hand with the growing emotional maturity of the child and the greater capacity to recognize the divergence of interests and directions among the different family members. As the anger gives way, the young person is able to obtain both closure and relief. Only in this way are the narcissistic injury of the divorce and the sense of powerlessness engendered in the child finally resolved. A significant aspect of forgiveness is a child's capacity to forgive himself or herself for having wished the divorce to happen or having failed to restore the intact marriage. And, indeed, it may well be that there is a profound connection between children's capacity to forgive themselves and the capacity to forgive one or both parents. Further, the close relationships and friendships between parents and children that Weiss[16] and others have described as emerging out of this crisis may have their roots in part in a triumph over anger.

Among the distinguishing attributes of some of the parent–

child relationships at the 10-year mark is a growing closeness between youngster and parent which seems to have the hallmarks of a significant, long-delayed reconciliation:

> *Barbara reported at age 17, ten years after the marital rupture, "My mom and I are real close now. I stopped being angry at her when I was 15 when I suddenly realized that all of the kids who lived in tract houses with picket fences were not any happier than I was. It took me a long, long time to stop blaming her for not being in one of those houses."*

Task 5: Accepting the Permanence of the Divorce

Closely related to all of the foregoing tasks, and particularly to the task of successfully mastering the distress evoked by the father's departure, is the child's gradual acceptance that the divorce is permanent and will not be undone. Time and again we have been impressed with the tenacity of the fantasy that the divorced family will be reunited. We have observed children, adolescents, and adults decades after the divorce persisting in this expectation that the intact family will be restored, weeping for the father that they hardly knew, finding omens of reconciliation in a harmless handshake or a friendly nod. Even the remarriage of both parents sometimes did little to diminish the intensity of this persistent fantasy, wish, hope, or expectation. Our clinical experience includes a middle-aged woman patient who sought help from two therapists simultaneously, a man and a woman, and who finally confessed to each her central preoccupation: that she wished to bring both therapists together within the same room so that they could hold hands and restore the intact family that she had lost as a preschool child. It proved difficult to dissuade this functioning, nonpsychotic woman that the actualization of her enduring childhood fantasy with the participation of both therapists would not immediately cure her recurrent severe depressions.

We have concluded that the child of divorce faces a more difficult task in accepting permanence than does the bereaved child. The bereaved child, despite intense hopes to the contrary, knows full well that death can never be undone, whereas the living presence and availability of two parents gives continuing credence to the child's wish to restore the marriage. In effect, the reality that both parents are alive and that divorce is always possible, as is remarriage, fuels the fantasy and permits it, even encourages it to flourish. It is by now quite clear that the fantasy of restoration taps into deep wellsprings within the child's functioning and yields to reality only very gradually, perhaps only when the child finally makes and consolidates a clear psychological separation between self and parent during the adolescent years.

Developmental factors seem relevant to the resolution of this task. It may well be that the younger children encountered greater difficulty in relinquishing the restoration fantasy than their peers who were older at the time of the marital breakup. Another factor of importance was the extent to which one or both parents also continued to long for the restoration of the marriage. Such adult fantasies reinforced the fantasies of the children. We did not find, however, that the adult wishes to restore the marriage governed the widespread fantasies and hopes of the children.

Task 6: Achieving Realistic Hope Regarding Relationships

Finally we come to the task that is perhaps the most important both for the child and for society, namely the resolution of issues of relationship in such a way that the young person is able to reach and sustain a realistic vision regarding his or her capacity to love and be loved. This is the task that occupies the child of divorce during the adolescent years and lends its particular cast and additional burden to the many developmental tasks that the adolescent confronts. It is also the task that brings together and integrates the coping efforts of earlier years and provides in this way an opportunity for the full-dress reworking of the impact of the divorce experience.

In this task we come full circle in comparing the child of divorce with his or her counterpart in bereavement. In the same way that the child who loses a parent through death must learn to take a chance on loving with the full and reinforced knowledge that humans are mortal and that all relationships will indeed end, so too the child of divorce must learn to take a chance on a loving relationship that may fail but with the realistic hope that it will flourish and endure.

As the adolescent youngsters examined their parents and themselves and considered their future, many were frightened at the possible repetition of marital or sexual failure in their own lives:

> *Pamela, at age 24, told us at the 10-year follow-up, "I'm afraid to use the word love. I tell my boyfriend that I love him, but I can't really think about it without fear."*

A significant number of young people during late adolescence turned away from a parent's behavior in anger, having measured it and found it wanting. As expressed at the 10-year follow-up by one 26-year-old young man who had elected to follow an entirely different life-style from that of his father:

> *"Some day I will say to my dad, 'Are you proud of what you have done with your life?' But," he said bitterly, "what can he answer me?"*

We have reported earlier[15] the pointed and poignant comments of the youngsters during the adolescent years and their sober efforts to evolve strategies that might safeguard them from failure and help consolidate a separateness from the parents' experience:

> *My parents cheated and lied, but I decided never to do that. I will live with a guy for a long time. I won't rush in. They should both have been more considerate. My mother is selfish, and my father should never have married. The trouble with my parents is that they each gave too little and asked too much.*

Nevertheless, it seems evident that youngsters whose adjustment was otherwise adequate foundered on this last task. Sometimes the cynicism expressed was startling:

> *Jay, at age 14, told us, "Dad left because Mom bored him. I do that all the time."*

Others insisted that they would never marry because they were convinced that their marriages would fail. Still others were caught in a web of promiscuity and low self-esteem and spoke cynically and hopelessly of ever achieving a loving relationship or other goals. And, we have noted, we have been concerned at the emergence of acute depression during adolescence, especially what appears to be a delayed depression among adolescent girls many years following the marital rupture.[15]

Unfortunately, we lack the long-term findings that would enable us to gauge success or failure of the efforts of these young people to select a different or a better direction for their lives. Our own findings from the 10-year follow-up are still in the preliminary phase. And it might well be argued that even tentative conclusions would need to await the time when the child of divorce becomes, in turn, a parent as well as a marital partner.

Bearing in mind that the resolution of life's tasks is always relative and probably never complete, it nevertheless appears that this last task is built on the successful negotiation of those that went before. For in order to trust in the reliability of relationships and maintain the capacity to love and be loved, the child of divorce will need to have acquired confidence in his or her lovability and self-worth. He or she will have had to consolidate separateness from the parental orbit and conflicts and establish an independent direction; will have had to master the depression, the anxiety, and the conflicts stirred by the divorce that have remained residually over the years; will have had to complete the mourning over the loss of the intact family or the departed parent; will have had to resolve early issues of intense anger and guilt stirred by the marital rupture and arrive at some forgiveness, understanding, and compassion for the parents and for self; and will have had to come to terms with the permanence of the parental divorce and relinquish longings for the restoration of the childhood family. All of the tasks come together for reworking within the context of the many tasks of adolescence. And it is this last task, in the "second chance" that Blos[1] has proposed adolescence beneficently provides, that enables the child of divorce to reach or restore a sense of wholeness and integrity by rescuing a realistic vision of love and constancy in human relationships to which the developing youngster can aspire in adulthood and, in turn, transmit to children.

References

1. Blos, P. *On Adolescence: A Psychoanalytic interpretation.* New York: Free Press, 1962.
2. Caplan, G. (Ed.). *Emotional problems of early childhood.* New York: Basic Books, 1955.
3. Erikson, E. *Childhood and society.* New York: Norton,1950.
4. Hetherington, E., Cox, M., & Cox, R. The aftermath of divorce. In H. Stevens & M. Mathews (Eds.), *Mother–child relations.* Washington, D.C.: National Association for the Education of Young Children, 1978.
5. Kelly, J., & Wallerstein, J. The effects of parental divorce: Experiences of the child in early latency. *American Journal of Orthopsychiatry,* 1976, *46,* 20–32.
6. Kelly, J., & Wallerstein, J. Part-time parent, part-time child: Visiting after divorce. *Journal of Clinical Child Psychology,* 1977, *6,* 51–54.
7. Lindemann, E. Symptomatology and management of acute grief. *American Journal of Psychiatry,* 1944, *101,* 141–148.
8. Wallerstein, J., & Kelly, J. The effects of parental divorce: The adolescent experience. In E. Anthony & C. Koupernik (Eds.), *The child and his family.* New York: Wiley, 1974.
9. Wallerstein, J., & Kelly, J. The effects of parental divorce: The experiences of the preschool child. *Journal of the American Academy of Child Psychiatry,* 1975, *14,* 600–616.
10. Wallerstein, J., & Kelly, J. The effects of parental divorce: Experiences of the child in later latency. *American Journal of Orthopsychiatry,* 1976, *46,* 256–269.
11. Wallerstein, J. Some observations regarding the effects of divorce on the psychological development of the pre-school girl. In J. Oremland & E. Oremland (Eds.), *Sexual and gender development of young children.* Cambridge, Mass.: Ballinger, 1977.
12. Wallerstein, J. Responses of the pre-school child to divorce: Those who cope. In M. McMillan & S. Henao (Eds.), *Child psychiatry: Treatment and research.* New York: Brunner/Mazel, 1977.
13. Wallerstein, J., & Kelly, J. *Surviving the breakup: How children and parents cope with divorce.* New York: Basic Books, 1980.
14. Wallerstein, J., & Kelly, J. Effects of divorce on the visiting father–child relationship. *American Journal of Psychiatry,* 1980, *137*(12), 1534–1539.
15. Wallerstein, J. Children of divorce: Stress and developmental tasks. In N. Garmezy & M. Rutter (Eds.), *Stress, coping and development.* New York: McGraw-Hill, 1983.
16. Weiss, R. *Going it alone.* New York: Basic Books, 1979.

3

Children's Bereavement Reactions Following Death of the Father

ESTHER ELIZUR and MORDECAI KAFFMAN

This is the second report from a longitudinal study designed to assess the effects of the father's death on children aged 2 to 10 years. In the first report we described the bereavement reactions of 22 out of a study group of 25 kibbutz children 2 to 6 months after their father's death in the Yom Kippur War of 1973.[2] We found that about half of these children, who previously had no special psychological problems, reacted severely, with a variety of behavior problems that so disturbed their daily functioning in the family, the home, and school that professional help was considered indispensable. There were considerable individual differences from one child to another, not only according to his or her age, but also to family, individual, and circumstantial variables.

It is clear that in the kibbutz as in the normative Western family, the parent remains the most important and stable emo-

This chapter appears in abridged form from *Journal of the American Academy of Pediatrics*, 1982, *21*, 474–480. Copyright 1982 by the American Academy of Child Psychiatry. Reprinted by permission of The Williams & Wilkins Company.

ESTHER ELIZUR, Senior Research Associate, and **MORDECAI KAFFMAN,** Medical Director • Kibbutz Child and Family Clinic, Derech Haifa 147, Tel Aviv 62507 Israel.

tional attachment for the child,[3] but in the kibbutz there exist conditions that appear to ease the child's encounter with the trauma of his or her parents' death. The complementary interaction of three important attachment centers—parents, educators, and children's group—usually assures continuity in daily life and satisfaction of the child's basic security needs even in stress situations that affect one of these centers. The availability of emotional surrogate models along with the provision of the child's material needs and the daily care by the commune reduce dependence on parents and should ease—at least from a theoretical standpoint—the kibbutz child's reaction to the loss of a father. However, this was not the case. Contrary to our expectations regarding the supportive potential of the kibbutz, we found evidence of serious psychological disturbance in the early months of bereavement.

In view of this, we felt it important to continue the follow-up study of this group of bereaved children. For this purpose, we investigated the nature and course of the emotional problems of these children $1\frac{1}{2}$ years after the father's death. We were especially interested in the fate of the children (45% of the sample) who reacted severely during the first months of bereavement in order to learn if the severity of reaction during the early period is a prognostic index of later adjustment. We were also interested in examining whether in those children who did not show initially any noticeable emotional disturbance, clinical evidence pointing to delayed pathological responses appears at a later date.

Population

The 25 children included in the study represented all the children (ages 1 to 10) in seven kibbutzim whose fathers died in the Yom Kippur War. The sample included 15 widowed mothers and 10 pairs of siblings. Eight of the children were girls; 17 were boys. Two children were under 2 years old, 15 were between the ages of 2 and 6, and 8 were between 6 and 10 years old when the father died.

This is a representative sample of "normal" children within the community with no special problems before the loss. All the children lost a father in war under similar circumstances (in battle) and during the same period of time. All the families belong to the middle class, and all the mothers had at least a high school education. The specific framework of the kibbutz was common to all the children. It is this similarity of circumstances that strengthens the internal validity of the study. Furthermore, because this study concentrated on the consequences of the loss of a father, it provides a contrast to the extensive literature on the importance of a disrupted mother–child relationship.

Conduct of the Research

Although psychiatric interviews and psychological tests were conducted for all the children, data for this chapter were drawn exclusively from interviews with the widowed mothers and the children's teachers. To prevent ambiguity in listing and assessing mourning reactions of the children, we recorded only symptomatic reactions expressed by manifest behavior change that appeared or worsened since the fathers' deaths.[2] In each phase of the study, a bimodal distribution of the children's "problem score" around the average was found. Thus two distinct groups could be identified: children whose exceptional difficulties impaired their daily functioning ("pathological bereavement"), and children who succeeded, despite the stress, to adjust to the new reality ("normal bereavement").

Incidence and Duration of Emotional Disturbances

There was a significant increase in the average number of behavior symptoms per child after the loss, as compared with the prebereavement period. The marked raise in the rate of behavior problems observed in the early months of bereavement and the high percentage of "pathological bereavement" remain almost unchanged 18 months and even 42 months after the father's death. In fact, the highest prevalence of behavior problems—an average of nine handicapping problems per child—appear in the course of the follow-up period, reaching a peak in the second year after the father's death.

There is no substantial change throughout the follow-up period in the severity of the behavior problems. Three and a half years after the loss, 65% of the total clinical symptoms are still rated as medium to severe in degree. The percentage of children with marked impairment and severe emotional problems ("pathological bereavement") remains high during the total follow-up period—almost half of the children in all phases of the study. About 40% of the children were included in the category of "pathological bereavement" in at least two of the three stages of the investigation, that is, throughout a 1½-year period of observation. Nearly 70% of the children showed signs of severe emotional disturbance in at least one of the stages. Thus, only a minority of children—less than a third—did not show overt signs of emotional impairment and were able to achieve satisfactory family, school, and social adjustment throughout the entire 3½ years of follow-up.

Regarding the influence of the child's sex on the type and severity of bereavement reactions, we did not find significant differences between boys and girls except for the augmented prevalence of aggressiveness and outbursts of rage in boys at all stages of the investigation. We were unable to corroborate the generally accepted assumption that the psychological disturbance is greater if the death involves the parent of the same sex as the child because of the relatively small number of girls, who comprised only one-third of the sample.

The findings indicated no uniform psychological syndrome that might be considered "typical" of childhood bereavement. The range of symptomatic responses was very wide, whereas the specific combination of various reactions and their intensity and duration differed from child to child. Nevertheless, a number of general reactive tendencies could be identified in most of the children.

Mourning Reactions

Mourning reactions are related to the specific event of death. They included grief reactions (sobbing and crying, expressions of sadness and longing); remembering the deceased father (recalling shared experiences, imitating him, talking to his photographs, using his personal effects); denial of the fact of death; avoidance of the subject of death; or other coping reactions such as continuous preoccupation with the theme of nature and meaning of death, and search for a "substitute father" (demanding a new father, clinging to available male attachment figures).

In the early months after the loss, this type of affective response made up about a third of the total number of bereavement reactions. Gradually, these mourning reactions, especially the crying, denial, and remembering responses, decreased during the second year. The only exception was the phenomenon of search for a substitute father, which was found in about half of the children throughout all the phases of the study.

Nature and Course of the Bereavement Reactions

Generally, our findings point to the fact that the bereavement reaction is not a set of symptoms that start after the loss and gradually fade away. Rather, it involves a succession of clinical pictures that blend into and replace one another.

The First Months

The child's immediate reaction to the sudden stress of his or her father's death was expressed by a clear emotional response of pain and grief. In contrast to those studies that underscore the "absence of grief" in childhood mourning,[1,4] in this study it was found that the majority of children aged 2 to 10 reacted by crying, moodiness, and varied expressions of longing. Only two children (under age 3) showed indifference and continued their daily activities as usual. Expressions of anger and protest were also quite frequent in the immediate reaction of the child to the loss. They did not replace manifestations of grief and sorrow, as some authors suggest,[5] but appeared together with them.

The children utilized various defensive measures that helped them to mitigate the acute pain of grieving and enabled them to "gain distance and time" so that they could assimilate the shock gradually. The most common means was maintaining the impression that the deceased father was nearby although he might not be seen or heard. This was achieved by (1) intensive revival of the image of the lost father from the past (recalling joint experiences) and (2) by denying the finality of death and expecting the father's return in the future. In contrast to the younger children who denied the loss and tended to talk about the father, most of the older children (ages 7 to 10) tended to gain distance by withdrawal, restraint, and ignoring the subject of death directly.

At the same time, and to an increasing extent throughout the first year of bereavement, the children began to examine the meaning and, after that, the implications of what had happened. Attempts to understand the concept of death were expressed in various ways in the early months of bereavement either by translating the concept of death to concrete and familiar situations or by asking many realistic questions to gain understanding of the difference between *dead* and *alive*. During the first months the children oscillated between the two opposing tendencies: the inhibitory tendency that by denial, postponement, avoidance, and the like limited or disturbed the perception of disturbing stimuli and the reality testing tendency that enhanced perception and thought about the father's death. The delicate interplay between these two tendencies enabled the children to accept the fact of death and to make familiar the numerous areas of uncertainty that appeared in their world.

The Second Year

A year and a half after the father's death, the children usually had achieved a certain understanding and acceptance of the loss. Together with the decrease of the primary defensive measures (especially denial) and the painful understanding of the finality of the loss, there was a significant increase in the children's levels of anxiety. This was expressed by the appearance of various fears among more than half of the children studied. Usually, these were fears about being left alone, apprehension that the mother might suddenly disappear or be inaccessible, and fears of injury and danger to oneself. Other reported fears concerned darkness, medical treatment, terrorists, and various external threats and animals, but the most common fear was the fear of being left alone.

The notable increase in the children's level of anxiety at this phase appears to be connected with the greater realistic perception of the permanent loss. Only now does the child perceive the full implications of the traumatic event. Eighteen months after the loss, it was clear that many children sensed the world as dangerous and threatening and had many fears of being abandoned or injured. Dreams, compositions, and drawings about the subject of death were frequent and may have served as one of the children's ways to master their anxiety.

The most common coping reactions at this period of anxiety and uncertainty were augmented dependency and demandingness. About two-thirds of the children showed increased dependence on the mother. This was expressed by their difficulties in parting from their mother, clinging to her, looking for her at irregular hours, and constant requests for assistance and attention. Some children also showed overdependence on teachers or other significant adults.

During each phase of the study, a greater incidence of fear (especially night fears), difficulties in separation from the mother, and other expressions of dependence were found among the preschoolers. Obviously, the younger the child, the greater his or her dependence on the parent as the principal object for satisfying physical, emotional, and developmental needs.

Increased aggressive behavior, discipline problems, and restlessness characterized more than one-third of the children 2 to 3 years after the father's death—three times more than the prebereavement period. In about half these cases the aggressive reactions were rated in the medium to severe degree of intensity. During all the postbereavement period, expressions of hyperaggressiveness were significantly more frequent among boys and among children over the age of 6.

The increased incidence of eating problems (vomiting, poor appetite, or overeating) and regressive symptomatic behavior (thumbsucking, enuresis, encopresis) that was observed during the early months remained stable throughout the follow-up period. They appeared among 25% of the children, especially the younger ones, usually as combined symptoms.

The Third and Fourth Years

For many of the children, we found at the last stage of the study some evidence of symptomatic improvement and adjustment to the changed life circumstances. Compared to the former two stages, there was a drastic decline in the rate of grief reactions. Manifestations of overdependence still typified about two-thirds of the sample, but there was a clear reduction in the anxiety level, separation difficulties, and severity of fears. The augmented aggressiveness and the concentration difficulties were also reduced. Many of the children were reported to have returned to normal integration in the school and social frameworks. For many, there was also further adjustment to the new family situation, either to a new set of roles in a single-parent family or to the extended family or to a stepfather. The attachment to an adult male figure was now more permanent and stable, as opposed to the tendency of changing the object frequently that characterized the first two stages after the loss. Most of the children "nagged" the mother less about finding a new husband and getting married; they usually succeeded in finding an identification male figure within the existing family framework or in the immediate surroundings. In four families where the mother remarried, mothers and teachers reported that the relations with the stepfather were quite satisfactory.

During the 4 years of study, there was a gradual rise in the frequency of two other phenomena: general emotional restraint (including restraint on the subject of the father's death) and "exemplary behavior." These two reactions had characterized the older age group in the sample. The pattern of "good behavior" was expressed by the child's beginning to undertake new responsibilities and functions in the family and outside (care for a younger brother, helping the mother in household chores, diligence in studies, and social obligations, etc.). In most cases this pattern did not become rigid or neurotic and was the child's way of coping with the new situation by "accelerated maturity," which assured the mother and other adults' approval and strengthened the child's self-esteem and independence. In some cases, this reaction also reflected a certain type of identification with the father by taking on family roles that had been his.

It should be remembered that despite the general trend toward symptomatic improvement and adjustment during the third and fourth years after the father's death, still more than one-third of the children (39%) showed signs of marked emotional impairment.

These adverse reactions reflect the severity of the shock and the prolonged psychological consequences of the death of a father. The symptoms are clearly connected with the loss of a beloved object but are also associated with the child's difficulties in coping with a stressful new reality created by the drastic changes in the family structure, in the daily routines, and in the functioning of the mourning mother. Although from the second half of the first year of bereavement onward there is a considerable reduction in the amount, intensity, and frequency of affective grief reactions, the increased number and severity of the behavioral symptomatic reactions remain quite stable through the fourth postbereavement year.

The findings in this study do not give a definitive answer to the questions of the "normal course and duration" of childhood mourning. The range of symptomatic responses and the individual variability make it very difficult to recognize a normative model. The great variations in the quality and severity of the bereavement reactions call for a more thorough analysis of the factors influencing the child's ability to cope with the trauma. We shall deal with this subject in subsequent papers. Of course, the lack of a control group may open the way for some reservations as to the significance of the correlation between the loss of the father by death (and subsequent events) and the psychopathological states found in this sample. We found that in a high percentage of cases, normal children in early and middle childhood reacted to the loss of a father with psychological disturbance and an emotional upheaval of a prolonged and severe nature. The common assumption that "time will heal" and the problems will disappear seems to be misleading and may prevent indispensable help and intervention at the critical stages of the first years of bereavement. The central conclusion of our follow-up study remains that the death of a parent in childhood should be regarded as a crisis situation with long-term consequences.

References

1. Deutsch, H. The absence of grief. *Psychoanalytic Quarterly,* 1937, *6,* 12–22.
2. Kaffman, M., & Elizur, E. Children's bereavement reactions following death of a father. *International Journal of Family Therapy,* 1979, *1,* 203–229.
3. Kaffman, M., Elizur, E., & Sivan-Sher, A. Personal choices of kibbutz children in simulated situations of distress and joy. *International Journal of Family Therapy,* 1980, *2,* 57–71.
4. Nagera, G. Children's reactions to the death of important objects. *The Psychoanalytic Study of the Child,* 1970, *25,* 360–400.
5. Wolfenstein, M. Loss, rage and repetition. *The Psychoanalytic Study of the Child,* 1968, *28,* 433–456.

III

Developmental Life Transitions
Adolescence and the High School Years

The metamorphosis of adolescence brings an end to childhood and ushers in adulthood. As adolescents leave childhood behind, they face the transition to junior and senior high school and the challenges of establishing heterosexual relationships, getting their first job, and making decisions about college. Despite changes in many life spheres, Daniel Offer[6] and his associates found that teenagers see themselves as competent people who can manage the problems that come their way without much difficulty. They face life's challenges with confidence, optimism, and a willingness to work to achieve their goals. (For an interesting study of the daily experiences of normal, modern teenagers, see Csikszentmihalyi & Larson.[2])

The interplay of physical, emotional, and environmental factors is especially striking in the adolescent. Adolescents must accomplish the developmental tasks of acquiring a stable ego and sexual identity, becoming independent from family, and exploring new roles within the context of the dramatic physical changes precipitated by puberty. The transition to high school is notable in that the adolescent confronts a new school environment, new peers and teachers, and role expectations at a time when the self-image is influenced by bodily changes associated with puberty. Roberta Simmons[8] and her associates explored physical and emotional development during the transition to high school and found that early-adolescent girls who enter a junior high school have lower self-esteem than girls who have not yet changed schools. Girls who experienced multiple changes, that is, reached puberty, started to date, and changed schools, had the lowest self-esteem. In contrast, Dale Blyth[1] and his associates found that early puberty in junior high boys is linked to increased self-esteem. In junior high school, where there are many pubertal boys, satisfaction with developing muscularity leads to increased self-esteem. However, in an elementary school where younger boys predominate, puberty has little impact on self-esteem.

For some adolescents, the challenge of normal developmental tasks is amplified by life crises that abruptly hurl them into the world of adult responsibilities. A crisis such as the death of a sibling may temporarily delay adolescents' efforts toward increased independence from their nuclear family, whereas the freedom to pursue different roles may be restricted when adolescents accept some responsibility for their divorced or bereaved parents or become parents themselves. But these crises may also promote mature behavior and an increased sense of mastery and competence. Adolescents growing up in such families are expected to do their share to help their overloaded parent with daily chores and household management. Additionally, these adolescents may be the primary source of emotional support for depressed or grief-stricken parents.

In Part II, we saw how children cope with divorce and death of a parent. In the first chapter in this section, Robert Weiss describes the impact on children of living in a single-parent family. In most instances, children rise to the challenge and become reliable and responsible family helpers and at times "substitute parents" who cook and care for younger siblings. Single parents often consult with their children about family decisions and confide in them about household and personal problems. As a result, parents and children develop an increased closeness and friendship, and children come to see themselves as peers of their parents.

Single parents viewed their children's added responsibilities as positive but wished that a more "carefree" adolescence was possible. Although the adolescents took pride in their accomplishments, they also regretted the added duties and wistfully longed for more freedom. As confidants of their parents, they were privy to family financial information and were able to develop a realistic understanding of their parents' weaknesses. But this new information sometimes led to more tension and insecurity. Nevertheless, adolescents living in single-parent families may experience special benefits. They may acquire greater self-reliance and independence and a heightened sense of competence. Younger children can also successfully cope with the added responsibilities of a single-parent household. However, their needs for nurturance are less likely to be met.

Illness in the family is another situation that may trigger early psychological maturity in adolescents. Sibling relationships are, for the most part, supportive despite the bickering that typically occurs, and so, when a serious illness strikes, healthy siblings may experience considerable stress. They must cope with disruptions in their relationships with their ill sibling, parents, and peers. In addition, they face changes in the routines of family life because parents spend much of their time at the hospital. Healthy older siblings may take on responsibility for younger brothers or sisters, and like the children in single-parent families, the added responsibilities may provide an impetus for growth. Siblings also have been found to show increased empathy for their parents and greater respect for their ill sibling.[4]

Death of a sibling is a less common but especially devasting crisis that adolescents may confront. In the second article, David Balk describes the grief reactions and self-perceptions of adolescents whose sibling had died. These adolescents initially experienced shock, confusion, depression, anger, guilt, and loneliness. The adolescents frequently thought of their dead sibling; their sleeping habits were disturbed, and their schoolwork suffered. Many of these responses were tempered by time, but some of the feelings of confusion and sadness persisted. Painful feelings of loss recurred on anniversaries of the death and on holidays (see also Chapter 3).

When a sibling dies, the remaining children must cope not only with their own grief but also with that of their parents. Anita Morawetz[5] found that adolescents who lost their brother in war coped in a variety of ways. Some assumed emotional responsibility for their grief-stricken parents and tried to shield them from their own grief. Other adolescents took pride in the fact that their brother had died in the war and found solace in the idea that his death was not in vain. Still others used schoolwork as a retreat from emotional pain and tried to come to grips with the death by writing essays about war.

David Balk found that family characteristics had an impact on the course of adolescents' bereavement reactions. Children from more cohesive families experienced more depression at first. For these adolescents, the rupture of close family ties that occurred with the death made it more of a shock. However, family cohesion ultimately proved to be a resource that facilitated long-term adjustment. Adolescents from less cohesive families experienced less emotional pain initially, but they were more likely to be troubled by guilt feelings and confusion later. However, like the adolescents in single-parent families, some benefits ultimately accrued to these adolescents. They saw themselves as more mature than their friends and learned to value each day because they realized that tragedy could strike suddenly.

Another developmentally vulnerable group of adolescents are those who become parents. Their developmental needs may conflict with the tasks of parenthood. For example, the self-concern that normally occurs in adolescence may interfere with the adolescent mother's ability to form an empathic relationship with her infant. Adolescents' needs to explore new roles may be stifled by the responsibilities of parenthood, and the physical changes accompanying pregnancy may interfere with sexual-identity formation.[7] Adolescent parents face such challenging problems as financial hardship, isolation from peers and school friends, and difficulty of finding affordable child care so they can work or finish their education. Marriage may follow quickly on the heels of an unplanned pregnancy, requiring the adolescent partners to cope with yet another set of developmental tasks.

In the third article, Susan Panzarine and Arthur Elster explore the coping behaviors of adolescent expectant fathers. The expectant fathers used a variety of problem-focused coping strategies. They took direct action by assuming the role of provider and helped to prepare for the baby by buying clothes, toys, and supplies. The unemployed fathers-to-be tried to find jobs, others left school to work full time or sought second jobs or ones with higher pay. The fathers-to-be also coped by seeking advice and reassurance from married friends, and talking with their partners about issues of child rearing and child-care responsibilities. In addition, they read about fatherhood and child care, observed other parents' behavior with their children, and evaluated the parenting they had received. The adolescents saw themselves as "growing up." They spent less time partying and drinking with their single friends and established friendships with married peers. A few adolescents tried to reduce their tension by excessive drinking, avoiding thinking about the baby, and denying the changes that would occur in their lives following the child's birth.

The pregnant adolescent's immaturity and lack of resources increases the likelihood that she will experience psychosocial problems. Economic and social support from family members and community resources may facilitate coping with the crisis of parenthood and help adolescent parents successfully accomplish the task of identity formation.[3] For example, young mothers living at home have certain advantages over young mothers on their own. Their parents may provide advice, food, clothing, and help with child care. This assistance allows young women to continue their education and work, facilitates their transition to parenthood, and enhances their life chances.

References

1. Blyth, D. A., Simmons, R. G., Bulcroft, R., Felt, D., Van Cleave, E. F., & Bush, D. M. The effects of physical development on self-image and satisfaction with body image for adolescent males. In R. G. Simmons (Ed.), *Research in community and mental health* (Vol. 2). Greenwich, Conn.: JAI Press, 1981.
2. Csikszentmihalyi, M., & Larson, R. *Being adolescent: Conflict and growth in the teenage years.* New York: Basic Books, 1984.
3. Friedman, S. B., & Phillips, S. Psychological risk to mother and child as a consequence of adolescent pregnancy. In E. McAnarney (Ed.), *Premature adolescent pregnancy and parenthood.* New York: Grune & Stratton, 1983.
4. Iles, J. P. Children with cancer: Healthy siblings' perceptions during the illness experience. *Cancer Nursing,* 1979, *2,* 371–377.
5. Morawetz, A. The impact on adolescents of the death in war of an older sibling: A group experience. In C. D. Spielberger & I. G. Sarason (Eds.), *Stress and anxiety* (Vol. 8). New York: Academic Press, 1982.
6. Offer, D., Ostrov, E., & Howard, K. I. *The adolescent: A psychological self-portrait.* New York: Basic Books, 1981.
7. Sadler, L. S., & Catrone, C. The adolescent parent: A dual developmental crisis. *Journal of Adolescent Health Care,* 1983, *4,* 100–105.
8. Simmons, R. G., Blyth, D. A., Van Cleave, E. F., & Bush, D. M. Entry into early adolescence: The impact of school structure, puberty, and early dating on self-esteem. *American Sociological Review,* 1979, *44,* 948–967.

4

Growing Up a Little Faster

The Experience of Growing Up in a Single-Parent Household

ROBERT S. WEISS

The Single-Parent Family and the Absence of an Echelon Structure

In most well-functioning two-parent households, there is not much opportunity for children to enter into household decision making. Young children and even adolescents generally have little influence on familial matters. The children may decide on the decorating scheme for their rooms, select their own clothes, choose their friends and their hobbies. But household issues, such as when mealtimes are scheduled and which household jobs are assigned to the children, and familial issues, such as where the family will go on the parents' vacation, tend to be decided by the parents, perhaps after limited consultation with the children. The maintenance and direction of the family unit is a parental responsibility.

This chapter appears in abridged form from *Journal of Social Issues,* 1979, *35,* 97–111. Copyright 1979, the Society for the Psychological Study of Social Issues. Reprinted by permission.

ROBERT S. WEISS • Department of Sociology, University of Massachusetts, Boston Massachusetts 02115.

Because the parents are jointly responsible, each parent feels pledged to support the other. Should there be no prior agreement on a particular issue, each parent is expected to respect the position assumed by the other, at least while the parents are in the presence of the children. In reality, one parent may countermand the other's directives or may collude with the children to frustrate the other's wishes, but behavior of this sort is understood as irresponsible and, perhaps, hostile in intent. In a well-functioning two-parent household, each parent can count on the other to support that parent's rulings.

Goffman[2] has given the name *echelon structure* to an authority structure in which a partnership agreement, not necessarily explicit, exists among those on a superordinate level which has the effect of giving anyone on that level authority in relation to anyone on a subordinate level. The army maintains this sort of authority structure; so do hospitals; so do two-parent families. One-parent families do not. The parent in the one-parent family need not check with the second parent before acceding to the children's wishes in an area in which the second parent is known to have strong commitments. The parent in the one-parent family need not avoid alliances with the children which might prove embarrassing should it become necessary to back up the second parent. No longer is there a structure in which the parent is unable to make common cause with the children for fear of betraying a prior understanding with the other parent. Without a second parent in the household, the echelon structure of the two-parent family dissolves.

Although the collapse of the echelon structure does not require that a parent's relationship to the children undergo change, it makes certain types of changes possible. In particular, it makes possible the development of a new relationship in which the children are defined as having responsibilities and rights in the household not very different from the parent's own. Children now can be asked not only to perform additional chores—this would have been possible within an echelon structure as well—but also to participate in deciding what is to be done.

If a single parent is working full-time, and, especially, if the parent has more than one child to care for, then the parent is likely to find that sharing responsibility with the children is very nearly necessary to maintain the functioning of the household. Some single parents report having called their children into a family council at which they announced to the children that now, with only one parent in the household, the family would have to be run in a new way, with every member of the family assuming a full share of responsibility. The following is from an interview with a mother of four children who ranged in age from about 10 or 11 to about 16:

> As soon as I was on my own, I sat down with the children—I always had a good rapport with the children—and I told them, "Now things are different. Instead of, more or less, it being a family of mother and four children, we're all one family with all equal responsibility, and we all have a say, and we're all very important. And if it is going to work right, we all have to be able to cooperate with each other."

But the single-parent household is different from the two-parent household not simply because children are likely to be asked to do more household tasks. It is different because children are held responsible, not only for the chores themselves, but also for the continued functioning of the household. They are asked to accept that the functioning of the household is as much dependent on their contributions as on the contributions of the parent. They are asked, in a way, to assume some of the concerns of management, to move from the role of subordinate member of the household to that of junior partner.

One way in which a single parent may share managerial responsibility with a child is by making the child responsible for younger children in the family. This delegation of parental responsibility may happen even though the older child is still quite young. Another way in which a single parent may share managerial responsibility is by asking a child to assume responsibilities that might, in a marriage, have been assumed by the spouse. Thus, a single father may rely on an elder daughter to act as hostess and housekeeper as well as to keep an eye on the other children; and a single mother may rely on an elder son to do the heavy work around the house. One mother said:

> I expect my 17-year-old son to understand that even if his friends don't explain to the plumber what happened, that in his particular situation he should do it, because a plumber will pay more attention to another male.

Parents are sometimes brought up short when others remark on the shift that has taken place in their relationships with one or more of the children. One woman found it entirely natural to consult her 6-year-old son, her only child, about when they would have supper, until a friend remarked that few other 6-year-olds were treated by their parents as though they were peers. Occasionally parents are forced by a sudden sense of incongruity to recognize the shift themselves. One woman described wondering, on being criticized by her 15-year-old son for being late with dinner, whether she had encouraged her son to assume the prerogatives of man of the house.

Single parents sometimes report that one of their children competes with them for the leadership role within the family. The child may intrude, challenging the parent's authority, when the parent is talking with one of the other children. Or a child may attempt to play the role of parent in a helpful fashion, just as might the second parent in a two-parent household. One mother said:

> My oldest son has taken on the role of being a parent, telling the others what they should do and what they shouldn't do and how he will send so-and-so to bed if so-and-so doesn't do this or that. And he'll take on all kinds of responsibilities. And I don't think it's good for him, because he's only 11.

In a single-parent household, there may be no one other than the children for the parent to confide in or to turn to for advice or company, especially about household and family problems. In a well-functioning two-parent household, parents bring to each other their tensions and uncertainties. Even in a badly functioning two-parent household, the echelon structure of the household encourages parents to discuss central family-related issues with each other. Certainly it acts as a deterrent to either parent confiding in the children. In a one-parent household the children easily become friends and confidants. Thus there is often greater closeness between the single parent and the children than there was when the parent was married. (George and Wilding[1] also comment on this point.) In addition, the parent can justify sharing worries with the children because the children are understood as having some responsibility for the household. Said one parent:

You're hit with bills and who can you talk to about it but the kids? It's the only other people that you can really talk to. You have to have someone to share it with and so you share it with the people that you're doing it for. And, every so often, if they're bugging me for something that costs too much money, that's out of proportion to what I can afford, I take the bills out and show them the bills, show them what we get in monthly and say, "Now you make sense of it."

The ending of the echelon structure permits children to define themselves as peers of the parent—younger peers, but still peers—and the sharing of responsibility together with the development of companionship between parents and children encourages the children in this definition. But parents may go beyond simply being open and companionate with their children. Especially during the troubled months immediately following the ending of their marriages, single parents may rely on their children for comfort, reassurance, and the sort of nurturant caring that might be called parental.

Our respondents generally saw the changes produced in their children by the children's new responsibilities to have been largely beneficial, although they sometimes regretted that their children had not had a more carefree childhood and adolescence. With the exception of a few parents who worried that they had lost control of their children, parents were pleased that their children had proven so capable of rising to the challenge of increased responsibility.

Adolescents living within single-parent families, although they tended to agree with their parents that they had been required to move toward early maturity in a number of ways, seemed to see the experience as of mixed value. It meant less security; they learned to share their parents' worries. Several adolescents whose parents were separated or divorced said that they were constantly aware that their parents were financially pressed. Their fathers complained to them of their mothers' financial demands, and their mothers complained of their fathers' unwillingness to help. Or their mothers asked them to tell their fathers that they needed clothes or schoolbooks or money for orthodonture, while the father told them to tell their mothers to be more reasonable. A few children had shifted their residence from mothers' homes to fathers' homes and had then been made aware of disputes between the parents over whether their fathers remained liable for support payments. One adolescent girl, reviewing her childhood, said:

> *You don't have, not necessarily the childhood, but you don't have the freedom of not worrying about things, about money.*

Some adolescents report having been made quite insecure by their parents' concern about money. One girl told of checking her downstairs food pantry to reassure herself that it was filled with canned goods.

Awareness of their parents' problems and uncertainties led adolescents to recognize that their parents were people like themselves, with frailties as well as strengths. Further impetus to seeing their parents as vulnerable came from adolescents' observations of the parents' attempts to establish new cross-sex relationships. They learned that their parents could be elated when things went well in the parents' dating life, and depressed when they went badly, just as was true for them. They may also have been led to recognize their parents' uncertainty in sexual matters, and to see their parents as beset by some of the same conflicts that troubled them. This more realistic view of their parents was strengthened when the parents turned to them, as junior partners in the household or as confidants, for understanding and support. Recognizing the parents' frailties reduced the adolescents' ability to rely unquestioningly on them and led to feelings of insecurity as well as to resolutions to be self-reliant: indeed, adolescents implied that they had become self-reliant just because there seemed no one else on whom they could rely. Here is a comment by a 16-year-old girl that expressed this feeling:

> *I have become very independent. I am an independent person. I can probably get along by myself if I have to. Not completely. If my mother died, I'd be crying. But I'd get along. I think it's because I already do a lot of things by myself that, I suppose, if I had both parents, I wouldn't have to.*

These children sometimes describe themselves as "loners": not isolated, but not deeply enmeshed in the peer culture either. Other children sometimes see themselves as unusually serious and mature. One girl spoke of being used as "Dear Abby" by her friends. But most prominent in the self-description of these children is their sense of unusual competence. In contrast to children in two-parent homes, these children may regularly cook or clean the house, be responsible for their clothes, and be responsible for younger children. They are likely to take pride in being able to carry more responsibility than their friends from two-parent households who, in their view, have been pampered. Here is a comment by a 16-year-old girl:

> *I get very angry at times, like when I hear this girl, she said, "My mother yelled at me this morning because I didn't make my bed, and I am so upset today." And, I just think, "You little twerp! I have to make my bed, my mother's bed, I have to clean the whole house, I have to cook the dinner, I have to take trash out!" And I was just so angry.*

These children, on recognizing how much more capable they are in certain respects than other children, may feel enhanced esteem for themselves. But they may also feel some envy of children who have had fewer responsibilities. One girl said:

> *If there were two parents, it might be better. It would be kind of like when my grandmother comes. You come home, and there is Grandmother. You know she's going to be there, you know she's going to have the house cleaned up and the table set. I don't know, just silly little things, that you don't have to come home and worry about it and do it yourself or try to get your sisters help to do it, because Mother isn't there.*

It would seem accurate to say that most children of single-parent families, though they may be pleased that they proved able to meet the challenges of new expectations, also regret having had to do so.

Possible Long-Run Effects on Children of Growing Up a Little Faster

What difference does it make in the long run for a child to have "grown up a little faster"? The loss of a parent from a household is, for most children, a serious reverse which may for some time affect their development. And, if parents remain in conflict with each other after the ending of their marriages, their children may well be victimized in the process: no matter whether the children identify with one parent, attempt to maintain loyalty to both, or refuse to ally themselves with either, the children may find the parents' quarrel drains their energy, leaving them with too few resources for their own concerns. The changed role of the children in the household and the new responsibilities, rights, and obligations engendered by the end of the parental echelon structure, however, appear not in themselves to be injurious, at least not for adolescent children.

Adolescents appear capable of managing both greater responsibility and greater independence than they are ordinarily permitted. This is not to say that adolescents can forego parental support and investment, but rather that, so long as there has been no earlier deprivation of nurturance, and so long as some degree of parental support and investment remains available, adolescents can, in general, assume additional responsibility for their households and themselves without sustaining harm to their development. It seems well within adolescents' capabilities for them to assume genuine responsibility for the functioning of their households, to get through much of the day without adult supervision or control, to act as surrogate parents to siblings, and to act as junior partners, companions, and confidants to their parents, and, on occasion, as their parents' parents. Of course, should there be a withdrawal of parental emotional investment in an adolescent's well-being as an accompaniment to the change in the structure of the adolescent's family, the adolescent's trust in the reliability of apparently committed others may well be diminished, with some risk to the course taken by the adolescent's future life. But so long as both parents display continued concern and support, adolescents seem able to take in stride the new responsibilities of living in a single-parent family. Indeed, they may find their feelings of self-worth enhanced by the realization that the maintenance of the household depends on their contributions.

Those whose experience with children who have grown up in single-parent families comes primarily from working with children in trouble are likely to emphasize the pathogenic potential of the single-parent family. But for many children, both younger and older, the new demands on them for autonomy and responsibility may lead to growth. Although these youngsters may regret not having a more traditional family and a more care-free youth, they often respect themselves for having been able to respond to what they recognize as their family's genuine need for their contributions.

The single-parent family, insofar as it requires that the children within it behave responsibly, may, in this respect, be a better setting for growing up than the two-parent family. In many two-parent families genuine responsibility for the household is withheld from children. The children may be assigned a variety of chores, but the partnership of the parents prevents them from participating as full members of the household. Children in single-parent households often have no option; they must participate in their households as full members, with the rights and responsibilities of full members. And this can be a useful experience which leads to self-esteem, independence, and a genuine sense of competence. The last word may be given to a 17-year-old boy, the youngest of four children, who had been in a single-parent household for 5 or 6 years. He said:

In the long run—I feel sort of like I shouldn't say it—but a lot of kids are better off if their parents do get divorced, because you grow up a lot quicker.

References

1. George, V., & Wilding, P. *Motherless families.* London: Routledge & Kegan Paul, 1972.
2. Goffman, E. *Asylums.* New York: Doubleday, 1961.

5

Adolescents' Grief Reactions and Self-Concept Perceptions Following Sibling Death

DAVID BALK

Introduction

Few researchers have investigated sibling bereavement during adolescence.[2,12,25] The devastating potential of sibling bereavement on children has been noted, but none of the studies on this subject focused upon adolescents.

   Sibling death during adolescence very likely has an enduring effect on a surviving child.[23] At the same time, sibling death may provide teenagers the impetus for psychological growth. Offer[17] was impressed by the resiliency of his adolescent subjects in mastering serious crises such as death in the family and by their ability to profit developmentally from such events. Crisis theorists,[1,3,7] life-span developmental psychologists,[9,10,11] and psychiatric investigators of psychosocial transitions[18] have noted that certain crises present paradoxical prospects to human beings—vulnera-

This chapter appears in abridged form from *Journal of Youth and Adolescence*, 1983, *12*, 137–161. Reprinted by permission.

DAVID BALK • Director of Program Evaluation, La Frontera Center, Tucson, Arizona 85713.

bility to major behavioral disorganization as well as potential for growth. Crises involving psychological development, traumatic stress, or anticipated life transitions often present growth prospects.[1]

Uncertainty about the effects of sibling death on adolescents' psychological development, as well as the lack of systematic study of teenagers' reactions to sibling death, provided the motivation for conducting this investigation. What are the effects of sibling bereavement on teenagers who are, to all appearances, "normal adolescents"? Are teenagers likely to be impaired psychologically, or are they likely to successfully integrate sibling death into their lives? What do these teenagers report as their grief responses to a sibling's death?

Sample

Two national organizations that provide support to parents by means of local self-help groups assisted in obtaining all participants for this study. The Society of Compassionate Friends, a mutual support group for bereaved parents and the largest growing self-help organization in the United States, according to one study,[4] helped locate 90% of the teenagers interviewed; The Candlelighters, a mutual support group for parents of children who have cancer or who have died from cancer, helped locate the rest of the participants.

Forty-eight teenagers were interviewed, but two methodological restrictions permitted data from only 33 to be included in the sample. The restrictions were (1) to include only one interviewee per family and thereby prevent overrepresentation of a single family environment and (2) to include only persons between 14 and 19 years of age and thereby to obtain relative homogeneity of ages while allowing for both younger and older adolescents. Also, sibling death had to have occurred during the participant's adolescence.

The 33 teenagers in the sample were almost evenly divided between younger (14–16) and older (17–19) adolescents. Participants were white, from middle- to upper middle-income families, and predominantly from urban environments; 13 were male, and

20 female. Twenty were the opposite sex of their sibling who had died. Most siblings had died from accidents, and 10 had died from terminal illnesses; in most cases of death from terminal illness, the teenager interviewed had not anticipated the sibling's death.

Findings

These 33 teenagers had endured a life stress considerably greater than those that the majority of adolescents in the United States face. They had withstood this stress and demonstrated psychological adjustment equal to that of their peers. However, there was something qualitatively distinct about these teenagers when the author compared them in his mind with other adolescents with whom he is familiar. At the very least, this qualitative difference was summed up well by several of the participants who independently said their sibling's death made them "grow up fast."

All of the participants indicated that their sibling's death had considerably influenced their lives, but only in a few cases did there seem to be an adverse impact on psychological development. In the great majority of cases, sibling death during adolescence apparently had not impaired these 33 teenagers' psychological development. Some evidence gathered in this study would not support the notion that the serious life crisis of sibling death had facilitated psychological growth, as suggested by some researchers;[1,17] study data indicated that the teenagers were similar to their peers in terms of adjustment. Conservatively, it can be said that the crisis of sibling death presented obstacles the teenagers could surmount.

On the other hand, evidence from the interviews and from the author's interaction with these teenagers during the interviews suggests that the crisis of sibling death had been used as a means of growth. The teenagers perceived themselves as "more grown up" or "more mature" than most of their peers; they valued each day and its potential more than they had prior to their sibling's death; they had learned that some severe things can happen and have to be accepted because the outcome cannot be altered; they had an increasing sense of contrast with the selves they remembered prior to their sibling's death, and this contrast was a function of elapsed time since the death, rather than of age of participant. The participants' values development seems to have been influenced positively.

It would be erroneous to assume that everything had returned to normal over time for these teenagers or that they were exempt from ongoing struggles associated with sibling bereavement. Their grief symptoms, which were much like those reported typical of normal adult bereavement responses,[15,19,20] had a lingering quality. Emotional responses diminished on the whole, but one-quarter to one-half of the participants in this study reported what would be considered enduring grief reactions. These enduring effects of sibling bereavement are of clinical significance. Academic work continued to suffer for 25% of the participants. Other grief reactions seem to have run their course. Yet the adage *time heals* could hardly be considered appropriate for a significant minority of these teenagers. Silver and Wortman[23] aptly noted that "outsiders frequently underestimate the nature and duration of the distress encountered by victims" (p. 338) of serious life crises. Two or more years after the death of their sibling, many adolescents still recalled their sibling's death as a source of current pain: tears, shaking, shortness of breath, and periods of heavy sobbing were not uncommon during the interviews. One wonders if these teenagers encounter problems imposed by unrealistic societal expectations regarding recovery from bereavement.

The first year of bereavement may well be an important key to researchers' identifying the changes in bereavement resolution, as the literature has suggested.[19,20] This inference is based on the fact that dividing participants into three time periods since the death revealed very few differences in responses. If significant changes take place in the first 12 months after the death, a framework to identify the changes would examine key events that occur throughout this year as well as sampling across time at randomly selected points. These key events would include the funeral, the return to school, holidays, and the anniversary of the death. Identifying what responses to key events influence bereavement resolution would provide knowledge of the process whereby "time heals."

Sex differences were considered likely when this study was first conceived. Maccoby and Jacklin[16] pointed to sex differences in coping with stress and frustration, and Rutter[22] reported sex differences in response to family distress. Some sex differences did emerge in the present study.

One sex difference was the apparent insulation from shock at the time of the death among females older than the sibling who died. Would this reaction be found if a similar study of bereaved teenagers were conducted? What could account for this reaction, which was unlike that of all the other participants in this study? Perhaps as Maccoby and Jacklin believe, self-control mechanisms are learned earlier by females than by males. However, females younger than the sibling who died apparently did not manifest such self-control mechanisms. Are different self-control mechanisms operative for females older than the sibling at the time of death? If so, what are the sex self-control mechanisms, and how do they work?

A portrait could be tentatively drawn of probable reactions to sibling death during adolescence. In general, after a sibling's death a bereaved teenager will likely feel shocked, afraid, lonely, confused, depressed, and/or angry. Thoughts about the dead sibling will occur most or all of the time. Sleeping habits, but not eating habits, will be upset. Holidays and other special times of the year will be experienced as unpleasant. Hallucinations of the deceased sibling may occur, but this bereavement reaction is less likely than are others. Grades and study habits will almost certainly suffer. Thoughts of suicide may occur, which are primarily sparked by a desire to be reunited with the sibling and/or to get away from troubles. In time, emotional responses to the death will diminish, but feelings of confusion, shock, anger, depression, guilt, or loneliness may well persist. Thoughts of the dead sibling will occur less frequently, certainly not as obsessively. Sleeping habits will return to normal. Anniversary reactions will persist, and certain days or times of the year will present special difficulties because they will bring to mind the dead sibling. Suicidal thoughts will be unlikely, as will hallucinations. Grades and study habits will return to normal for most teenagers.

Bereaved teenagers younger than their sibling at the time of death are likely to feel shocked. For some reason, females older than siblings who die are not likely to feel shocked. However, females seem prone to a growing sense of confusion about their sibling's death. Teenagers who are depressed at the time of the death seem likely to feel confused about the death later on. Teenagers afraid at the time of death seem to feel confused about their sibling's death later on. Further research in this regard may explore if sex-related factors link fear and depression at the time of the death and later feelings of confusion about the death.

The preceding general portrait can be supplemented by the information provided by the examination of the family's influence on teenagers' emotional responses to sibling death. Tatsuoka[24] referred to this exercise as giving data derived from discriminant analysis a psychologically meaningful interpretation.

Following a sibling's death, a teenager with greater family coherency is faced with a shattered family environment; previously this environment was the source of security. The death leaves the teenagers shocked, numb, lonely, and scared; the intensity of these feelings convinces the teenager that the feelings will "never go away." Never having been plunged so deeply into painful emotions, the teenager believes that there will be no remission. Sources of comfort, strength, and support are suddenly absent, and the youth is hurting intensely. The teenager's prospects seem bleak, and the youth is filled with dread. As time passes, the teenager notices that these feelings change. The youth shares personal thoughts with family members, especially with his or her mother. Over time the teenager notices an enduring sense of depression about the sibling's death, but no longer reports feeling scared, lonely, or numb. Little confusion lingers about the death. The teenager does not feel guilty.

The profile that emerges for a teenager from a family with less perceived family coherency contrasts sharply with the portrait of a teenager from a family with greater coherency. In the less coherent families, personal conversations occurred infrequently, and feelings of emotional closeness prior to the death were minimal. The teenager, as would be expected from this history, talks to no one in the family about personal matters after the death. Threats to the family environment are not distressing to the teenager, however, because the family has not been a source of support or security. Immediate reactions after the death are guilt and anger, but teenagers from less coherent families are unlikely to experience shock, numbness, or fear. The distance already established with family members does not increase feelings of loneliness. Over time such teenagers feel confused about the death and their attitudes about it but feel relieved to be beyond the ordeal.

Family coherency differences among participants may be associated with bereavement resolution differences. The research literature suggests that the distinctions found between greater and less family coherency are related to a family's role in facilitating or inhibiting healthy bereavement outcomes.[5,6,8,13,14,21,22] The role of communication and of interpersonal bonds seems paramount in this regard. A tradition of greater family coherency tends to assist teenagers to work through problems by using the family as a resource; however, teenagers in such a situation report current feelings of depression, unlike their counterparts from families with less family coherency. Perhaps depression is the price for close personal sibling relationships severed by death. The lack of family coherency insulates youths from many troubling emotions, but they tend to feel guilty at first and later feel confused about the death. Perhaps guilt and confusion are prices paid for distant sibling relationships severed by death.

Two Case Descriptions

Two case descriptions will illustrate the impact of greater versus less coherent families on a teenager's experience and resolution of bereavement. In the first case, an intact family with extensive personal communication and close emotional ties enabled a young girl to gradually integrate her brother's death. The girl said she still hurts over her brother's death, finds her family and friends a source of support, and remembers her relationship with her brother as never having been better than in the weeks before he died. In the second case, an estranged family whose communication was marked by sarcasm and distrust, was incapable of providing mutual support during the months preceding and following its youngest member's anticipated death. Unable to help each other, the family provided no solace to its teenage boy.

This youngster still seethed with anger at his parents' handling of his sister's illness, and he remained haunted over being on poor terms with his sister before she died.

These teenagers' continued feelings of grief support the observation of Silver and Wortman[23] that outsiders underestimate the intensity and duration of feelings aroused by life tragedies. However, the boy's emptiness, confusion, guilt, and anger contrast sharply with the girl's clean sense of hurt and her lack of confusion regarding her brother's death.

The boy's major aim was to get away from his home and begin life on his own. What sort of life he wished to live remained unclear. The girl was involved in many school activities and planned to obtain a college degree in one of the helping professions, probably clinical psychology. One of her goals was to help youth experiencing a significant loss, for example, the death of a sibling.

Deborah

Deborah is a 15-year-old whose brother was killed in an accident 2 years before she was interviewed. She feels very close to her parents and her remaining brother. She talks with her mother about "practically everything" and respects her mother very much. She would like to talk with her brother about their sibling's death. Having gone through some rough times after her brother's death, Deborah has found clear direction for her life. She was very concerned that her family might not recover from her brother's death. However, not only did her family pull through well, they were a major source of help to one another. Her family spends a lot of time together. Throughout the interview, she struck me as being more mature than her years. Here are some of her comments:

> I talked often with my mom right after Ed's death. Talked about why. Why did he die. And what am I supposed to do. Nowadays we talk very often. Just about the way we both have taken it.
>
> Right after Ed died, it was somewhat difficult to talk. I was still at the stage where I wasn't sure at all, everything comes so quick, and I still wasn't sure that everything was true and that everything was real. It's not all that

difficult these days to talk. I've realized it's true, and I guess I've faced it. I've faced a lot of it. I'm pretty much a person that talks. I can't keep a lot in me. I've learned how to deal with it.

One guy I wanted to talk to seemed scared he would hurt me. If he had been willing, I would have just cried.

The death makes me value a lot more things. It's made me think a lot more in that it's changed some of my thoughts. It's changed a lot of things about my religion, and it's made me value life, 'cause my brother really enjoyed life and he did a lot in it and he helped a lot of people.

I'd really like to talk to my brother Mike about this. But I haven't. He keeps a lot of his feelings in and doesn't talk a lot. He's more quiet, and I'm more the kind that can't hold any kind of feelings in and needs to talk to somebody.

Right after Ed died, a bunch of his friends wanted to talk to me. Mostly about how I was. How I was and how the family was doing. Then next came what did I feel like and what really happened. I wanted to talk with them because they were the people we knew best and how I would react. And I felt comfortable with them. They were like—Ed's friends, because they knew him first.

I want to talk because it still hurts.

After Ed died, my folks wanted to know what they could do. My mom said, when the relatives started to come over, that she didn't want me to be pushed out of the way. "We're still here," she said, "but if you want to get away for a while you can go away." Now they encourage me to get involved in things. To know what's going on.

After Ed's death, school wasn't the most important thing. I had to get myself back together. I was more with people, and I don't believe that you get everything out of a book 'cause you have a lot more to learn out of life itself. I'm starting to study more again. I don't study as much as I used to. But I want to go to college. I know my directions better now, and I'm out of that shock. And I've faced a lot of things, and I've looked at more things and am gradually piecing my life back together.

The most important thing to know if your brother dies is that all these different stages of feelings you go through are normal. That you are not crazy.

Ralph

Ralph is a 16-year-old whose sister died of cancer a year and a half before the interview. He never talks to his family about personal matters and does not feel close to anyone in his family. However, he reports that he often talked to and felt very close to his sister who died. He prefers to be away from the house, and frequently comes home these days in the early morning hours when everyone else has gone to bed. His family does very little together. After his sister's death, Ralph spent hours in his bedroom listening to tape recordings he had made of her. This behavior is only one indication of how deeply affected he was by his sister's death. His parents had him see a psychiatrist after the death because "they thought I was sick or something, so I figured I'd get it out and let them know I am normal." It still bothers Ralph that his sister died at a time when the two of them were not getting along. As far as Ralph's family goes, Ralph seems detached, as though he could take them or leave them. However, he misses his sister very much. Here are some of his comments:

I never really talked to anybody in my family after Sally died. They thought I was crazy or something. They wanted to bring it up, but I knew she was going to die, and there was nothing I could do about it. So I accepted the fact, and when it happened, it happened. They all felt I should feel worse than I did or something. They thought there was something wrong with me because they didn't think I was acting normal. They wanted me to go to a psychiatrist. I told them, "Get out of here," but they made me go anyway. Seventy-five bucks to have them tell me I'm OK.

When she first died, I sort of moped around. And I didn't talk too much at school. Usually I'm a big mouth in class. I seem to get along better with kids at school now. I don't know why. I guess I just appreciated everything more. I'd never really thought about dying. It was just something that happened 80 or 90 years away. I never had it that close—just other relatives.

Right after she died, I wasn't dumbfounded. A little shocked. Numb. I knew when my mom first came in my room that Sally was dead. They hardly ever come in my room, and when they do it's to tell me breakfast is ready or something like that. My mom came in, and her eyes were all red. She sat down on the bed, and right away I knew it was over. I just figured—well, when I went to bed the night before I just thought I'd try to get on her good side tomorrow, and I never got the chance. I did feel sort of relieved. There were things that I could do now that I couldn't do then. Like we couldn't have no people in and had to be real quiet when she was asleep. Now I can come home at 1 o'clock and make as much noise as I want, and it doesn't matter. Yeah, I felt depressed. I had moped around a lot like my dad. Nowadays I feel alone because you could always hear Sally in the house, no matter where you were. I still wish it hadn't happened, but every time I think about it, I start feeling empty. I feel more guilty about the way I treated her at the end than that she died. I felt cheated when Sally died, and I was angry at mom. Because she could have kept giving her those drugs, even though they weren't doing anything. I never thought I'd get that mad at my mom. It's not the same, but it's not gone.

After Sally died, I had some dreams about her. Never nightmares. The dreams didn't start right away. I guess I'll always have them, but it's only occasionally.

The important thing to know if your brother or sister dies is, well, you've got to look at it from a reality point. You've got to face the fact. You can't ignore it. Try to live with it, that's the biggest thing. Try to become at peace with yourself, about how you felt. Sit down and think it out by yourself.

References

1. Baldwin, B. A paradigm for the classification of emotional crises: Implications for crisis intervention. *American Journal of Orthopsychiatry*, 1978, *48*, 538–551.
2. Balk, D. E. *Sibling death during adolescence: Self concept and bereavement reactions.* Unpublished doctoral dissertation, University of Illinois at Urbana-Champaign, 1981.
3. Bloom, B. L. *Community mental health: A general introduction.* Monterey, Calif.: Brooks/Cole, 1977.
4. Borman, L., Videka, L., Sherman, B., & Wax, M. *Feedback report to Compassionate Friends.* Unpublished manuscript, Department of Behavioral Sciences, University of Chicago, 1979.
5. Cain, A., Fast, I., & Erickson, M. Children's disturbed reactions to the death of a sibling. *American Journal of Orthopsychiatry*, 1964, *34*, 741–752.
6. Calhoun, L. G., Selby, J. W., & King, H. E. *Dealing with crisis: A guide to critical life problems.* Englewood Cliffs, N.J.: Prentice-Hall, 1976.
7. Caplan, G. *Principles of preventive psychiatry.* New York: Basic Books, 1964.
8. Cobb, B. Psychological impact of long illness and death of a child on the family circle. *Journal of Pediatrics*, 1956, *49*, 746–751.
9. Danish, J. J., & D'Augelli, A. R. Promoting competence and enhancing development through life development intervention. In L. A. Bond & J. C. Rosen (Eds.), *Primary prevention of psychopathology.* Hanover, N.H.: University Press of New England, 1980.
10. Danish, S. J., Smyer, M. A., & Nowak, C. A. Developmental intervention: Enhancing life-event processes. In P. B. Baltes & O. G. Brim (Eds.), *Life-span development and behavior* (Vol. 3). New York: Academic Press, 1980.
11. Datan, N., & Ginsberg, L. (Eds.). *Life-span development psychology: Normative life crises.* New York: Academic Press, 1975.

12. Feinberg, D. Preventive therapy with siblings of a dying child. *Journal of the American Academy of Child Psychiatry*, 1970, *9*, 644–688.
13. Hilgard, J. R., Newman, M. R., & Fisk, F. Strength of adult ego identity following childhood bereavement. *American Journal of Orthopsychiatry*, 1960, *30*, 788–798.
14. Krell, R., & Rabkin, L. The effects of sibling death on the surviving child: A family perspective. *Family Process*, 1979, *18*, 471-477.
15. Lindemann, E. Symptomatology and management of acute grief. *American Journal of Psychiatry*, 1944, *101*, 141–148.
16. Maccoby, E. E., & Jacklin, C. N. *The psychology of sex differences*. Stanford, Calif.: Stanford University Press, 1974.
17. Offer, D. *The psychological world of the teenager*. New York: Basic Books, 1969.
18. Parkes, C. M. Psycho-social transitions: A field for study. *Social Science and Medicine*, 1971, *5*, 101–115.
19. Parkes, C. M. *Bereavement: Studies of grief in adult life*. New York: International Universities Press, 1972.
20. Parkes, C. M. Unexpected and untimely bereavement: A statistical study of young Boston widows and widowers. In G. Schoenberg, I. Gerber, A. Wiener, A. H. Kutscher, & D. Peretz (Eds.), *Bereavement: Its psychosocial aspects*. New York: Columbia University Press, 1975.
21. Poznanski, E. O. Childhood depression: A psychodynamic approach to the etiology and treatment of depression in children. In A. P. French & I. N. Berlin (Eds.), *Depression in children and adolescents*. New York: Human Sciences Press, 1979.
22. Rutter, M. Sex differences in children's responses to family stress. In E. J. Anthony & C. Koupernik (Eds.), *The child in his family* (Vol. 1). New York: Wiley, 1970.
23. Silver, R. L., & Wortman, C. B. Coping with undesirable life events. In J. Garber & M. E. P. Seligman (Eds.), *Human helplessness: Theory and applications*. New York: Academic Press, 1980.
24. Tatsuoka, M. *Discriminant analysis: The study of group differences*. Champaign, Ill.: Institute for Personality and Ability Testing, 1970.
25. Vernick, J. (1980, June 17). Personal communication.

6

Coping in a Group of Expectant Adolescent Fathers

SUSAN PANZARINE and ARTHUR ELSTER

Adolescents represent a special subgroup of fathers who risk having parenting difficulties because of several situational and developmental factors.[1] Few studies have explored these factors in a group of expectant adolescent fathers. Although research has begun on the special needs and concerns of these young men,[2-5] few, if any, studies have been concerned with how adolescent fathers deal with the transition to parenthood. Since a significant number of these young fathers continue to be involved with their children,[6] investigations into how they cope with this new role are needed.

For our purposes, *coping* will be defined as "cognitive and behavioral efforts made to master, tolerate or reduce external and internal demands and conflicts among them."[7] In keeping with the work of Lazarus *et al.*,[7-9] coping has been conceptualized as multidimensional. Lazarus *et al.* describe two major foci of coping

From *Journal of Adolescent Health Care*, 1983, *4*(2), 117–120. Copyright 1983 by the Society for Adolescent Medicine. This article was originally entitled, "Coping in a Group of Expectant Adolescent Fathers: An Exploratory Study." Reprinted by permission.

SUSAN PANZARINE • School of Nursing, University of Maryland, Baltimore, Maryland 21201. **ARTHUR B. ELSTER** • College of Medicine, University of Utah, Salt Lake City, Utah 84132.

strategies: dealing with the problem itself and managing the stressful emotions that arise. Individual coping strategies can be categorized into four main modes that can be either problem- or emotion-focused: (1) *direct actions* are anything one does to deal with a stressful event or the emotions it engenders; (2) *information seeking* is any effort to gather knowledge that can be applied toward problem solving or reappraising the situation; (3) *intrapsychic processes* are the cognitive processes used in relation to a stressful encounter; and (4) *inhibition of action* is restraining oneself from taking actions that would affect a stressful transaction.

In this report we describe the coping strategies exhibited by 20 expectant adolescent fathers during a series of interviews. These results comprise part of the data from an exploratory study reported elsewhere concerning the identification of perceived stressors.[3,10]

Methods

Subjects

Prospective adolescent fathers were recruited from three obstetric clinics affiliated with the University of Utah Medical Center. The sample was restricted to males who were 18 years of age or younger and who planned to continue contact with their female partners and babies after the birth. Access to each prospective father was obtained through his partner, who was given written information about the purpose and demands of the study and a form for the boyfriend/husband to complete on which he could indicate his willingness to participate. Contact with potential subjects was not initiated directly so that confidentiality could be maintained.

A total of 20 adolescents volunteered. All were 17 or 18 years of age; 18 were white, and 2 were Hispanic. Eleven subjects were Mormon. Most of the 20 were actively involved in the pregnancy: 17 attended at least some of their partners' clinic visits and/or participated in preparatory classes for labor and delivery. Only three subjects expressed any negative feelings about either fatherhood or the baby. Three subjects did not complete the prenatal interviews: one withdrew because of divorce; one partner delivered before the third trimester interview; and one subject did not have a final interview because the study had ended.

Although all conceptions were premarital, 15 subjects had married by the time of their partners' delivery. This is consistent with state statistics which reveal that whereas approximately 70% of babies born to adolescents are conceived premaritally, only 20% are actually born out of wedlock.[11]

Procedure

All interviews were conducted by one of the authors (SP) or by a female graduate student in perinatal nursing. The subjects were interviewed in their homes or at the hospital, depending upon the adolescent's preference. Each session lasted approximately 1 hour and was audiotaped.

Interviews were conducted during the first, second, and third trimesters of pregnancy when possible. Since many of the female partners did not begin prenatal care during the first trimester, only 4 subjects were interviewed during this time period ($\bar{X} = 12$ weeks). Twelve subjects were interviewed during the second trimester ($\bar{X} = 22.2$ weeks), and 17 during the third ($\bar{X} = 32.7$ weeks). In all, a total of 33 prenatal interviews were conducted. Nine subjects were interviewed once, 9 subjects twice, and 2 subjects were seen three times before delivery.

Interviews were semistructured. The investigators explored the adolescent's current thoughts about the baby and fatherhood and discussed any actions that he had taken to prepare for parenthood. Coping strategies that were used to deal with other stressors generated by the pregnancy (i.e., educational problems, health concerns, etc.) were not assessed.

Results

Content analyses of the tape-recorded interviews by one of the investigators (SP) generated a list of 10 coping strategies used by these 20 subjects. A response was coded as a coping strategy if it was a thought or action directed toward dealing with the up-

coming transition to fatherhood or toward managing or controlling any negative feelings aroused because of this. These strategies were then grouped according to their primary focus (i.e.,
problem versus emotion) and subdivided according to coping
mode (i.e., direct actions, information seeking, intrapsychic processes, and inhibition of action).

Problem-Focused Strategies

The predominant focus of the following eight coping strategies is to deal with the upcoming event of fatherhood. These
adolescents mobilized a variety of techniques to prepare themselves for the assumption of their new role.

Direct Actions.   All 20 subjects used direct actions sometime
during the pregnancy to cope with impending fatherhood. These
centered mainly on assuming the role of provider and helping
with various preparations for the baby.

Assuming the Role of Provider.   All 20 subjects viewed the provider role as a major component of fatherhood. Each was involved in some activity to improve the financial situation of his
partner and baby. Those who were not working before the pregnancy found jobs. For many, the job was in addition to school.
Others left school to work full time. Those who were already
working sought better paying jobs, overtime, or a second job.
Most were concerned about paying hospital bills and saving
enough money to move into their own apartment. If they were
already living on their own, they saved to get a larger apartment
in a better neighborhood. Some sought new jobs specifically to
secure health insurance for the pregnancy and pediatric care.

Helping Prepare for the Baby.   Some variation of this activity
was reported by 18 adolescents. Some helped buy baby clothes,
supplies, and toys. Others focused mainly upon preparing the
physical environment by fixing up a room or a crib for the
newborn.

Information Seeking.   Fifteen subjects sought information
throughout the pregnancy. Most gathered information by turning to others, and only a few utilized prepared literature.

Talking with Others about Fatherhood.   Fourteen talked with
their partner, friends, or parents about some aspect of fa-

therhood. Discussions with the partner usually centered on exploring ideas about child rearing. Some tried to clarify their respective responsibilities regarding child care and the upkeep of the household.

Several adolescents asked married friends about their experiences with fatherhood. A small number of subjects talked with their own fathers about what it was like when they were new parents. This type of information seeking may also have been a means of eliciting reassurance from those who had already been through the experience. As such, this strategy may have served a secondary purpose, namely coping with some of the anxieties about fatherhood.

Observing and Evaluating Other Parents. Four adolescents observed and evaluated other people's interactions with their children. They seemed to use these experiences to identify behavior they wanted to either emulate or avoid.

Reading about Fatherhood and Child Care. Four young men read literature on parenthood and infancy in order to learn "what to expect." They used pamphlets they had received from the hospital clinics as well as books they had bought.

Intrapsychic Processes. Thirteen subjects reported using coping strategies that reflected some type of intrapsychic process, such as mental rehearsal, worrying, fantasizing about the future, and reviewing the past. These centered in the following two areas.

Fantasizing about Fatherhood and the Baby. Twelve adolescents reported fantasizing about fatherhood and/or the baby. Some thought about themselves in different situations with their children, outlining the kinds of things they would teach them. Although most had thought about the child only in terms of a preferred sex, others had more detailed visions. Some formulated plans and goals for the child that ranged from plausible to fantastic. Many of these fantasies concerned the teen's own career aspirations which might be realized by the child. One adolescent described it this way:

> I dream about him [the baby] every night. I dream that he'll be a good rock star and things like that. . . . And I know, for one thing, he'll have rhythm in his hands already, 'cause I was never taught by a teacher. The rhythm was just there, and I always wanted to play in a band.

Others thought about how they would do as parents. Some worried particularly about the role conflict of being an adolescent and a father simultaneously, and how this would affect their ability to be a good parent. One young man reported:

I've thought about it [fatherhood] a lot, and it scares me. Hell, I'll admit it—I'm not a full grown man, and I never try to pretend to be. I'm still, well, a child in a sense. . . . I'll love it, but I'm not sure I'll know how to teach it and guide it.

Reviewing and Evaluating How They Were Parented. Seven of the adolescents began to think more about how they had been raised and began to evaluate their parents' performance. When asked to share their thoughts about impending fatherhood, they spoke of it in terms of traits and child-rearing patterns they saw in their own parents.

Inhibition of Action. At times, holding back from taking certain actions can be a means of coping with a potential problem situation. In our study group, six adolescents used this mode of coping.

Settling Down. Six expectant fathers described how the pregnancy had "mellowed" them. They had ended their partying, drinking, and fighting. They often talked about how their usual contacts with single friends had diminished and about their desire to begin developing friendships with married peers. This strategy also involved an additional dimension. These teens tried to alter the meaning of the situation by casting it in a positive light. They denied the desire to do the sorts of things their single friends did, since they were "growing up" and getting ready to be fathers. Thus, an intrapsychic process was also mobilized to reduce the emotional discomfort accompanying the loss of peer contact.

Emotion-Focused Strategies

The major emphasis of these strategies is to minimize or eliminate the emotional discomfort arising from the anticipation of fatherhood.

Direct Actions: *Alcohol Abuse.* Two subjects reported an increase in alcohol abuse during their partners' pregnancy. Their situations were quite different: one adolescent expressed marked ambivalence about becoming a father, and the other was upset at the obstacles that might prevent him from assuming the father role. The latter had been forbidden to see his partner by her parents. His distress was compounded by his partner's mixed messages about her own desire to continue her involvement with him. He was particularly anxious to see the baby and participate in its care, but he feared that her parents would not allow this.

Intrapsychic Processes: Changing the Meaning of the Situation. Three adolescents denied ever thinking ahead about fatherhood or the baby, even when interviewed late in the partners' pregnancy. When asked specifically about the kinds of changes in their lives that they thought would accompany the birth of the baby, these young men maintained that no major changes would occur. This response is particularly striking since two of these young men were married.

Discussion

Our results are based on a small convenience sample, and, as such, cannot be generalized. However, the goal of this exploratory study was to provide an empirical basis for generating hypotheses for future studies.

The Lazarus paradigm was used as a framework within which the data were organized. The adolescents in our study used coping strategies that included direct actions, information seeking, intrapsychic processes, and the inhibition of action. These strategies were used to prepare themselves for their upcoming role as fathers and to deal with the emotions generated by their situation.

Problem-focused direct actions were reported most often by our sample of young expectant fathers. Specifically, these were activities related to assuming the role of provider and helping their partners with preparations for the baby. Information seeking was also prevalent. The most popular sources of information were the teens' partners, married friends, and parents, rather than prepared literature. This raises the question of whether there would be any effect on the adolescent's assumption of his new role if this mode of coping were not effectively used. Such a situation could arise if these sources of support were not available for some reason (i.e., a tenuous relationship, or the absence of married friends).

Problem-focused intrapsychic processes were also used by a majority of the adolescents in our sample. These processes included fantasizing about fatherhood and the baby and reviewing how they themselves had been parented. However, the three subjects who used emotion-focused intrapsychic processes avoided thinking ahead about fatherhood and denied that the baby might have an impact on their lives. The use of these strategies may have differing implications for the adolescent's transition to fatherhood. As suggested by May, the expectant father's ability to fantasize about and plan for the future may be an important factor influencing his ability to perform the paternal role.[12]

There is a need for further research to clarify how the use of certain coping strategies either aid or hamper the teen's transition to fatherhood. This knowledge might assist the clinician in assessing which adolescents risk having parenting problems as well as provide a basis from which the clinician could support the use of effective coping strategies in young men who are becoming fathers.

References

1. Elster, A., & Lamb, M. E. Adolescent fathers: A group potentially at risk for parenting failure. *Infant Mental Health Journal*, 1982, *3*, 148–155.
2. Elster, A., & Panzarine, S. Unwed teenage fathers: Emotional and health educational needs. *Journal of Adolescent Health Care*, 1981, *1*, 116–120.
3. Elster, A., & Panzarine, S. *Adolescent fathers—A trajectory of stress over time.* Paper presented at the Society of Adolescent Medicine, New Orleans, 1981.
4. Panzarine, S., & Elster, A. Prospective adolescent fathers: Stresses during pregnancy and implications for nursing interventions. *Journal of Psychosocial Nursing and Mental Health Services*, 1982, *20*, 21–24.
5. Hendricks, L. E., Howard, C. S., & Caesar, P. P. Black unwed adolescent fathers: A comparative study of their problems and help-seeking behavior. *Journal of the National Medical Association*, 1981, *73*, 863–868.
6. Furstenberg, F. F. The social consequences of teenage parenthood. *Family Planning Perspectives*, 1976, *8*, 148–164.
7. Folkman, S., & Lazarus, R. S. An analysis of coping in a middle-aged community sample. *Journal of Health and Social Behavior*, 1980, *21*, 219–239.

8. Cohen, F., & Lazarus, R. S. Coping with the stress of illness. In G. Stone, F. Cohen, & N. Adler (Eds.), *Health psychology—A handbook.* San Francisco: Jossey-Bass, 1979.
9. Lazarus, R. S. The stress and coping paradigm. In L. A. Bond & J. C. Rosen (Eds.), *Competence and coping during adulthood.* Hanover, N.H.: University Press of New England, 1980.
10. Elster, A., & Panzarine, S. The adolescent father. In E. McAnarney (Ed.), *Premature adolescent pregnancy and parenthood.* New York: Grune & Stratton, 1983.
11. Van Dyck, P., Brockert, J. E., & Heiner, C. D. *Outcomes of teenage pregnancy relating to the interval between marriage and birth.* Unpublished report, 1973.
12. May, K. A. Active involvement of expectant fathers in pregnancy: Some further considerations. *Journal of Obstetric, Gynecological, and Neonatal Nursing,* 1978, 7, 7–12.

IV

Developmental Life Transitions
Career Choice and Parenthood

Career choice and parenthood are major developmental tasks for young adults. However, marriage no longer is as central an event in the transition to adulthood as it once was. The scenario of marriage followed by parenthood, job commitment for the man, and homemaker responsibilities for the woman have been replaced by new options. The developmental tasks typically associated with marriage now frequently occur outside of it. Young adults have sexual relationships, leave their parents, set up households as singles or cohabit, and become parents. Birth control and more liberal sexual mores allow marriage and parenthood to be postponed.[1]

Many young adults benefit from their single life-style. They acquire skills in household management and develop a certain sophistication in sexual and interpersonal relationships. Couples who live together may discover basic incompatibilities and thus avert a disastrous marriage. Today, young adults who marry do so with skills and experiences that their parents acquired only after marriage.

Recent social changes complicate the developmental tasks associated with career choice, marriage, and parenthood. Greater sex-role equality is contributing to expanded career opportunities for women and altered roles for men. These changing expectations present young adults with new options and challenges never faced by their parents. Increasingly, young adults are engaged in rewarding but often painful struggles to abandon traditional gender roles and adopt new ones. Women delay marriage and child-bearing while they establish a career; men assume more responsibility for household and parenting tasks; and couples develop creative ways to balance family and career demands.

As more and more women enter the work force, dual-career couples are becoming quite common. This life-style offers many personal and financial rewards, but it also requires creative problem solving and the ability to obtain support from the environment. In the first article, Denise Skinner reviews the sources of strain in dual-career families and the coping strategies couples use to manage them. Work demands and household tasks overloaded couples and left them with little free time. Husbands and wives found it hard to cope with the identity shifts demanded by their dual-career life-style, especially when they had been raised in traditional families. The conflict between work and family demands generated stress as partners tried to coordinate their individual careers with having children.

Environmental factors had a significant impact on dual-career couples. Jobs that demanded geographic mobility or considerable time commitments made it difficult for dual-career couples to maintain an egalitarian life-style. Lack of time for social activities and the desire to spend free time with their children occasionally led to breakdowns in relationships with friends and relatives. Isolation from relatives added to the strain because family members were unavailable for child care.

Coping strategies varied. Couples reduced dissonance by emphasizing the benefits of their dual-career choice. They compartmentalized work and family roles and gave family needs the highest priority. Couples also compromised career goals and advancement opportunities in order to avoid role conflict. Schedules were instituted at home, household standards were lowered, and husbands and children assumed tasks that typically were done by the wife. Supportive marital relationships provided a stress buffer as did friendships with other dual-career couples. Job sharing and flexible schedules enabled couples to cope with time constraints. Finally, support from outside the family facilitated coping. Couples hired baby-sitters and cleaning people and bought time-saving devices.

Some dual-career couples cope especially well with the problems inherent in their life-styles. They move from traditional work and family roles to what Douglas and Francine Hall[4] describe as "protean" careers and relationships. These couples are flexible, emphasize personal autonomy and self-fulfillment, and have a sense of control over their lives. They devise new ways of managing their lives rather than following social norms. A dramatic example is when, in order to pursue career goals, dual-career couples set up two residences and commute to see each other. In these commuter marriages, couples give up the comfortable intimacy that comes from daily conversations and companionship, but they benefit from heightened communication, a sense of rediscovery, fewer trivial conflicts, and more romantic love.[2] Despite the stress of career and family demands, and the trade-offs dual-career couples must make, their relationships may be strengthened when they work together to manage the problems associated with their life-style.

Many modern couples postpone pregnancy until they establish themselves in their careers. However, once couples have satisfying, well-paying jobs and are accustomed to a life-style that is free of the demands and responsibilities of children, the decision to have a child can be difficult. Couples are confronted with the task of negotiating plans for parenthood that will meet each partner's needs. They may be concerned about the effect of a child on their careers, their relationship with each other, and finances.[7] Once a decision is made and pregnancy occurs, husbands face the task of supporting their wives during pregnancy, labor, and delivery. When the baby arrives, the new father may experience a loss of freedom and flexibility and less support from his wife because of the baby's demands. He needs to accept himself and his family and to integrate the child into his life.

In the second article, Katharyn Antle May focuses on first-time fathers and identifies three phases of their involvement during pregnancy. The announcement phase occurs when the couple first suspect the pregnancy and then has it confirmed. For some men, this is a wonderful period of excitement; others may be shocked. During this phase, the man may not be as aware of the pregnancy as the woman, who rapidly begins to experience physical changes. The second, or moratorium, phase occurs early in the pregnancy. After adjusting to the reality of the situation, the expectant father may feel little emotion and not think about the pregnancy often. During this period, the couple may experience marital strain due to the incongruence in their needs and coping strategies. The father-to-be may project emotional distance to help him cope with his ambivalence. This apparent indifference may conflict with his wife's needs for support as she copes with the physical and emotional demands of pregnancy. Men who are ready to be fathers as evidenced by a sense of financial security, stability in their marital relationship, and an acceptance of the end of the childless period of their marriage experience a shorter moratorium period.

Toward the end of the second trimester, men became more emotionally involved in the pregnancy, in part, because of the very noticeable physical changes in their wives and experiences such as listening to the baby's heartbeat or feeling the baby kick. Howard Osofsky[5] noted that some men wrote books or planted gardens. These creative activities relieved feelings that they were "bystanders" in the reproductive process.

The third, or focusing, phase begins when the man sees the pregnancy as real and starts to imagine himself as a father. The expectant father becomes interested in reading about parenting and children, prepares for the baby's arrival, and envisions what life will be like as a family. He also may worry about the birth and whether he can help his wife through labor and delivery. She may worry about losing control during labor, the pain of childbirth, and whether the baby will be normal. Task-oriented coping such as enrolling in childbirth classes and seeking information by reading about pregnancy and childbirth may help the couple master their emotions.[3]

Once the baby arrives, new parents are confronted with added responsibilities that tax their marital relationship. The physical and emotional demands of an infant may be overwhelming and difficult to anticipate until the parents find themselves alone at home with their baby. In the third article, Brent Miller and Donna L. Sollie examine the changes in well-being and personal and marital stress experienced by new parents. The well-being of new parents declined over time. Marital stress increased for mothers after the baby was born and rose again by the time the baby was 8 months old. New fathers, on the other hand, did not experience added marital stress after the birth of their child.

Most new parents used adaptive coping strategies. They learned to cope with the unpredictability their infant generated. Parents became more patient, flexible, and organized, and learned to accept changing schedules. Social support also facilitated coping. Couples turned to friends and neighbors for advice, information, and child care. New parents found that spending time away from the baby was helpful, as was looking forward to the future and anticipating the time when the baby's demands would lessen. Although they were ambivalent about it, some mothers found that thinking about returning to work was helpful. In general, couples with good personal resources and marital relationships have an easier time adjusting to the demanding postpartum period and early parenthood.[8]

Despite temporarily increased marital stress and lessened well-being, there are many positive aspects to being a parent. Families benefit from increased integration, closeness, and interdependence. Parents describe their baby as a source of happiness, joy, and love. Parenting also brings self-fulfillment and an increased sense of maturity and purpose in life. Couples comment that they are closer and that the baby is a bond that strengthens their marriage. Finally, new parents identify with their child. They obtain satisfaction from watching their child grow and develop and look forward to the child's future accomplishments.[6]

References

1. Furstenberg, F. F., Jr. Conjugal succession: Reentering marriage after divorce. In P. B. Baltes & O. G. Brim, Jr. (Eds.), *Life-span development and behavior* (Vol. 4). New York: Academic Press, 1982.
2. Gerstel, N., & Gross, H. *Commuter marriage: A study of work and family.* New York: Guilford Press, 1984.
3. Gloger-Tippelt, G. A process model of the pregnancy course. *Human Development*, 1983, *26*, 134–148.
4. Hall, D. T., & Hall, F. S. Stress and the two-career couple. In C. L. Cooper & R. Payne (Eds.), *Current concerns in occupational stress.* New York: Wiley, 1980.
5. Osofsky, H. Expectant and new fatherhood as a developmental crisis. *Bulletin of the Menninger Clinic*, 1982, *46*, 209–230.

6. Sollie, D. L., & Miller, B. C. The transition to parenthood as a critical time for building your family strengths. In N. Stinnett, B. Chesser, J. DeFrain, & P. Knaub (Eds.), *Family strengths: Positive models for family life.* Lincoln: University of Nebraska Press, 1980.
7. Potts, L. Considering parenthood: Group support for a critical life decision. *American Journal of Orthopsychiatry,* 1980, *50,* 629–638.
8. Valentine, D. Adaptation to pregnancy: Some implications for individual and family mental health. *Children Today,* 1982, *11,* 16–20, 36.

7

Dual-Career Family Stress and Coping

DENISE A. SKINNER

A significant influence on contemporary family living is the increasing rate of female participation in the labor force. Examination of Department of Labor statistics reveals that the married woman is the key source of this growth and helps explain the growing interest in dual-career families reflected in both the professional and popular literature. Although it is difficult to assess the number of married *career* women in the work force, it seems reasonable to assume that the percentage for this group is positively related to the general increase in labor force participation rates of women.[12] As more and more women seek increased education and training, along with an increased demand for skilled labor and a greater awareness of sex-role equality, the dual-career life-style is likely to increase in prevalence and acceptability.[21]

A significant feature of the dual-career life-style is that it

DENISE A. SKINNER • Department of Human Development, Family Relations, and Community Educational Services, University of Wisconsin-Stout, Menomonie, Wisconsin 54751.

103

produces considerable stress and strain. The often competing demands of the occupational structure and those of a rich family life
present a number of challenges for dual-career family members.
Much of the literature implies that the stress is inherent in a dual-
career life-style. However, some of the constraints of the life-style
might be explained by the fact that it is a relatively new and
minority pattern. In coping with the pressures of this variant
pattern, dual-career couples have been forced to come up with
individual solutions as no institutionalized supports exist.[11]

The research on dual-career families has been primarily descriptive in nature and has focused on women. Rapoport and
Rapoport, who coined the term *dual-career family* in 1969, were
pioneers in the study of the impact of career and family on each
other. Their research was followed shortly thereafter by other
definitive studies on the dual-career life-style.[6,7,11,18] More recent
dual-career research has focused heavily on the stresses of the life-
style and on the management of the strains by the participants.[23]

The purpose of this paper is to delineate the source of dual-
career strain and summarize the coping patterns employed by
dual-career couples in managing stress. Hopefully, this summary
will benefit family practitioners as they assist individuals in making adaptive life-style choices as well as aid dual-career participants in effective stress reduction and in developing coping
strategies.

The Etiology of Dual-Career Stress

Rapoport and Rapoport[23] in reviewing the 1960s' studies of
dual-career families have noted that the stresses of this pattern
have been differently conceptualized by various researchers.

> The concepts include *dilemmas* [such as] overload, . . . network, identity;
> *conflicts* between earlier and later norms . . . , *barriers* of domestic isolation,
> sex-role prejudices . . ., and *problems* such as the wife finding an appropri-
> ate job. (p. 5)

Although there is a considerable degree of variation in dual-
career stress, there are also common patterns. In the review that
follows, an adaptation of the Rapoports'[20] delineation of strains
confronting dual-career families will be used as an organizing

framework in highlighting these common patterns reported in the literature. Although interactive and cyclical in nature, strains have been classified as primarily (a) internal: arising within the family; or (b) external: the result of conflict of the dual-career family and other societal structures.[1]

Internal Strain

Overload Issues

The problem of work and role overload is a common source of strain for dual-career families.[6,7,10,11,18,21,24] When each individual is engaged in an active work role and active family roles, the total volume of activities is considerably increased over what a conventional family experiences.[19] In dual-career families, this can result in overload, with household tasks generally handled as overtime.

The feelings of overload and the degree of strain experienced varied for couples in the Rapoports' study.[21] The Rapoports suggested that overload was affected by four conditions, which were, in part, self-imposed:

> (a) the degree to which having children and a family life (as distinct from simply being married) was salient; (b) the degree to which the couple aspired to a high standard of domestic living; (c) the degree to which there was satisfactory reapportionment of tasks; and (d) the degree to which the social-psychological overload compounded the physical overloads. (pp. 302–305)

There was a positive relationship between the conditions in Items A, B, and D and the degree of strain experienced. Satisfactory reapportionment of tasks was a coping strategy that helped alleviate strain.

Identity Issues

The identity dilemma for dual-career participants is the result of discontinuity between early gender-role socialization and current wishes or practices.[21] The essence of masculinity in our culture is still centered on successful experiences in the work role, and femininity is still centered on the domestic scene.[10,11] The internalized *shoulds* regarding these traditional male and female roles conflict with the more androgynous roles attempted by many dual-career couples, resulting in tension and strain.

Bernard,[2] focusing on professional women, observed that intrapersonal integration of work and domestic roles and the personality characteristics associated with each, do *not* constitute the "psychological work" of the career mother. Rather, the major difficulty, according to Bernard, is that the woman *alone* is the one who must achieve this identity integration.

Role-Cycling Issues

The dilemma of *role cycling*, identified by Rapoport and Rapoport,[21] refers to attempts by the dual-career couple to mesh their different individual career cycles with the cycle of their family. Bebbington[1] noted that role cycling, unlike other sources of strain, has a developmental pattern. Both employment and family careers have transition points at which there is a restructuring of roles that become sources of "normative" stress.

Dual-career couples attempt to avoid additional strain by staggering the career and family cycles such that transition points are not occurring at the same time. Many couples establish themselves occupationally before having children for this reason.[1,11,21] Stress may also result when the developmental sequence of one spouse's career conflicts with that of the other.[1] The structural and attitudinal barriers of the occupational world, yet to be discussed, further contribute to the difficulty in role cycling for many dual-career couples.

Family Characteristics

Holmstrom[11] identified the isolation of the modern nuclear family as a barrier to having two careers in one family. The difficulty of childrearing apart from relatives or other such extended support systems is a source of strain.

The presence or absence of children as well as the stage of the family life cycle seems to affect the complexity of the dual-career life-style.[1,11,21] Heckman, Bryson, and Bryson[10] found that it was the older professional couples and those who had not had children who saw the life-style as advantageous. The demands of childrearing, particularly the problem associated with finding satisfactory child-care arrangements, are a source of strain for younger dual-career couples, especially for the women.[3,8,11,16,20,24] In relation to this, a child-free life-style has been noted by Movius[15] as a career-facilitating strategy for women.

External Strains

Normative Issues

Despite changing social norms, the dual-career life-style still runs counter to traditional family norms of our culture. Rapoport and Rapoport[21] have explained that, although intellectually the dual-career pattern is approved, internalized values from early socialization are still strong and produce tension, anxiety, and guilt. Pivotal points such as career transitions or the birth of a child can activate these normative dilemmas.

One of the more frequently cited problems by dual-career professionals is the expectation on the part of others that the dual-career husband and wife behave in traditional male/female roles.[10] This is consistent with the earlier findings of Epstein[6] who indicated that dual-career individuals experienced guilt because they were not conforming to the socially approved work–family structure. Furthermore, the women often had to deal with the implied or overt social controls placed on them by their children, according to Epstein's study.

Occupational Structure

Holmstrom[11] has commented on the inflexibility of professions noting that "pressures for geographic mobility, the status inconsistencies of professional women because the professions are dominated by men, and the pressure for fulltime and continuous careers" (p. 517) are a source of strain for dual-career couples.

The demand for geographical mobility and its effect on dual-career couples noted earlier by Holmstrom[11] was also examined by Duncan and Perrucci.[5] They found that the egalitarian orientation toward decision making promoted in dual-career living was not carried out in job moves with the wives experiencing more of the stress. However, Wallston, Foster, and Berger,[25] using simulated job-seeking situations, found many professional couples attempting egalitarian or nontraditional job-seeking patterns. These authors have suggested that institutional constraints are in part responsible for highly traditional actual job decisions.

Finally, the demands of particular professions for single-minded continuous commitment, for other family members' needs to be subordinated to the job, and for a "support person" (typically the wife) to be available for entertaining, and so forth are a source of stress for dual-career couples. The "two-person career"[17] that depends heavily on an auxiliary support partner is incompatible with the dual-career orientation, according to Hunt and Hunt.[13] Handy,[9] in a study of executive men, found that the dual-career relationship was infrequent and difficult when the husband was in such a "greedy occupation."

Social Network Dilemmas

Maintaining relationships outside the immediate family is a problem for dual-career members for a variety of reasons. The general dilemma exists because of the overload strain discussed earlier, which creates limitations on the availability of time to interact with friends and relatives.[19]

Rapoport and Rapoport[21] found that the dual-career couples whom they studied reported problems in sustaining the kinds of interaction that their more conventional relatives and friends wanted. Not only was there less time for socializing, but also, kin were at times asked by the dual-career couples to help out, which sometimes produced tension. St. John-Parsons[24] reported that kin relationships deteriorated when dual-career couples could not meet some of the expected social obligations. The husbands in his study experienced the greater loss as ties to their families of orientation lessened.

The study by St. John-Parsons revealed that none of the dual-career families maintained extensive social relationships. According to the author,[24] "a salient reason for their social dilemma was their sense of responsibility for and devotion to their children" (p. 40).

Coping Strategies

Just as the type and degree of strain experienced varies for dual-career families, so do the strategies employed for managing the stress. As was mentioned earlier in this chapter, Bebbington[1] suggested that "stress optimization," the acknowledging of dual-career stress as inevitable and preferable to the stress of alternative life-styles available, is an orientation of many dual-career couples. Defining their situation as such may serve as a resource in successful adaptation to the stress. Dual-career couples also employ stress-mitigating strategies. These coping behaviors are aimed at maintaining or strengthening the family system and at securing support from sources external to the family.

Coping Behavior within the Family System

Poloma[18] outlined four tension-management techniques used by the dual-career women in her study. They reduced dissonance by defining their dual-career patterns as favorable or advantageous to them and their families when compared to other alternatives available. For instance, the career mother noted that she was a happier mother and wife because she worked outside the home than she would have been if she were a full-time homemaker. Second, they established priorities among and within their roles. The salient roles are familial ones, and if a conflict situation occurs between family and career demands, the family needs come first. A third strategy employed was that of compartmentalizing work and family roles as much as possible. Leaving actual work and work-related problems at the office would be one way to segregate one's work and family roles. Finally, the women in Poloma's study managed strain by compromising career aspirations to meet other role demands.

Compromise is a common coping strategy noted in much of the dual-career literature as a way of reducing stress and making the life-style manageable. Women, in particular, compromise career goals if there are competing role demands.[2,6,10,11] However, men in dual careers make career sacrifices also, for example, compromising advancement opportunities in an attempt to reduce role conflict.

Prioritizing and compromising are coping strategies employed not only to deal with conflicts between roles but also in resolving competing demands within roles. Domestic overload, for instance, may be managed by deliberately lowering standards. One compromises ideal household standards because of constraints on time and energy in achieving them. Structurally, the domestic overload dilemma can also be managed within the family system by reorganizing who does what, with the husband and children taking on more of what traditionally has been the woman's responsibility. In these instances dual-career families are *actively* employing coping behaviors within the family aimed at strengthening its functioning and, thus, reducing the family's vulnerability to stress.[14]

Some dual-career individuals take a more reactive orientation toward stress and cope by attempting to manage and improve their behavior to better satisfy all of the life-style's demands. Holmstrom[11] reported that the couples in her study adhered to organized schedules and that the women, in particular, were very conscious of how they allocated their time and effort. Flexibility and control over one's schedule are highly valued by career persons in attempting to meet overload and time pressures.

Finally, the presence of what Burke and Weir[4] have labeled a *helping component* in the marital relationship can serve a stress-mitigating function within the dual-career family. Qualities such as open communication, empathy, emotional reassurance, support, and sensitivity to the other's feelings characterize this therapeutic role; the presence of these qualities would serve to strengthen the relationship. Related to this, Rapoport and Rapoport[22] reported that couples established "tension lines," "points beyond which individuals feel they cannot be pushed except at risk to themselves or the relationship" (p. 6). Couples organized their family lives with sensitivity to these tension lines.

Coping Behaviors Involving External Support Systems

Dual-career couples also employ coping strategies aimed at securing support outside the family to help reduce stress. Holmstrom[11] reported that couples were quite willing to use money to help resolve overload strain. Hiring help, especially for child care, is a common expense in this life-style. Couples also buy time in various other ways such as hiring outside help to do domestic work and purchasing labor- and time-saving devices.

Outside support in terms of friendships were also important to the couples in the Rapoports' study.[21] The dual-career couples formed friendships on a couple basis, associating with other career couples.

> Friendships, while gratifying, are also demanding, and in many of the couples there was a relatively explicit emphasis on the mutual service aspects of the relationship as well as the recreational aspect. (p. 316)

Thus, establishing friendships with couples like themselves helped to validate the life-style for these dual-career couples and provided a reciprocal support structure.

The literature suggests that dual-career couples are increasingly interested in negotiating work arrangements that will reduce or remove some of this life-style's stress. Flexible scheduling, job sharing, and split-location employment are used by some dual-career couples as coping mechanisms to reduce the family's vulnerability to overload stress.

Finally, most of the researchers noted that achieving a balance between the disadvantages and advantages of the life-style was the overriding concern of dual-career couples. Although noting the numerous strains associated with the life-style, dual-career couples were equally aware of the gains—things like personal fulfillment, increased standard of living, pride in each other's accomplishments, and the like. The goal for most dual-career couples, then, is to "plan how to manage the meshing of their two lives so as to achieve an equitable balance of strains and gains" (p. 298).[21]

References

1. Bebbington, A. C. The function of stress in the establishment of the dual-career family. *Journal of Marriage and the Family*, 1973, *35*, 530–537.

2. Bernard, J. *The future of motherhood.* New York: Penguin, 1974.
3. Bryson, R., Bryson, J. B., & Johnson, M. F. Family size, satisfaction, and productivity in dual-career couples. In J. B. Bryson & R. Bryson (Eds.), *Dual-career couples.* New York: Human Sciences Press, 1978.
4. Burke, R. J., & Weir, T. Relationship of wives' employment status to husband, wife and pair satisfaction and performance. *Journal of Marriage and the Family,* 1976, *38,* 279–287.
5. Duncan, R. P., & Perrucci, C. Dual occupation families and migration. *American Sociological Review,* 1976, *41,* 252–261.
6. Epstein, C. D. Law partners and marital partners: Strains and solutions in the dual-career family enterprise. *Human Relations,* 1971, *24,* 549–563.
7. Garland, N. T. The better half? The male in the dual profession family. In C. Safilios-Rothschild (Ed.), *Toward a sociology of women.* Lexington, Mass.: Xerox, 1972.
8. Gove, W. R., & Geerken, M. R. The effect of children and employment on the mental health of married men and women. *Social Forces,* 1977, *56,* 66–76.
9. Handy, C. Going against the grain: Working couples and greed occupations. In R. Rapoport & R. N. Rapoport (Eds.), *Working couples.* New York: Harper & Row, 1978.
10. Heckman, N. A., Bryson, R., & Bryson, J. Problems of professional couples: A content analysis. *Journal of Marriage and the Family,* 1977, *39,* 323–330.
11. Holmstrom, L. L. *The two-career family.* Cambridge, Mass.: Schenkman, 1973.
12. Hopkins, J., & White, P. The dual-career couple: Constraints and supports. *The Family Coordinator,* 1978, *27,* 253–259.
13. Hunt, J. G., & Hunt, L. L. Dilemmas and contradictions of status: The case of the dual-career family. *Social Problems,* 1977, *24,* 407–416.
14. McCubbin, H. Integrating coping behavior in family stress theory. *Journal of Marriage and the Family,* 1979, *41,* 237–244.
15. Movius, M. Voluntary childlessness—The ultimate liberation. *The Family Coordinator,* 1976, *25,* 57–62.
16. Orden, S. R., & Bradburn, N. M. Working wives and marriage happiness. *American Journal of Sociology,* 1969, *74,* 382–407.
17. Papanek, H. Men, women and work: Reflections of the two-person career. *American Journal of Sociology,* 1973, *78,* 852–872.
18. Poloma, M. M. Role conflict and the married professional woman. In C. Safilios-Rothschild (Ed.), *Toward a sociology of women.* Lexington, Mass.: Xerox, 1972.
19. Portner, J. *Impact of work on the family.* Minneapolis: Minnesota Council on Family Relations, 1219 University Avenue SE, 55414, 1978.
20. Rapoport, R., & Rapoport, R. N. *Dual-career families.* Harmondsworth, England: Penguin, 1971.
21. Rapoport, R., & Rapoport, R. N. *Dual-career families reexamined.* New York: Harper & Row, 1976.
22. Rapoport, R., & Rapoport, R. N. (Eds.). *Working couples.* New York: Harper & Row, 1978.

23. Rapoport, R. N., & Rapoport, R. Dual-career families: Progress and prospects. *Marriage and Family Review,* 1978, *1*(5), 1–12.
24. St. John-Parsons, D. Continuous dual-career families: A case study. In J. B. Bryson & R. Bryson (Eds.), *Dual-career couples.* New York: Human Sciences Press, 1978.
25. Wallston, B. S., Foster, M. A., & Berger, M. I will follow him: Myth, reality, or forced choice—Job seeking experiences of dual-career couples. In J. B. Bryson & R. Bryson (Eds.), *Dual-career couples.* New York: Human Sciences Press, 1978.

8

Three Phases of Father Involvement in Pregnancy

KATHARYN ANTLE MAY

Mounting evidence indicates that a woman who is well-supported by her male partner during pregnancy and birth experiences fewer complications during labor and birth and may have an easier postpartum adjustment.[1,2] Less well-substantiated are claims that father participation in pregnancy and birth benefits father–child attachment. Some research indicates that men who participate actively in pregnancy and birth experience greater closeness with their infants and spouses and heightened self-esteem and esteem for their spouses.[4,6,9,13]

Most of this research focuses on father participants, that is, fathers attending prenatal classes or clinic visits. Therefore, these findings probably reflect traits of men who choose active participation rather than the effects of such participation. Most research questions have focused on fathers' responses to birth rather than to pregnancy. In spite of increased interest in expectant fatherhood and father involvement, we know very little about

This chapter appears in abridged form from *Nursing Research*, 1981, *31*(6), 337–342. Copyright 1981, American Journal of Nursing Company. Reprinted by permission.

KATHARYN ANTLE MAY • School of Nursing, Department of Family Health Care Nursing, University of California, San Francisco, California 94143.

men's experiences of pregnancy prior to the last trimester, or how they came to be with their partners in birth classes or the delivery room. This study focused on the concept of father involvement and presents findings from a qualitative study of first-time expectant fatherhood. The evidence indicates that among first-time expectant fathers, feelings of involvement develop in three phases, and the man's readiness for pregnancy may significantly influence the emergence of father involvement.

The Literature

Despite current interest in father involvement in childbearing, relatively little research has been published, and the existing literature poses several problems. Many studies on men and pregnancy present only data collected in the last weeks of pregnancy, with little information on the early phases of expectant fatherhood. The term *father involvement* appears frequently, but its meaning is inconsistent. Father involvement can mean behavioral involvement such as attendance at birth classes, clinic visits, and the birth. It can also mean emotional involvement or how emotionally invested the man feels in the pregnancy and reports himself to be. Other findings[11,15] showed that behavioral involvement and emotional involvement among expectant fathers may not always be related.

Colman and Colman[3] stressed that the resurgence of the man's unconscious feelings and his earliest memories of childhood play an important part in his emotional reaction and adjustment to pregnancy. They stated that the expectant father would become "actively involved" to the extent that he was able to deal with and work through this emotional stress. They added that his identification with, and active involvement in, the pregnancy and birth promoted nurturance and a closer tie with the infant. Although their findings offered no evidence to support this conclusion, the statement appears plausible and has gained much acceptance.

Wapner's[15] study of 128 expectant fathers who attended Lamaze classes highlighted the discrepancy between behavioral and emotional involvement. He constructed a set of questions to assess behavioral involvement and asked how often the expectant father (1) talked to his wife's doctor; (2) spent more time with his wife because of the pregnancy; (3) did extra housework; (4) read about pregnancy and birth; and (5) helped prepare the house for the baby. Men rated themselves very low on all of these activities except the last. However, when interviewed, most fathers reported that they felt very involved in the pregnancy. Apparently, the activities selected to measure behavioral involvement had little relationship with the emotional involvement the men experienced.

Evidence indicates that to some extent the female partner controls the man's involvement in childbearing. Reiber[14] found that if, during pregnancy, women wanted their spouses to be involved actively in child-care activities, the men were likely to hold the same expectation. If women wanted to keep these activities to themselves, the men expected that they would be less involved in child care. Fein's study supported these findings, showing that "women's pre-birth expectations predicted men's actual involvement even more strongly than did men's expectations" (p. 346).[5] Logically, the woman would play an important role in shaping the man's involvement during pregnancy. Zussman[16] substantiates this. In all study cases where fathers participated in labor and birth, the women initiated discussion of their participation during pregnancy. In no case did the husband or obstetrician first suggest the idea.

Few studies encompass the entire experience of expectant fatherhood. Inconsistency prevails about the use and meaning of the term *father involvement,* and no research is reported that examined the development of father involvement over the course of pregnancy.

Methods

The present study examined the social-psychological experience of first-time expectant fatherhood, and the progression of pregnancy from the father's perspective. The primary sources of data were interviews conducted with 20 expectant fathers and their spouses; 11 of the men were interviewed two to four times during the pregnancy, and 9 were interviewed once, intensively.

This core sample was primarily Caucasian (13, Caucasian; 3, Filipino; 3, Latino; and 1, black), middle to lower middle class by income and occupation, and all residents of the San Francisco Bay Area. Subjects met the following criteria: (1) their partners were experiencing an uncomplicated pregnancy; (2) the pregnancy was the first for both partners, excluding previous early abortions; and (3) the couple were living together (although not necessarily married) at the time of conception and intended to parent the child together. Nursing personnel in clinics and private offices and childbirth educators recruited subjects for the study.

Semistructured interviews focused on the man's perception of the impact of the pregnancy on his life and his subjective experience as the pregnancy progressed. The man's perspective of change over time was a major focus in both the repeated and one-time interviews. In cases where core subjects were interviewed once, special attention was given to obtaining a detailed description of the man's pregnancy experience to date and his expectations for the future. Interviews lasted 2 hours and were taped and transcribed. Several other data-collection strategies were also used. These included brief interviews with 80 other expectant fathers at various stages of their partners' pregnancies, participant observation in two series of prepared childbirth classes in which subjects were enrolled, and content analysis of materials written for and about expectant fathers. Data were collected for a 2-year period.

Data from all sources were analyzed for recurrent themes and for emergent concepts, using comparative analytic techniques for qualitative data.[7,8] Three phases in the development of father involvement in pregnancy among first-time expectant fathers were identified. These phases mark shifts in the father's emotional and behavioral involvement in a first pregnancy and reflect the importance of the man's readiness.

Results

Expectant fathers typically stated they felt more involved in pregnancy as the birth approached, which led to the concept of a characteristic pattern of development of father involvement. Data suggested a pattern consisting of three phases. Benchmarks showed increasing emotional and behavioral involvement, signaling movement from one phase to another. The term *father involvement* refers to the subjective state of the father, that is, how close to or emotionally invested he felt in the experience of pregnancy and what were the consequences that he saw of that investment in his own behavior. Father involvement was defined by the subject himself; it could be primarily emotional or behavioral, or both. The three phases were (a) the announcement phase; (b) the moratorium; and (c) the focusing phase.

The *announcement phase* is the period during which the pregnancy was first suspected and then confirmed. This phase varies in length from a few hours to a few weeks. It can be characterized by great joy and excitement for the man if he desired a pregnancy; pain and shock if he did not. The length of this phase depends on how soon both partners suspect pregnancy, what initial impact that suspicion has on the father, and how soon the pregnancy is confirmed to the father.

The common myth that most men are oblivious to early signs of pregnancy and astounded by the news that they are going to become fathers was not substantiated. Most men noticed or were advised of early signs. Typically, they reported feeling stressed and uncomfortable in situations where the diagnosis of pregnancy was in doubt, regardless of whether the pregnancy was wanted or not. One man who very much wanted a pregnancy said, "I surprised myself when we thought that she was pregnant and then she got her period. I was *much* more disappointed than I expected I would be." Another man who did not want a pregnancy said:

> I was finally beginning to warm up to the idea that she was pregnant, but when . . . the first test [showed] she wasn't, I was relieved. She kept having all these symptoms. She went in for another test . . . it was positive, and it all came right back in our faces. I was really upset. It took me about 2 weeks to calm down and try to accept it. The second time was even worse.

The man's involvement in the pregnancy remains of little concern for the couple for several weeks after the pregnancy is confirmed. Since the woman has not yet begun to believe that she is pregnant, she does not expect to see any change in her partner.

Within a few weeks, the pregnancy begins to have a noticeable impact on the woman and assumes more importance in her life than in his. One man described this realization at 14 weeks and attributed it to his ambivalence about the pregnancy. He said:

> *I have to admit there are times when I get away from it. I know she's pregnant, but I'm not as enthusiastic about it as she is. It's like you're waiting for this spectacular moment, but you can't really respond to it until it happens. I feel like there is a state of limbo here.*

Another couple interviewed at 16 weeks began to argue in the course of the interview about whether or not the woman needed to begin wearing maternity clothes. She insisted that she did, and he was not convinced. He remarked that "the pregnancy is not something that is obvious in our lives every day." She responded, "It's not obvious in *your* life—people don't go around patting you on the stomach every day. They do to me." The man's awareness of the pregnancy is lagging behind at this stage, which marks the beginning of the next phase in the development of father involvement in pregnancy.

The *moratorium* is the phase when, adjusting to the reality of the pregnancy, many men put conscious thought about the pregnancy aside for a time. Most men in this study experienced this at some point in early pregnancy. The length of this phase was individual and ranged from just a few days following the announcement to several months. Most often, men remained in this phase from the 12th week of pregnancy until about the 25th week. A large part of this phase corresponds to the period during which the man cannot see much evidence of pregnancy. As his partner becomes more visibly pregnant, the moratorium usually ends.

The man's emotional distance from the pregnancy characterizes this phase. Frequently men said that the pregnancy was not real to them. They did not expect to feel much emotional impact until later, when "she begins to show more." Men regarded this as normal. They concentrated on other life concerns and forgot, sometimes for days at a time, they were expecting a child. The moratorium can be a stressful time for the couple because the man's experience and his partner's seem so different. He feels no change in his life, yet his partner is experiencing definite physical and emotional changes and must adjust to the pregnancy in a variety of ways. She may need more reassurance and support from her partner, yet he may be unable to provide any because he does not experience the pregnancy as a real stressor. Men established an emotional distance from the pregnancy in relation to the amount of ambivalence they experienced. Women often sensed this distance and attempted to involve their partners more closely. Often the man responded by withdrawing more.

This emotional distance appears to allow the man to work through the ambivalence he feels about the pregnancy. Even though women frequently feel ambivalent early in pregnancy, such ambivalence may be more pronounced among men and may have a greater impact on their overall pregnancy experience. The reasons for this include the man's lack of preparation for fatherhood and the fact that many men in this culture have negative connotations of pregnancy. One such negative connotation can be called the "male subculture," presented in a book of humor entitled *How to be a Pregnant Father*.[12] Mayle says, "For the first-time father, pregnancy can be puzzling, tiring, and sometimes hurtful, and a frequent strain on the patience and the digestion" (p. 1).[12] This image reflects the stereotypical expectant father, who worries over his wife's every complaint, is deprived of sexual attention, is run ragged by his wife's peculiar dietary cravings, and is confused by her mood swings and unusual behavior. Expected or actual feelings of jealousy, either of the wife's ability to conceive and bear a child, or of the attention pregnancy takes away from men as husbands may contribute to first-time expectant fathers' ambivalence about pregnancy.[3]

Other findings substantiate the impact of ambivalence in the male pregnancy experience and appears to support the existence of a moratorium phase. Heinowitz found that early in pregnancy men felt so uprooted by the news and experienced enough ambivalence even when the pregnancy was desired, that for a time they had to withdraw emotionally. He stated that

> pregnancy seems to emphasize the disparity in the couple's life pace and life focus. Feeling resigned to the situation, the man decides to back off and take care of himself. Reality compels him to face the isolation of his own transformation. He is thrown back on his own resources. (p. 337)[10]

The man may not consciously focus on the pregnancy during

this period, but some emotional adjustment is apparent. One man in the present study talked about "doing triage" as he tried to order his thoughts and emotions in terms of the pregnancy. Other men expressed inner turmoil and changes in themselves. The following comment was made by one man during the moratorium phase:

> *There are so many other things playing along, too many other issues. You will be sitting there thinking "How is this child going to be?" Then all of a sudden you're thinking "What about the mortgage? How is this class going to be? How's this job going to be a year down the line?" You're preoccupied with all these things.*

For men, the pregnancy is separate, not yet integrated into their lives, yet it is pressing them to confront the future. At this point they can imagine the future only globally but recognize they must begin to organize and adapt as best they can.

The couple must begin to negotiate a level of father involvement satisfactory to both partners. One couple reported their negotiation this way:

> BILL: *I can do this much, but I can't do more than that!*
> ELAINE: *Fine, I need this much. Some days I need more, but I can handle it. We just worked it out.*

Other couples did not negotiate as successfully. The following are typical comments from women who were not able to negotiate with their emotionally distant partners during this period: "He really let me know nonverbally that he didn't want to talk about the baby, and I needed to talk. I was really nervous about it, and I was talking to everyone else." "It's very hard to get feedback from him. I am going through certain feelings, and it is alone at this point. He does not grasp it yet, so it is like the adjustment to the pregnancy is really on our own. I'll say something and I don't get feedback mainly because he doesn't seem to understand where I am right now."

Marital tension and disrupted communication characterized this phase. The man's emotional distance may lead to arguments, with the woman claiming, "You don't care!" and the man not understanding her complaint.

The length of time a man spent in this adjustment period depended largely on his readiness for pregnancy. The more ready he felt, the shorter, less stressful a moratorium he experienced. Expectant fathers defined readiness for pregnancy in terms of three major areas: (1) a sense of relative financial security; (2) stability in the couple relationship; and (3) a sense of closure to the childless period in the couple relationship. Men who perceived a problem in any one of those areas tended to describe themselves as somewhat unready for pregnancy and required a period of emotional distance to adjust. These men gradually redefined the pregnancy more positively and moved into more involvement, although at a slower pace than men who described themselves as ready for pregnancy.

One man described that he could not feel involved until late in pregnancy because he felt the pregnancy had interrupted other life plans. He said,

> *I really don't think that the father should be rushed. Men are not insensitive. It's not that they don't care about the baby early in pregnancy just they are going to care at the right time, when it is right for them. That shouldn't make us bad guys. . . . If [the man] is forced to respond to the pregnancy before he is ready, by the time the child comes, the father may almost resent the child. I am grateful that my wife hasn't pushed me. I think I had enough time in that waiting period to adjust.*

A few men had great difficulty accepting a pregnancy and remained emotionally distant well into the last trimester. These men described themselves as completely unready for pregnancy because they perceived serious problems in more than one of the areas described. One man, who had planned on a childless marriage, avoided any involvement in the pregnancy. The pregnancy ended his expectations of childlessness and, in his opinion, his wife's pressure to allow her to conceive introduced instability into their relationship. He did not participate in any of the preparations for the child, stating emphatically that the pregnancy was "her business." He left the country on business voluntarily late in pregnancy and did not attend the birth. In a phone conversation with the investigator two months after the birth, the man never mentioned the child by name, instead he referred to "her kid" or "the child."

The findings in this study show that men who balk at the first news of a pregnancy usually come around and eventually become enthusiastic. Men who are mildly rushed into or opposed to a pregnancy probably with time will redefine the situation more positively. Unfortunately, such men tend not to become as enthusiastic as their spouses may wish and may act uninvolved in the experience and be unable to support their spouses emotionally until late in the pregnancy. The couple will likely encounter marital strain during the period in which he adjusts. Men who are strongly ambivalent about or opposed to pregnancy are unlikely to become willing participants. Such men may be unable to support their spouses effectively. They may experience feelings of alienation and resentment, and the couple may be at risk for continued marital and parenting problems.

Such extreme cases appear rare. Most men resolve their ambivalance without much difficulty, and as they do the moratorium ends, marked by an experience one man described as taking hold or getting caught up in the pregnancy. Men connected these emotional experiences with noticing for the first time the dramatic physical changes in their wives' bodies, late in the second trimester; hearing the baby's heartbeat; or feeling the baby move for the first time. For some men, the physical reality of the baby moved them into more emotional involvement. For others, more concrete experiences such as painting the nursery or building a crib triggered a sense of emotional investment. Most men reported such a change in their relationship to the pregnancy near the end of the second trimester, or around 25 weeks. This marked the beginning of the focusing phase.

The *focusing phase* ends the "not real–not mine" quality of the moratorium. The man's conversation shows he perceives the pregnancy as real and important in his life. One man described his experience as follows:

> A few weeks ago, there was a sale of baby furniture and she wanted to buy some things. So we went. Then it really dawned on me that I was going to be a father. I got to thinking "Wow," and we bought a crib and a stroller. I pictured myself—me—pushing a stroller down the street. I kept seeing that all day!

The focusing phase begins around the 25th to 30th weeks (although it may begin sooner for men who are particularly ready for pregnancy) and extends until the onset of labor. The expectant father's attitudes and feelings about the pregnancy change. The man focuses on his own experience of pregnancy, and, in doing so, he feels more in tune with his wife. He begins to re-define himself as a father and the world around him in terms of his future fatherhood.

These two processes of focusing on the pregnancy and re-defining himself as a father are apparently linked, as if the man must accept the pregnancy and its impact on him before he can begin to see himself as a future father. One man reported "being pregnant is like getting the measles. You get exposed, but it takes a while before you catch on that you've got it." Once men make this transition, they find themselves reading or hearing about parents and children and suddenly feeling the pregnancy more personally. They think about what the pregnancy means to them day to day. Their spouses notice these changes and comment on how much more understanding and sensitive their husbands have become. The couple may experience a sense of being in tune with the pregnancy and with each other.

If the expectant father has resisted participation previously, generally, he will become more involved in preparations for the birth at this point. One father who had felt unconnected to the pregnancy at 20 weeks was difficult to interview at 34 weeks because he kept asking the investigator questions about stretch marks, nonviolent birth, and proper weight gain during pregnancy. Men may channel much energy into preparing for the birth, physical preparations in the nursery, or making purchases for the baby.

During this phase, expectant fathers begin to redefine themselves and their worlds in terms of their future status. Men report they feel more fatherly and have a mental image of their child. They construct their image of "self-as-father," remembering how they were fathered and comparing those memories with their expectations of themselves. The expectant father redefines others in this way. Frequently, men commented on their surprise when first they realized their parents were going to be grandparents.

Men reported a change in their circle of friends. Those who did not fit the picture of the man's future life fell away, and those with children or who liked children became closer.

The process of redefining themselves as future fathers includes constructing an image of a man's future life with his wife and child. Men may experience some fear about the birth. These feelings may be intensified among men who have prepared to support their spouses during labor and birth and who feel responsible for a successful birth.

This study focused exclusively on pregnancy. One can only speculate about possible connections between the emotional preparation for fatherhood that occurs during this phase and later fathering behavior. It seems logical that men who begin their emotional preparation for fatherhood early by focusing on their experience of pregnancy and redefining themselves as future fathers long before the birth might adjust more easily in the weeks and months of early parenthood. Fein[5] reported that men in couples who had worked out congruent parenting roles before the birth made an easier postpartum transition than men in couples who did not. Preparation during the focusing phase may relate to establishing congruent parenting roles and to constructive parenting later. If this relationship exists, the importance of men's readiness for pregnancy is underscored because the longer the man needs to resolve his ambivalence, the less time he may have for emotional preparation during pregnancy.

References

1. Block, C., & Block, R. Effect of support of the husband and obstetrician on pain perception and control in childbirth. *Birth and the Family Journal*, 1975, *2*, 43–50.
2. Cogan, R., & Henneborn, W. The effect of husband participation on reported pain and probability of medication during labor and birth. *Journal of Psychosomatic Research*, 1975, *19*, 215–222.
3. Colman, A., & Colman, L. *Pregnancy: The psychological experience.* New York: Herder and Herder, 1971.
4. Cronenwett, L., & Newmark, L. Fathers' responses to childbirth. *Nursing Research*, May–June 1974, *23*, 210–217.
5. Fein, R. Men's entrance to parenthood. *Family Coordinator*, October 1976, *25*, 341–348.

6. Gayton, R. *A comparison of natural and non-natural childbirth fathers on state-trait, anxiety, attitude and self-concept.* Unpublished doctoral dissertation, United States International University, San Diego, California, 1975.
7. Glaser, B. *Theoretical sensitivity.* Mill Valley, Calif.: Sociology Press, 1978.
8. Glaser, B., & Strauss, A. *The discovery of grounded theory.* Chicago: Aldine, 1967.
9. Greenberg, M., & Morris, N. Engrossment: The newborn's impact upon the father. *American Journal of Orthopsychiatry,* 1974, *44,* 520–531.
10. Heinowitz, J. *Becoming a father for the first time: A phenomenological study.* Unpublished doctoral dissertation, California School for Professional Psychology, 1977.
11. May, K. A. A typology of detachment and involvement styles adopted during pregnancy by first-time expectant fathers. *Western Journal of Nursing Research,* 1980, *2*(2), 445–461.
12. Mayle, P. *How to be a pregnant father.* Secaucus, N.J.: Lyle Stuart Publishing, 1977.
13. Peterson, G., Mehl, L. & Leiderman, P. The role of some birth related variables in father attachment. *American Journal of Orthopsychiatry,* 1979, *49*(2), 330–338.
14. Reiber, V. Is the nurturing role natural to fathers? *MCN,* November 1976, *1,* 336–371.
15. Wapner, J. The attitudes, feelings and behaviors of expectant fathers attending Lamaze classes. *Birth and the Family Journal,* Spring 1976, *3,* 5–13.
16. Zussman, S. *A study of certain social, psychological and cultural factors influencing husbands' participation in their wives' labor.* Doctoral dissertation, Columbia University, 1970.

9

Normal Stresses during the Transition to Parenthood

BRENT C. MILLER and DONNA L. SOLLIE

For a large majority of married adults one of the sharpest expected changes is the transition to parenthood. Although pregnancy is a harbinger, the roles and tasks of parenting are acquired abruptly. As soon as the first infant is born, and certainly by the time parents go home from the hospital, they *have* parental roles—there are social expectations about what they should do. By comparison, later normative changes during the parental career occur much more gradually as children become toddlers, schoolchildren, teenagers, and then leave home. There is, then, a point in time when parental roles are abruptly acquired, but there is also a more gradual transition into the skills and routines of parenting. Although the transition to parenthood is considered a "critical role transition *point*," it is also a *phase* or span of time.[1]

This chapter appears in abridged form from *Family Relations*, 1980, *29*, 459–465. Copyright 1980 by the National Council of Family Relations, Fairview Community School Center, 1901 West County Road B, Suite 147, St. Paul, Minnesota 55113. Reprinted by permission.

BRENT C. MILLER • Department of Family and Human Development, Utah State University, Logan, Utah 84322. **DONNA L. SOLLIE** • Department of Home and Family Life, Texas Tech University, Lubbock, Texas 79409.

129

Previous Studies

Based on Hill's[6] conceptualization that *accession,* or adding a family member, would constitute a sharp change for which old patterns were inadequate, LeMasters[13] conducted the first study of parenthood as a *crisis.* He found, as did Dyer,[4] that a majority of middle-class parents experienced "extensive or severe" crisis as previously defined. Both of these studies can be faulted for small unrepresentative samples, and the LeMasters study for probable experimenter effects[18] because he helped the couples decide how much crisis they had experienced.

The term *crisis* has also been criticized because the transition to parenthood is generally considered to be a normal event. Because of this, Rapoport[16] suggested the term *normal crisis,* and Rossi[17] advocated dropping references to crisis altogether: "There is an uncomfortable incongruity in speaking of any crisis as normal. If the transition is achieved and if a successful reintegration . . . occurs, then crisis is a misnomer" (p. 28). After Rossi's classic essay, the use of the term *crisis* declined, but comparisons with earlier studies continued to be based on amounts of "crisis" experienced.

Hobbs[7,8] and Jacoby[11] reported much lower levels of crisis experienced by new parents than either LeMasters or Dyer had found. More recent studies[9,10,11] have arrived at similar conclusions. Part of the discrepancy between the earlier and later studies seems to be due to focusing on different aspects of the transition; recent studies have focused more on *reactions* to changes (feelings and attitudes) rather than on the *changes* (behavior patterns) themselves. The Hobbs checklist, for example, asks questions about how "bothered" parents were about various problems of new parents; only small amounts of crisis have been found when operationalized in this way. It would probably be accurate to say that the behavioral changes accompanying new parenthood are typically extensive, but most new parents are only slightly or mildly bothered by these changes, and a large number report gratifications arising from first parenthood as well.[19]

The present research was designed to (a) study the same couples as they *changed* over time; (b) measure *stresses* during the transition more directly; and (c) avoid *socially desirable* responses by not overtly connecting children with the new parents' evaluations of their personal and marital feelings. Based on the previous studies, it was expected that stresses would increase after having a baby, more so among mothers than fathers.

Methods

Sample and Design

The 120 couples who began the present study were recruited from one of three different hospital-based parenthood preparation classes in Knoxville, Tennessee. Couples volunteered to participate after hearing a brief overview of what would be required; they were not randomly selected. The majority of couples had middle-class occupations, incomes, and life-styles. Both husband and wife in 109 couples completed and returned questionnaires at three points in time: first, when the wife was in midpregnancy; second, when the baby was about 5 to 6 weeks old; and finally, when the baby was between 6 and 8 months old. Eleven couples were lost from the sample because of such diverse reasons as divorce, disinterest, and moving without forwarding addresses.

The longitudinal design of the present study made it possible to objectively describe changes in stresses that occurred during the transition to parenthood, rather than relying on the remembered or recalled experiences of new parents studied retrospectively. Couples were studied twice after becoming parents because of the "baby honeymoon" idea expressed by Feldman (as cited in Hobbs[8]). When babies were only 5 to 6 weeks old, few and/or slight changes were expected, but changes were expected to be more pronounced by the time babies were 8 months old.

Measures

At all three points in time, measures of personal well-being, personal stress, and marital stress were included in the questionnaires along with many other measures not reported here. The measures of personal well-being and personal stress came from a national survey of the quality of American life.[2] Before and twice after having their first child, husbands and wives rated how they felt about their present lives on nine semantic differential adjective pairs, such as boring/interesting, enjoyable/miserable, and so on. When factor analysis was utilized in the present study, seven of these nine items were very strongly associated with each other as Campbell, Converse, and Rodgers found. These seven items were used in a summated scale to measure *personal well-being*. The two remaining items were highly intercorrelated but less related to the other seven items. These two semantic differential items "easy/hard," and "tied down/free" were summed to create a scale of *personal stress* for husbands and wives at each of the three points in time.

The measure of *marital stress* was previously developed by Pearlin.[15] Respondents indicated the degree to which they felt bothered, bored, tense, frustrated, unhappy, worried, and neglected in their day-to-day marriage relationship.

Results and Discussion

Both new mothers and fathers reported higher scores on personal stress items ("hard/easy" and "tied down/free") after they had become parents. The magnitude of these changes is especially interesting; wives' personal stress scores during pregnancy were lower than their husbands' scores, but new mothers ended up with higher personal stress scores than their husbands. The fact that seven of the nine significant differences were between 1 month and 8 months postpartum, and pregnancy and 8 months postpartum, provides some support for the notion of the "baby honeymoon" in the early postpartum period.

Personal well-being scores of new mothers were lower at Time 3 than at Time 2, and personal well-being for fathers was lower at Time 3 than during pregnancy observation or when the baby was about 1 month old. The most interesting sex difference in the changes was evident on the marital stress scale. New mothers reported higher stress in their marriages after the baby had been born than before, and even higher marital stress by the time the baby was about 8 months old. New fathers' marital stress scores, by contrast, remained essentially the same across the year of the study. These data coincide with Ryder's[20] finding that new mothers were more likely than fathers to report that their spouses were not paying enough attention to them.

Although we should be cautious about generalizing from volunteer samples, the agreement of these findings with previous research suggests that the typical new parenthood experience probably includes a slight to modest decline in personal well-being and some increase in personal stress over the first year or so of parenting. New mothers feel these changes more keenly than fathers, and wives are more likely than husbands to view their marriages as changing in a negative way. The changes noted previously were statistically significant (not likely to be due to chance) in the present study, but it must be pointed out that they were not huge changes. Even in the moderate changes of these new parents, however, a number of coping strategies seem to be brought into play.

Adaptation to Stress

Preparation for parenthood through reading, attending classes, or caring for infants probably increases the prospective parent's feelings of preparedness and self-confidence, but no amount of preparation and rehearsal can fully simulate the constant and immediate needs of an infant. The sometimes overwhelming demands of new parenthood usually result in some degree of personal and marital stress.[21] So, the question of how new parents cope is especially appropriate.

McCubbin, Boss, and Wilson[22] noted that successful adaptation to stress involves at least two major kinds of family resources. The first of these includes the internal resources of the family, such as adaptability and integration. The second includes coping strategies that can strengthen the organization and functioning of the family, including the utilization of community and social supports. McCubbin[14] has also emphasized the need for interpersonal support systems, noting that families have the capacity to organize a variety of supports to respond to stresses in adaptive ways.

Although the parents in this study were not directly asked to identify coping behaviors that they used, they were asked to write an open-ended response about the positive and negative aspects of having a baby in their lives. Several strategies that they relied on were evident in their replies.

Adaptability appeared as a major strategy utilized by these first-time parents in coping with the stresses they experienced. For example, a theme that appeared frequently in their comments was the change from an orderly, predictable life to a relatively disorderly and unpredictable one. As one father said, "I certainly don't try to keep rigid schedules anymore! And I'm becoming a more flexible person." A new mother wrote,

> *One of the hardest adjustments for me was the unpredictableness of my day. I couldn't be sure of anything—that I would be able to take a nap after her next feeding, that I would have time to clean the house on a certain day, that I would have time to fix supper, etc.*

Other coping strategies of new parents which reflect adaptability included learning patience, becoming more organized, and becoming more flexible.

Integration of the family was also evident in the responses of these first-time parents, especially in the emphasis by some respondents on parenthood as a shared responsibility. Another example of integration was the attempt to continue some activities that were engaged in before the birth of the child—that is, to maintain a sense of continuity, and to recognize the importance of the husband–wife relationship. Husband–wife discussions of feelings were utilized by some couples during this period. One wife wrote of her husband, "He's been very understanding of my feelings and doubts and because we're very open with each other I can express a lot of what I feel, which helps." Many respondents indicated that the child brought them closer together, increased their feelings of unity and cohesion. In this sense, integration of the family is a coping resource that may be present before the birth of the child but which can increase afterward. Husband–wife integration could be enhanced through discussing each spouse's expectations of their own and the other's roles after the birth of the child. Fein[5] found that husband–wife negotiation of roles was an important factor in the adjustment of first-time fathers.

Other coping strategies seemed to be directed toward

strengthening individual responses to some of the stresses experienced. These included utilizing social supports and looking to the future. For example, support from neighbors and friends in the form of advice, information, and caretaking was reported as being helpful. Taking time away from the baby was also beneficial, both during day and at night. One husband noted that a positive aspect of parenthood was "my being able to help with the baby, giving my wife time to herself—therefore giving myself personal satisfaction." This statement also reflects family integration. Just realizing that ambivalent feelings are also experienced by others can be reassuring. One mother said,

Because an infant is so demanding, there are days when one wishes the baby did not exist. Knowing these feelings are normal, however, makes coping with the day-to-day routine possible.

Looking to the future was also a personal coping strategy. One mother commented, "Most of the time I realize that she will get better as time goes on. This isn't as hard during the day, but at night I find I can't deal with her as objectively." Another mother who missed her teaching career wrote, "I have applied to do some teaching on a homebound basis and just knowing that I might soon be working has lifted my spirits." A father expressed some of his negative thoughts about the present and hopes for the future as follows:

Care of the baby has been somewhat tiring for both of us. I expect my thoughts to become positive again after the baby grows some more, becomes more predictable, and can be played with.

One aspect of motherhood that appeared to be stress-producing did not seem to have any ready solutions—the problem of balancing motherhood and a career. This dilemma was identified over 20 years ago in LeMasters'[13] classic study of parenthood as crisis. Although only a small number of the women in this sample were strongly career-oriented, this issue is becoming increasingly salient as more and more women make career commitments outside the home. The comments of some mothers expressed their doubts and the lack of easy answers to this dilemma. One mother said,

> *My baby is a new individual in my life whom I love dearly, but at this point I am not personally fulfilled in simply being a mother. I am finding it difficult to cope with the boredom and lack of intellectual stimulation in my life. I gave up my career in teaching because I felt it would be unfair to take my baby to a daycare center or babysitter. I'm very undecided as to what I should do.*

Another mother wrote, "Like many new mothers I am faced with hard decisions about the future of my career since my baby was born. I am full of doubts, and I'm uncertain how to maintain my career and raise my child satisfactorily." When a mother does interrupt her career, she may experience both intellectual and social voids in her life. Additionally, she may feel tied down and find it difficult to adjust to the changes in the husband–wife roles in her marriage. Lamb[12] noted that a change from egalitarian roles to more stereotyped roles could be a cause of stress for some couples, and it would seem especially likely to be stressful for career-minded but homebound mothers.

Considered as a normal developmental event in the individual and family life cycle, the birth of the first child can be both a source of stress and an event to test the family's coping strategies. That is, the baby can cause certain stresses arising from lack of sleep, tiredness, less time for self and spouse, and feelings of overwhelming responsibility and being tied down. At the same time though, the baby can provide a sense of fulfillment, new meaning in life, and can strengthen the bond between husband and wife, thus contributing to a sense of family cohesiveness.[21] This cohesiveness or integration is one of the intrafamily resources identified by McCubbin, Boss, and Wilson[22] which facilitates adaptation to stress.

Families not only rely on their own internal resources, but they also develop coping strategies by utilizing community and social supports. In addition to relying on extended family or friends during the transition to parenthood, many new parents are taking advantage of preparenthood classes offered by local hospitals, community agencies, and other organizations. Unfortunately, most of these classes are really prenatal or childbirth preparation classes which fall short in helping prospective parents *after* the child is born. New parents are probably in greater need of information and support during the months after their baby is born than during the months leading up to delivery.

Although there are logistical problems in bringing new parents together, it would seem that postparenthood classes have a relatively untapped potential for providing support systems after the birth of the child.[3] Such classes could teach basic skills, provide an opportunity for observing others with their infants, provide an outlet for expressing feelings, and an opportunity to share ideas, experiences, and problems of adjusting to parenthood. Since the negotiation and resolution of marital and parental roles may be an important factor in adjusting to parenthood,[5] husband and wife integration might also be enhanced by discussing role expectations after the baby is born.

It is our general impression that romantic conceptions about having children are declining in our culture. People seem to be more realistic about the impacts children have on parents and marriage. This realization, in and of itself, might be another way of better coping with the stress of parenting. Knowledge about the probable effects of children, both positive and negative, and a less romantic definition of infants, might help new parents cope more easily with the usual stresses that accompany this normal life event.

References

1. Aldous, J. *Family careers: Developmental change in families.* New York: Wiley, 1978.
2. Campbell, A., Converse, P., & Rodgers, W. *The quality of American life.* New York: Russell Sage, 1976.
3. Cowan, C. P., Cowan, P. A., Cole, L., & Cole, J. D. Becoming a family: The impact of a first child's birth on a couple's relationship. In W. B. Miller & L. F. Newman (Eds.), *The first child and family formation.* Chapel Hill, N.C.: Carolina Population Center, 1978.
4. Dyer, E. D. Parenthood as crisis: A restudy. *Marriage and Family Living,* 1963, *25,* 196–201.
5. Fein, R. A. Men's entrance to parenthood. *The Family Coordinator,* 1976, *25,* 341–350.

6. Hill, R. *Families under stress.* New York: Harper, 1949.

7. Hobbs, D. F., Jr. Parenthood as crisis: A third study. *Journal of Marriage and the Family*, 1965, *27*, 367–372.

8. Hobbs, D. F., Jr. Transition to parenthood: A replication and an extension. *Journal of Marriage and the Family*, 1968, *30*, 413–417.

9. Hobbs, D. F., Jr., & Cole, S. P. Transition to parenthood: A decade replication. *Journal of Marriage and the Family*, 1976, *38*, 723–731.

10. Hobbs, D. F., Jr., & Wimbish, J. M. Transition to parenthood by black couples. *Journal of Marriage and the Family*, 1977, *39*, 677–689.

11. Jacoby, A. P. Transition to parenthood: A reassessment. *Journal of Marriage and the Family*, 1969, *31*, 720–727.

12. Lamb, M. E. Influence of the child on marital quality and family interaction during the prenatal, perinatal, and infancy periods. In R. M. Lerner & G. B. Spanier (Eds.), *Child influences on marital and family interaction: A life-span perspective.* New York: Academic Press, 1978.

13. LeMasters, E. E. Parenthood as crisis. *Marriage and Family Living*, 1957, *19*, 352–355.

14. McCubbin, H. I. Integrating coping behavior in family stress theory. *Journal of Marriage and the Family*, 1979, *41*, 237–244.

15. Pearlin, L. I. Status inequality and stress in marriage. *American Sociological Review*, 1975, *40*(June), 344–357.

16. Rapoport, R. Normal crises, family structure, and mental health. *Family Process*, 1963, *2*, 68–80.

17. Rossi, A. S. Transition to parenthood. *Journal of Marriage and the Family*, 1968, *30*, 26–39.

18. Rosenthal, R. *Experimenter effects in behavioral research.* New York: Appleton-Century-Crofts, 1966.

19. Russell, C. S. Transition to parenthood: Problems and gratifications. *Journal of Marriage and the Family*, 1974, *36*, 294–302.

20. Ryder, R. G. Longitudinal data relating marriage satisfaction and having a child. *Journal of Marriage and the Family*, 1973, *35*, 604–607.

21. Sollie, D. L., & Miller, B. C. The transition to parenthood as a critical time for building family strengths. In N. Stinnett, B. Chesser, J. DeFrain, & P. Knaub (Eds.), *Family strengths: Positive models for family life.* Lincoln, NE: University of Nebraska Press, 1980.

22. McCubbin, H. I., Boss, P. G., & Wilson, L. R. *Developments in family stress theory: Implications for family impact analysis.* Paper presented at the Preconference Theory and Methodology workshop of the National Council on Family Relations, Philadelphia, October, 1978.

V

Developmental Life Transitions

Divorce and Remarriage

Divorce and remarriage are increasingly common among modern couples. Many couples recognize the fragility of marriage and worry about their ability to succeed where others have failed. Perhaps it is understandable that some partners react to these uncertainties by signing prenuptial agreements designed to minimize conflict if their marriage fails. Nevertheless, the dissolution of a marriage is often painful even for individuals who yearn for freedom from marital strife and constriction.

Divorcing couples face a complex set of tasks. They must find meaning in their broken marriage, understand the reasons for it, and accept the loss of their relationship. Couples need to master feelings of grief, anger, and personal failure and overcome doubts about their ability to sustain a lasting relationship. Family roles must be restructured and new identities forged. Women in traditional marriages confront abrupt identity shifts as they move from being wife and mother to head of household. Noncustodial parents face drastic changes in relationships with their children and need to find ways to maintain meaningful bonds with them. Couples must negotiate satisfactory custody arrangements, help their children cope with the breakup, and develop ways of relating to their children, mutual friends, and in-laws individually rather than as a couple (see Chapter 2 on children of divorce). Finally, the harsh economic realities of divorce may compel wives to find a job and force husbands to cope with burdensome alimony and child-support payments.

In the first article, Kenneth Kressel describes the psychological issues associated with divorce and stages in individuals' and couples' coping responses to divorce. After a period of denial, there is an increasing awareness that the marriage will not survive. Individuals mourn and may try to deal with their grief and sense of failure by withdrawing from social contacts. At this point, persons in the throes of divorce may experience "separation distress" that stems from lingering attachment to their partner. Anger at the spouse gradually replaces feelings of failure. A period of readjustment follows eventually as hostility toward the spouse wanes. Individuals make plans for the future and may acquire some insight into the causes of marital problems.

Four stages in a couple's coping are identified. The predivorce decision period is marked by efforts to reconcile, seek counseling, and obtain advice from friends and family. In the second stage, one partner makes a clear decision to divorce. However, uncertainty about the separation may lead couples to vacillate between periods of intimacy and dependency and bouts of increased marital discord. Once a definite decision to divorce is made, the couple enters the third stage or period of negotiation. During this time, they work out emotion-laden issues of custody, child support, division of property, and alimony. Efforts to achieve equitable divorce settlements may be hampered by personal ambivalence and anger, unsophisticated negotiating skills, lack of knowledge about family and financial matters, and limited economic resources. The final coping stage is one of reequilibration in which the partners see their relationship more objectively, stabilize their feelings toward each other, and work out custody and parenting relationships.

The psychological upset that occurs following a divorce is a normal response to a difficult life event that is influenced by demographic, personal, and social factors. David Chiriboga[2] notes that older persons experience more emotional distress following divorce. Men tend to be more unhappy and troubled by separation, whereas women experience more psychological symptoms. Steven White and Bernard Bloom[9] found that men with weak social networks or continuing intense relationships with their wife showed poor adjustment to divorce. Men fared better when they were able to distance themselves from their spouse, find a new job, and take the opportunity to meet new people. Similarly, William Berman and Dennis Turk[1] noted that divorced persons who became involved in social activities, developed new friends, and engaged in pursuits that promoted autonomy were less lonely and experienced fewer problems in the postdivorce period.

When divorce ruptures a family, there is a loss of the sense of belonging and meaning that an intact primary group provides. This loss can be especially wrenching for women whose identity and status are tied to being a wife and mother. Life after divorce for a woman with children frequently involves becoming head of the household, a role she may be ill-prepared to assume. However, Kenneth Kressel notes that some women experience increased self-confidence in the wake of changes generated by a divorce. They obtain a full-time job or a degree or establish credit in their own name for the first time. Benefits also can accrue to divorced men. Henry Friedman[4] found that divorced fathers, especially those with joint custody, had more opportunities to nurture their children. This led to increased attachment and improved relationships with their children, which helped them cope with their sense of loss.

In the second article, Jean Baker Miller describes how a group of single mothers changed their self-perceptions, formed meaningful new relationships, and learned to function successfully as head of the household. The women established links with social resources through activities with their children and pursued such community goals as trying to get better schools, housing, and playgrounds. The women bolstered their self-esteem by obtaining part-time jobs or returning to school. They also established a network of friends and neighbors whom they counted on for company and help with errands, baby-sitting, and driving. Overall, these women became more independent and learned to find happiness in their own accomplishments instead of relying on men to fulfill their needs. Basically, the single mothers diversified their emotional ties and began to believe in themselves.

In another study, Janet Kohen[6] found that women who were able to maintain some continuity in their lives, such as by being able to stay in their own home or not having to change jobs, did not experience a serious emotional crisis after divorce. These

women's personal and social resources—job skills, supportive social networks, and financial support from ex-husbands—contributed to their success in building their identity as head of the
household. Like adolescents who become more mature as they
take on the added responsibilities of living in a single-parent family (see Chapter 4), these women experienced personal growth and
increased self-confidence as they successfully tackled the problems associated with single parenthood.

As divorce rates have increased, so have remarriages. Couples who embark on a second marriage encounter a unique set of
tasks that involve undoing some of the adaptations made to divorce. Ann Goetting[5] describes six developmental tasks associated
with remarriage: (1) emotional remarriage; (2) psychic remarriage, changing one's identity from an individual to a couple; (3)
community remarriage, altering friendships and losing some
close relationships established during and after the divorce; (4)
parental remarriage, working out discipline issues and role expectations regarding the spouse's children; (5) economic remarriage,
dealing with financial instability due to sporadic child support
payments and the changeable needs of the husband's children;
and (6) legal remarriage.

In the third article, Jane Ransom, Stephen Schlesinger, and
Andre Derdeyn describe the developmental phases and tasks of
reconstituting families. In the first phase, the new family must
recover from loss and cope with a new set of relationships. The
tasks during this phase include mourning the loss of the predivorce family and establishing the reconstituted family. These
tasks are difficult to achieve because stepparents have little or no
time to form an exclusive relationship with each other prior to
assuming parental responsibilities.

The second phase, planning the new marriage, involves three
major tasks. The partners need to master doubts about their abilities to sustain an intimate relationship and to be stepparents, invest in their new family members, and resolve the loss of the first
partner and the predivorce family. Phase 3 focuses on reconstitution of the family and the need to work out a satisfactory relationship with the divorced parent. Finally, family roles must be
restructured, especially with regard to nurturance and discipline.
Couples' efforts in this direction may be hampered by lack of

clear-cut roles, rights, and obligations for new spouses with regard to their stepchildren.[7] As reconstituting families struggle with these tasks, children may become the focus of conflicts. In a case study of two single parents who married, Jane Ransom and her associates illustrate the difficulties of negotiating these stages and the scapegoating of an adolescent daughter.

With time and effort, stepparents can establish rewarding relationships with their stepchildren. Emily and John Visher,[8] the parents of eight stepchildren and the founders of the Stepfamily Association of America, have developed guidelines to help stepparents anticipate and cope with the pitfalls of stepfamily life. They provide ideas for managing such practical problems as helping stepchildren adjust to a new family, figuring out what stepchildren should call their stepparents, dealing with former spouses and stepgrandparents, and handling the added sexuality in the household.

In an insightful account of her experience as a stepdaughter and as a stepmother to two sets of children, Elizabeth Einstein[3] chronicles the painful interpersonal struggles her stepfamilies experienced as they tried to establish a new family with a separate identity of its own. She also writes of the opportunities and rewards that flow to stepchildren and stepparents. Children can be enriched by exposure to the different personalities, values, skills, and parenting styles of their stepparents. Stepchildren may become more flexible as a result of learning how to live with stepparents and stepsiblings. Successful remarriage can allay the guilt stepchildren have about causing their parents' divorce and change their negative attitudes about marriage. For stepparents, the rewards come from knowing that they have had a positive impact on the lives of their stepchildren and from the close parental relationships that evolve over the years.

References

1. Berman, W. H., & Turk, D. C. Adaptation to divorce: Problems and coping strategies. *Journal of Marriage and the Family*, 1981, *43*, 179–189.
2. Chiriboga, D. A. Adaptation to marital separation in later and earlier life. *Journal of Gerontology*, 1982, *37*, 109–114.

3. Einstein, E. *The stepfamily: Living, loving, and learning.* New York: Macmillan, 1982.

4. Friedman, H. J. The father's parenting experience in divorce. *American Journal of Psychiatry,* 1980, *137,* 1177–1182.

5. Goetting, A. The six stations of remarriage: Developmental tasks of remarriage after divorce. *Family Relations,* 1982, *31,* 213–222.

6. Kohen, J. A. From wife to family head: Transitions in self-identity. *Psychiatry,* 1981, *44,* 230–240.

7. Messinger, L. *Remarriage: A family affair.* New York: Plenum Press, 1984.

8. Visher, E., & Visher, J. *How to win as a stepfamily.* Chicago: Contemporary Books, 1982.

9. White, S. W., & Bloom, B. L. Factors related to the adjustment of divorcing men. *Family Relations,* 1981, *30,* 349–360.

10

Patterns of Coping in Divorce

KENNETH KRESSEL

Psychological Sources of Stress

Clearly, a central psychological stress for those undergoing a divorce arises from a perception of oneself as "unlovable" or wanting as a spouse or parent. At a less conscious level, perhaps a major stressor is what Rice[15] has called "narcissistic injury"—the damage inflicted by the loss of the spouse to one's primitive fantasies of infantile greatness.

A related concept is what Weiss[17] has referred to as "separation distress," that intense, painful, and persistent focusing on the former partner long after the physical separation and divorce has occurred. As yet we have little empirical documentation on the frequency and severity with which separation distress occurs. However, some figures from the recent—and only—longitudinal investigation of postdivorce adjustment[8] are instructive. In the 2-month period following their divorce 17% (8 of 48) of the husbands helped with home repairs, 8% babysat while their former

This chapter appears in abridged form from *Family Relations*, 1980, *29*, 234–240. Copyright 1980 by the National Council of Family Relations, Fairview Community School Center, 1901 West County Road B, Suite 147, St. Paul, Minnesota 55113. Reprinted by permission.

KENNETH KRESSEL • University College, Rutgers University, Newark, New Jersey 07102.

wives went out on a date, and 13% of the couples had sexual intercourse. Fully 70% of the wives and 60% of the husbands said that the spouse was the first person they would contact in a personal crisis and that the divorce had either been a mistake or that they should have tried harder to resolve their differences. With time, of course, these indexes of continuing psychological attachment declined. Even so, 2 years later one-fourth of the women and one-fifth of the men still expressed strong regret about the divorce.

Nonpsychological Sources of Stress

The numerous concrete changes in life circumstances occasioned by the marital disruption add additional stress to the task of postdivorce adjustment. For the husband, a divorce typically involves a change in residence and, occasionally, in job. What is most important is that as the noncustodial parent, he must adapt to seeing his children less frequently and often on a schedule not of his own choosing. His lessened involvement in his children's lives combined with his children's lessened involvement in his life may occasion an extremely painful and continuing emotional injury.

For the wife, the changes entailed by divorce are usually more radical. Often she must adjust to the new responsibilities of working while simultaneously playing the role of both mother and father. Divorced mothers report having significantly less contact with adults than other parents and often comment on a sense of being locked into a child's world.[8] Establishing a satisfying dating and sex life may be retarded by inexperience, uncertainty as to the prevailing norms, and fear of being an inappropriate model of social behavior for her children. Compared to her ex-husband, the ex-wife with custody often has a more narrow range of possibilities for remarriage.

It is in the economic sphere, however, that the stresses of divorce are likely to be most severe. The situation is typically more acute for the divorced mother. Bane[1] has documented the severe decline in economic status that divorced women undergo. She cites data, for example, that indicate that in the same 5-year period

(1967–1971), intact families experienced an average rise of 35% in income. Men who had lost a wife and did not remarry showed some overall rise in earnings. However, women in the same situation showed a net economic decline of nearly 17%. There are several reasons for this precipitous decline in the economic fortunes of divorced women, among which we may list the greater expense incurred in supporting two households; economic discrimination against women; and the generally poor compliance of husbands with alimony and child-support payments.

The economic aspect of divorce deserves emphasis because marriage counselors and psychotherapists frequently overlook such seemingly mundane factors in the emotional conflicts of their patients. The following remark from an experienced therapist illustrates this tendency:

> I think where people have had no conflicts around money prior to the divorce, they don't have them in the divorce process. The kinds of quarrels that go on around money have nothing to do with the realities of money and how much there is to be shared. It has to do with the feelings people have about money. (p. 424)[12]

Compare this with the perspective of a lawyer interviewed as part of our research:

> There are typical cases where the man makes $18,000 a year and there are three or four children and a nonworking wife. There you have complete chaos, and anybody who tried to introduce so-called "equity" would be much better off introducing money, because it's the only thing that's going to solve this insoluable problem. (p. 251)[14]

Although approximately 75% of divorced women and 80% of divorced men remarry, there are data that suggest that second marriages are less satisfying for women than men.[3,6] One possible explanation is that because of the numerous economic problems of remaining single the divorced woman is more likely to accept a new match that she would otherwise regard as less than optimal.

Individual and Interpersonal Patterns of Coping

Although while every divorce and every divorcing person's experience is unique, certain general patterns of coping appear to exist. These patterns may be described from two perspectives: that of the individual partners and that of the marital dyad considered as an interactive unit. The accounts that follow draw heavily from our initial series of in-depth interviews conducted with over 50 lawyers, judges, psychotherapists, and clergy, all of whom were highly experienced in divorce work; and an intensive study of 17 couples participating in an experimental program to assist divorcing spouses in negotiating their divorce settlements.[13,14]

At both the individual and dyadic levels the pattern of coping may be generally characterized as follows. First, through much of the coping process, decision making and rational planning are markedly impaired. Second, the experience of the initiator of the divorce, although basically similar to that of the noninitiator, is less difficult. Much of the difficulty in adjustment attributed to the noninitiator can be viewed as a consequence of a lack of psychological preparedness and intense feelings of diminished self-regard. Some of our professional respondents noted that the noninitiator could not be expected to recover for as long as 3 years or more after the physical separation. Third, legal divorce may, and frequently does, occur in the absence of true emotional divorce. The worst examples of postdivorce bitterness and general mayhem may be most often ascribed to a failure of successful emotional coping in one or both of the former spouses. Finally, the coping process occurs in distinguishable stages. These stages embody powerful swings in mood and in quality of marital interaction. On balance, the more painful moods and conflictual types of relating predominate.

Stages in the Individual's Coping Response

For the individual, the process of coping may be divided into four broad stages:

1. An initial *period of denial* during which the individual refuses to face the possibility that the marriage may be dying or engages in behaviors that suggest a strong unconscious wish that the marriage still be intact
2. A *period of mourning* involving withdrawal from social contacts and intense feelings of personal failure and confusion
3. A *period of anger* involving feelings of betrayal and hostility

directed at the spouse and perhaps members of the opposite sex generally

4. A gradual *period of readjustment* during which the person begins to start planning realistically and (ideally) gains psychological insight into himself/herself and the dynamics of the relationship with the former spouse

These stages are similar to accounts of coping responses in a variety of stress situations, such as those caused by bereavement, loss of a body part, the prospect of one's own impending death, and the impact of natural disasters.[5] These similarities suggest that the reactive process described for divorce may best be viewed as part of a general human adaptive mechanism, rather than the reaction of a neurotic few.

There is some question as to whether men or women suffer more in divorce. It has been suggested from some of the representative national surveys that it is women who experience more distress.[3,7] Summarizing the data on psychiatric hosptial admissions, however, Bloom, Asher, and White[2] noted that males with disrupted marriages have substantially higher admission rates than females.

Our own interviews with divorced couples are consistent with what others with extensive clinical contact with marital dissolution have observed: compared to women, men appear much more cut off from the emotional side of divorce. Typically, the men we interviewed denied that they or their children had any great difficulty in adjusting psychologically. They also seemed less able to articulate plausible psychological explanations for the divorce, and, in general, seemed far more bewildered by the entire experience. To a large extent this may be attributable to what Komarovsky,[10] in another context, has referred to as the "trained incapacity" of American men to fully experience and express the emotional and interpersonal side of life.

Ironically, women may benefit in terms of postdivorce adjustment by the subordinate economic, educational, and vocational status they occupied while married. Compared to their former husbands, the women with whom we spoke could identify more concrete postdivorce accomplishments: purchase of a house, establishment of their own credit, completion of a degree, or obtainment of full-time employment. These achievements were visible demonstrations of their coping abilities and imbued them with a sense of pride and self-confidence.

Stages in the Couple's Coping Responses

From the perspective of the couple, the process of coping may also be divided into four major periods:

1. *A predivorce decision period.* The predivorce decision period begins with increasing marital dissatisfaction and tension on the part of both spouses, but it is often felt more acutely by one than the other. This is often followed by attempts at reconciliation that may include frantic efforts to recapture a sense of mutual caring and the seeking of advice from friends or relatives. Psychotherapeutic help may be sought for the first time. Next, there is a clear decline in marital intimacy. One or both spouses may take a lover as psychological "insurance" for the impending separation. Finally, there is a break in the facade of marital solidarity. There is open fighting; lawyers may be contacted; one party may move out of the family home. The fact that the marriage is in serious trouble becomes public knowledge. The predivorce decision period may last for weeks, months, or years. In some cases, the coping process neither moves to the next period nor attains resolution in the form of a return to marital harmony.

2. *A decision period.* In this period the decision to divorce is firmly made by at least one partner. The initiator may feel a sense of relief or even exhilaration—a difficult but liberating step has been taken. This euphoria is quickly followed, however, by anxiety and fear at the prospect of permanent separation. The outgrowth for the marital relationship is a stage of renewed intimacy and/or a mutually dependent clinging. This stage is soon superseded by renewed outbreaks of marital fighting, which ultimately lead to a final acceptance of the inevitability of divorce. The entire decision period may also be marked by what one of our professional respondents referred to as the "marital flip-flop," that is, the partners take turns alternately pushing for and opposing the divorce.

3. *A period of negotiations.* This is the complex, critical period

during which custody, visitation, child support, alimony, and division of property are decided upon. The difficulties of the negotiation period appear to be a function of four primary factors: the emotional reactivity of the partners, their naiveté as negotiators, the scarcity of divisible resources, and the discrepancy in relative power between husbands and wives.[13]

The emotional ambivalence of the parties about the divorce may be a serious impediment to a rational process of negotiation. Anger, humiliation, grief, jealousy, and guilt are among the powerful emotions that may be competing with the spouses' desire to end the marriage. If, as is frequently the case, one of the parties is psychologically less accepting of the idea of divorce than the other, their resistance may find expression in unyielding and unrealistic demands, which are frequently couched in terms of the needs of the children. In addition, dysfunctional styles of interaction that characterized the marriage do not disappear during settlement negotiations; the couple that was never able to disagree openly and constructively during the marriage is unlikely to develop that ability now that the marriage is ending.

Negotiating naiveté on the part of both spouses is a common occurrence. In the cases that we have studied, neither spouse easily took a negotiating stance based on compromise or developed an ability to see the other party's needs and perspective. The search for a viable settlement was further impeded by ignorance about basic details of family finances. One and frequently both spouses were uncertain about such matters as annual net income, family debt, monthly cash flow, and so on.[13]

When the spouses confront the necessity of supporting two households with resources that previously supported—or barely supported—one, their anxiety and chagrin is likely to fuel the flames of conflict even higher. Negotiations are particularly likely to be prolonged and difficult where there has been a previous history of debt and financial strain during the marriage, in part because there are no extra resources with which to arrange trade-offs (e.g., "I'll pay you a high rate of alimony while you seek vocational training if you agree to a decreasing scale of payments tied to your earnings").

There is abundant empirical and anecdotal evidence that any negotiation is more difficult when one party exceeds the other in its access to and knowledge about existing tangible resources.[11,16] In our case studies, the imbalance-of-power issue was prominent, and generally stemmed from the disadvantaged position of wives who had given up college or career for the role of homemaker. Moreover, the husbands, in comparison to their wives, were paragons of financial expertise. The financial ignorance of the wives combined with their poor postdivorce economic prospects created a climate in which guilt and/or coerciveness toward the wife on the part of the husband were dysfunctionally high.[13]

4. *A period of reequilibration.* In this period, the parties' relationship and attitudes toward one another assume a more or less stable form after the roller-coasterlike ups and downs of the preceding periods. If the coping process has been successful, the relationship between the former partners will be marked by a balanced view of the good as well as the bad aspects of the marriage and an objective view of the former spouse. The co-parenting relationship will be handled smoothly and tactfully on both sides. As yet, there is little empirical data on the degree to which reequilibration fully occurs among divorcing couples. There is some evidence to suggest that relatively high degrees of conflict prevail, particularly around issues of child care and child support.[4,8,9]

Some Implications for Clinical Practice

The coping process in divorce has several implications for marriage counselors and clinicians. Clinicians need to be wary of diagnostic fallacy. For most people the psychological disequilibria surrounding a divorce represent a *normal* and *temporary* reaction to a stressful life event. The diagnosis of psychopathology is likely to be misleading and should be regarded skeptically, particularly for individuals in the acute stages of coping.

The therapeutic priorities are likely to be somewhat different for men and women patients. With women, practical areas such as finances, vocational planning, and coping with the world outside the home may require extended therapeutic attention. For men, support in uncovering and dealing with the emotional pain of divorce may be more difficult and therefore constitutes a more critical and arduous therapeutic task.

References

1. Bane, M. J. Marital disruption and the lives of children. *Journal of Social Issues*, 1976, *32*, 103–117.
2. Bloom, B. L., Asher, S. J., & White, S. W. Marital disruption as a stressor: A review and analysis. *Psychological Bulletin*, 1978, *85*, 867–894.
3. Campbell, A., Converse, P. E., & Rodgers, W. *The quality of American life: Perceptions, evaluations and satisfactions.* New York: Sage, 1976.
4. Eckhardt, K. Deviance, visibility and legal action: The duty to support. *Social Problems*, 1968, *15*, 470–477.
5. Falek, A., & Britton, S. Coping: The hypothesis and its implications. *Social Biology*, 1974, *2*, 1–7.
6. Glenn, N. D., & Weaver, C. H. The marital happiness of remarried divorced persons. *Journal of Marriage and the Family*, 1977, *39*, 331–337.
7. Gurin, G., Veroff, J., & Feld, S. *Americans view their mental health.* New York: Basic Books, 1960.
8. Hetherington, E. M., Cox, M., & Cox, R. Divorced fathers. *The Family Coordinator*, 1976, *25*, 417–428.
9. Jones, C. A., Gordon, N. M., & Sawhill, E. V. *Child support payments in the United States.* Washington, D.C.: The Urban Institute, 1976.
10. Komarovsky, M. *Blue-collar marriage.* New York: Random House, 1962.
11. Kressel, K. *Labor mediation: An exploratory survey.* Albany: Association of Labor Mediation Agencies, 1972.
12. Kressel, K., & Deutsch, M. Divorce therapy: An in-depth survey of therapists' views. *Family Process*, 1977, *16*, 413–443.
13. Kressel, K., Jaffe, N., Tuchman, B., Watson, C., & Deutsch, M. Mediated negotiations in divorce and labor disputes. *Conciliation Courts Review*, 1977, *15*, 9–12.
14. Kressel, K., Lopez-Morillas, M., Weinglass, J., & Deutsch, M. Professional intervention in divorce: The views of lawyers, psychotherapists and clergy. In G. Levinger & O. Moles (Eds.), *Separation and divorce.* New York: Basic Books, 1979.
15. Rice, D. G. Psychotherapeutic treatment of narcissistic injury in marital separation and divorce. *Journal of Divorce*, 1977, *1*, 119–128.
16. Rubin, J. Z., & Brown, B. R. *The social psychology of bargaining and negotiation.* New York: Academic Press, 1975.
17. Weiss, R. S. *Marital separation.* New York: Basic Books, 1975.

11

Psychological Recovery in Low-Income Single Parents

JEAN BAKER MILLER

Mental health literature has tended to characterize the single mother in concepts steeped in loss, grief, separation, defects, deficiencies, and the like. The single-parent family is frequently discussed in terms of "broken homes" and with a concern for "problem children."[5] Recently, a small but significant body of literature has countered these prevalent assumptions.[1,2,4,7] In utilizing this newer material, it is important to study the parents' own sources of strength. A significant number of the single women studied have solved many extraordinary problems in the face of formidable obstacles. Their single parenthood has led to personal growth for many. In adulthood they have made major revisions in their roles in life, and in their self- and object-representations. Many have become contributors to their community, and their children are often a source of strength rather than difficulty.

This chapter will examine the process by which a small group of low-income single mothers arrived at a new definition of self,

This chapter appears in abridged form from *American Journal of Orthopsychiatry*, 1982, 52, 346–352. Copyright 1982, the American Orthopsychiatric Association, Inc. Reproduced by permission.

JEAN BAKER MILLER • Stone Center, Wellesley College, Wellesley, Massachusetts 02181.

developed the ability to function well on their own, and went on to form meaningful new relationships after an experience that had left most destitute at every level, economic through psychic. The group consisted of eight women of working-class origin, most in their late 20s to early 30s, who had married and had their children during or immediately after high school, a common working-class pattern.[6] Most had two to three children, ranging from 3 to 11 years of age. One woman was black, one Puerto Rican, and the rest were of Irish, Italian, or Greek extraction. All were on welfare for the first time because of marital separation or their husbands' prior psychological decline.

All except one woman had been separated from 3 to 9 years, most for 3 or 4 years. The causes of separation were generally reported as gross defections or deficiencies of the husband, including alcoholism, desertion, wife beating, infidelity, and sometimes combinations of these. All the women portrayed the separation as a last resort, after all their other efforts had failed. Despite the obvious defect of the husbands, the women all said that, at the time of marital disruption, they had felt like failures in their main purpose in life.

These women were very verbal, direct, crisp, often witty, and very responsive on a personal level. When they saw a need, particularly among other single parents, they reacted immediately and with feeling (e.g., to a woman new in the community: "Why don't you come skating on Sunday?"; or, to a woman in the midst of an anguishing custody battle: "Call me anytime, I'll be here."). They were also psychologically sophisticated, with an appreciation for subtleties: a woman who had difficulty disciplining her child was told,

> *You're too damn guilty. And you're making your child suffer for it. . . . I think we feel our children have been hurt already* [by divorce and prior discord]. *Children need love and discipline. It's easier to give them love, but if you don't give them discipline, you're really depriving them.*

Links to Community

The women were engaged in many forms of activity. They involved their children in events through the schools and community agencies, as well as in their own projects such as skiing, museum visits, camping, and the like. They included other people's children, often nieces and nephews, much more so than when they were married. Despite their added responsibilities as single parents, the women somehow had more time and freedom; they seemed to spend less time on the rigidities of family organization. They were flexible and directed their energies to the more interesting things; chores could always wait.

In addition to self-initiated activities with their children, the women had contact with many community resources, such as the school system, the Scouts, Head Start, and so on. Spurred on by their concern for their children, some had moved into leadership on community issues. Their activities included struggles to obtain better housing, better school placements, safer playground facilities, and the like. Many of the women were adept at dealing with difficult bureaucracies and agencies, and showed evidence of sophisticated acumen regarding local agencies such as the recreation board or the housing authority.

Self-Development

Almost all had a job, most part-time. Because they had married during or just after high school, most had begun to work for the first time following marital separation. All their jobs were low paying and involved domestic work or the occupationally segregated pink-collar market.[3]

Four women had returned to school since marital separation. For two, this meant finishing high school; for one, starting college; for another, medical assistant's training. Success in school was exceedingly meaningful, creating a change in their conception of themselves. They said they had not thought of themselves as capable of scholastic accomplishment, either before or during marriage. Their explanations seemed to indicate that, previously, they had looked to marriage as their goal in life. School had not seemed relevant; it had made them feel insignificant and incapable, and had offered no attractive career prospects. After marital separation, they had been forced to look in directions other than marriage. Motivated by the need to provide financially for their families, they hoped to increase their earning capacity. In addition, school success enhanced their image of themselves and their worth.

Networks

In general, there appeared to be more permeability of family boundaries than in most two-parent families, a flow of relationships with friends and neighbors. A readily assumed and readily offered aid system seemed to operate, based on an already existing level of understanding. The mutual aid revolved around baby-sitting, driving, errands, medical emergencies, and just providing company for each other, often on the spot and when one felt the need.

Most agreed that they were more involved in such mutual aid than their married friends and relatives. In fact, they provided more help to friends and relatives than they received from them. As one woman put it:

> *Married women have to worry more about being home at certain times, to get their husbands' dinner or just to be there when their husbands are, like evenings and weekends.*

Although their husbands seem not to have done much for the children prior to marital separation, these women did not feel as free when they were wives. As married women, they had not even thought of pursuing the activities that now involved them.

With a few exceptions, the women did not look to members of their families of origin for practical aid or more intimate sharing and support but rather to friends and community agencies. Most had contact with parents, siblings, and other relatives, but they did not count these relationships as most significant. The reasons for this were several and had deep reverberations. They involved disappointment at family members' past criticism, lack of understanding and of help at crucial periods. It appeared easier to turn outward for relationships, rather than work through these family issues. But they had arrived at close and viable relationships.

Relationships with Children

Almost all the women described the fun they have with their children. They clearly give and receive love and enjoy close emotional interactions. Many poignant moments of exchange of intimate thoughts and feelings were described as well as many accounts of children's remarks and escapades which illustrated qualities they admired such as skill, perceptiveness, intelligence, and humor. It was clear that the children provide a major stronghold and are central to the development of the mothers' newfound strengths and skills.

It is often stated that women, especially women who are seen as deprived, are dependent on their children. This was not the case among these women. They were clearly competent in many ways and provided extensive care for their children and others. It would be more accurate to say that the children had given them a "reason for living," as they said, during a period when they felt like unwanted failures, without direction or purpose. Many of the women were particularly gratified that they had been able to change in ways that might benefit their children.

In explaining to their children the marital separation or their husbands' behavior, all agreed that it is best to reiterate that they and their husbands "just didn't get along." They felt that they didn't have to tell the children more than was necessary and that it would be bad to disparage the father excessively "even if he deserves it." The multiple reasons were portrayed in such comments as:

> *A child feels he is part of both parents. If you make the father seem so bad, the child will feel that badness is in himself, too. The child knows things anyhow. She saw him beat me. You can't cover it up. But you don't have to keep talking about it and adding to it. It's hard to explain to a child why his father doesn't show any interest in him but it's no use tearing the father down further.*

Relationships with Men

All seemed to have some current relationships with men; most had a steady or semisteady friend, but only one saw this friend as a candidate for marriage. What they wanted now from men varied ("A good time; someone to go out and have fun with." "Sex, that's all." "Maybe it's just the feeling that there's someone there.").

In general, current relationships with men seemed to have two characteristics that differed from prior relations: first, the women now took a major hand in setting the terms of the relationship; second, they no longer looked to men for fulfillment of all their needs. As a consequence, they no longer saw themselves or their functioning as defined by these relationships. The women were especially determined not to admit men into their relationships with their children, although they all said that if they met a man they could accept and respect more completely, they might then allow him to play a more significant role in their lives and families.

Another aspect of this topic was the women's concern for their "reputations." Most were aware that they were likely subjects for the varied fantasies of neighbors, both women and men—and, on the part of men, some suggestive actions. While the women maintained that they were not as concerned with gossip as they used to be, the discussion suggested that it still affected them—but not enough to dissuade them from living as they wished.

Becoming a Single Parent

All had gone through a period of anguish, despair, and depression. In discussing the alleviation of this distress, three concrete factors were cited: children, jobs, and personal counseling. The intrapsychic tasks were the conquest of resentment, the realization that they could do more than they had thought possible, and the overcoming of a sense of failure. The women pointed to the rock-bottom knowledge that they had to try to do the best they could for their children as the factor that sustained them during the most difficult periods:

It finally came to me when I wasn't eating or sleeping and was walking the floors all night that I just had to stop it and do something for the children.

In addition, several said that getting a job "saved" them:

> *Just having to get up and get out of the house. . . . Talking to people who didn't always have the same things on their minds as I always did.*

Almost every woman had seen a counselor, usually a social worker, and this definitely had been helpful:

> *She made me see things I hadn't been seeing. She made me realize that I could do something. She stuck by me through everything.*

Other factors were observed which the women did not, themselves, delineate, but which were impressive. One was the support of friends and neighbors, as mentioned previously.

All of these women experienced a sense of profound failure following the breakup of their marriages, no matter how much they perceived their partners to be at fault. But the situation in which these poor, young mothers found themselves forced them to take on a number of new activities and roles. Having done so successfully, they went on to take further steps, increasingly exercising their own will and building a sense of self-worth. Eventually they recognized that they were able to cope, and even enjoy their own abilities. It appeared certain, from their accounts of their experience, that they would not readily relinquish this hard-won competence and new sense of self-esteem.

Discussion

Perhaps the changes that these women made can be summarized under two headings: first, they "diversified their emotional investments" rather than sinking them more totally into a relationship with one person or into "the family" as a relatively self-contained institution; second, a major part of this diversification was the investment in themselves, the development of the belief that they could play a major role in generating their own goals and bringing about their fulfillment, rather than looking to a husband to define these goals or to the existence of "a family" to provide these life satisfactions.

In regard to the first point, they sought several people for different things, rather than one person for all. A concomitant of this was the implicit notion that they, themselves, had to determine whom to seek. As mentioned before, a woman might have a relationship with a man but would no longer look to the man for guidance about child rearing or other areas of life. For this guidance, she consulted the school counselor, the social worker, or respected friends. For companionship, sharing of baby-sitting, and help with a variety of household tasks, she looked to women friends rather than to a husband. "Fighting city hall" she undertook herself, along with anyone who joined in—again, rather than "expecting the man in the family to do it."

An obvious result is that the women did not seek material or emotional returns where they were not likely to find them. Thus, they were more inclined to gain satisfaction, rather than go on hoping for gratification from a person not likely to provide it. Similarly, they have arrived at a belief in their own ability to generate action and gratification. They do not wait for others to provide solutions or satisfactions, again avoiding the possibility of dissatisfaction and frustration.

These women did not consciously choose this path. They were forced to it by a series of steps, each arising out of the exigencies of the time. Their success may provide some hints about the kinds of guidance we might offer others. Beyond this, their development after the breakup of the marriage may point to the kinds of limitations that marriage, or that society's and women's own conceptions about marriage, produce in the first place. These women accomplished things they never would have considered before or during marriage. It seems clear that they did not feel possessed of the abilities to do these things. They now attribute these negative feelings to both their internal estimate of themselves based on home and school experiences and to their husbands' perceptions of them. All said that they "felt more like a person now than I ever did before." Aside from the topic of single parenthood, these points have obvious implications for women's conceptions of self and for the kinds of expectations they bring to marriage.

The observations cited here indicate that these women freed themselves from many of the restrictions imposed by traditional values, although only after an inner psychological struggle. In so doing, they were able to utilize untapped potentials, thus altering a number of deep-seated beliefs (e.g., "School wasn't important for me, I'm only a women"; "I believed that everything had to center around the man"; "I really believed I couldn't do anything; it took a long while to see how duped I was"; "I definitely thought that you just got married and acted right to your husband and children, and everything else would be taken care of"; etc.). As Ladner[4] noted, the values upon which the minority-group woman acts may be of a higher level than those upon which the dominant group operates, and thus may contain lessons that the dominant group can ignore only at its peril. A situation of oppression can foster the development of a form of creativity unavailable to the dominant group. In a form that differs in its specifics but follows from Ladner's basic analysis, the experience of the single parents described in this chapter may offer important guides for us all.

References

1. Brandwein, R., Brown, C., & Fox, E. Women and children last: The social situation of divorced mothers and their families. *Journal of Marriage and the Family*, 1974, *36*(3), 498–514.
2. Guttentag, M., Salasin, S., & Belle, D. *Mental health of women: Fact and fiction.* New York: Academic Press, 1980.
3. Howe, L. *Pink collar workers.* New York: Avon, 1977.
4. Ladner, J. *Tomorrow's tomorrow.* New York: Doubleday, 1971.
5. Moynihan, D. *The Negro family: The case for national action.* Washington, D.C.: U.S. Government Printing Office, 1965.
6. Rubin, L. *Worlds of pain.* New York: Basic Books, 1976.
7. Spurlock, J. *Special issues of concern for the black single parent family.* Paper presented to the American Psychiatric Association, Chicago, 1979.

12

A Stepfamily in Formation

JANE W. RANSOM, STEPHEN SCHLESINGER, and ANDRE
P. DERDEYN

The rising divorce rate and the high incidence of remarriage
among both divorced and widowed persons has resulted in the
stepfamily becoming an increasingly common family form in our
modern society. The problems of integration of families that include children from the parents' prior marriages is one of increasing importance to clinicians.

The reconstituted family, comprised of two spouses and the
offspring of at least one of them, has been described as

> a family consisting of parts that have already participated in disparate and
> usually unhappy family experiences.[4] (p. 434)

The literature attests to the hurdles faced by stepfamilies in the
process of integrating these "disparate parts." These hurdles include family acceptance of the new spouse in parental discipline
and nurturing roles, sustaining generational boundaries, and coping with the impact of the absent biological parent. Formidable
integrative tasks are involved in melding a new family unit out of

From the *American Journal of Orthopsychiatry*, 1979, *49*, 36–43. Copyright 1979 by
the American Orthopsychiatric Association, Inc. Reprinted by permission.

JANE W. RANSOM • The Department of Social Services, Charlottesville, Virginia
22908 • STEPHEN SCHLESINGER and ANDRE P. DERDEYN • Division of Child and
Adolescent Psychiatry, University of Virginia Medical Center, Charlottesville, Virginia
22908.

the fragments of former families. Anthony[1] suggested that the all-too-frequent psychological reality continues to be "two broken families living together." Fast and Cain[3] cautioned, however, against viewing the reconstituted family solely in terms of its deviance from the normative biological family. They proposed that

> the stepfamily can be conceptualized as a structural variation of importance [whose] potentially soluble problems [deserve our attention]. (p. 490)

It is important for mental health clinicians to better understand the reconstituted family as a family form in its own right, and to develop clinical skills in helping adults and children involved in remarriage to establish a workable family system. In this chapter we describe our concept of developmental stages of the reconstituting family, and discuss the stepfamily's need to project family problems upon a scapegoated child. Clinical material illustrates the developmental stages of one such stepfamily and highlights the manner in which a single symptomatic child serves as the focus of conflict and ambivalence for the new family.

Developmental Stages

Solomon[7] has conceptualized the normal growth of the biological family in a framework of developmental stages comparable to Erikson's schema for individual development. Each stage presents the family with a developmental crisis resulting in some degree of distress and disorganization. Specific tasks characterize each stage, the adequate resolution of which is necessary in order for the family to cope with the next step. Failure to effectively accomplish these tasks, however, renders a family more vulnerable to the stresses of future stages.

Solomon's scheme conceptualizes the family as having five developmental stages: (1) the marriage; (2) the birth of children; (3) the individuation of family members; (4) the actual departure of the children; and (5) the integration of loss. The biological family has the potential luxury of a number of years for negotiating each of these stages. The reconstituting family, by contrast, has the challenge of simultaneously coping with the equivalent of the first two stages. Unlike Solomon's broad outline of family development over many years, our concept of the developmental phases of the reconstituting family is limited to the relatively short period prior to and immediately surrounding the initial family formation.

We have found it helpful to conceptualize the developmental phases of the reconstituting family as follows: *Phase 1:* recovery from loss and entering the new relationship. *Phase 2:* conceptualization and planning of the new marriage. *Phase 3:* reconstitution of the family.

Phase 1

The preliminary task of those individuals who will later comprise the reconstituted family is "mourning the loss of the predivorce family."[9] Feelings of anger, guilt, sadness, and anxiety due to the loss of the former familial relationships are experienced by both parents and children in the process of adjusting to the loss. The final relinquishment of the original family, if achieved at all, is accomplished only with difficulty, over a period of time.

Unlike the biological family, the reconstituted family lacks the usual opportunity for successful negotiation of the early family tasks outlined by Solomon.[7] The presence of children at the earliest stages prevents the establishment of an exclusive spouse-to-spouse relationship which predates the undertaking of parenthood. The unique history of the reconstituted family gives rise to resistance from both parent and child to the adult task of setting up new relationships outside the family. The parent's reluctance springs from such concerns as lowered self-esteem or frank depression after a failed marriage, and guilt about withdrawing investment from the children in order to seek satisfactions from other adults. The children resist the mother or father's new sexual relationship out of jealousy and anxiety about abandonment by their remaining parent.

Phase 2

The first task of the partners in the planned marriage is to come to terms with lack of self-confidence regarding their ability to sustain relationships, and fear of repeating the mistakes and unhappiness of the past. Goldstein[4] has called attention to the uncertainty with which parents contract their second marriage, doubtful of their capacity to participate in a healthy family life. Reentry into marriage arouses conflict in both parents and children regarding the children's acceptance of a stepparent. In addition, doubts are experienced on all sides about the stepparent's capacity to fulfill a parenting role toward the partner's children.

A second task revolves about investment in the new family members as primary sources of emotional gratification. Overly close relationships between single parent and child, brought about by loneliness and mutual need, are obstacles to the development of a necessary "primary bond" between the new spouses.[3] Not only must the parent relinquish an exclusive role with the child, but the child is likely to feel scorned and rejected in his or her "displacement" by the stepparent. The child's consequent anger, combined with feelings of disloyalty to the absent biological parent, mitigate against the child's acceptance of the new spouse as a source of parental gratification, particularly when the child is an adolescent.

A third task during this phase is final resolution of the loss of the first partner and the former family system. We have noted heightened feelings of loss and abandonment in some divorced people not only when an ex-spouse weds but also around the time of their own remarriage. Children of the first marriage may signify to their parent a "reincarnation" of the former spouse and may complicate the resolution of the loss by serving as the target of parental anger or ambivalence toward the previous partner.[4,10] Children often experience significant difficulty in resolving the loss of their biological parent and the former family unit. They will continue to yearn for the reuniting of their family, even after one or both parents have remarried.[2,9]

Phase 3

The reconstitution of the "combination family"[6] involves the task of restructuring family roles. Discipline and nurturance are two basic areas in which the newly formed family is suddenly confronted with the need to redefine roles.[4] The acceptance by spouse and child of the stepparent's right to function in these realms is crucial to resolution of this task. Children of both spouses must also come to terms with their new roles and relationships. Implicit in the task of restructuring roles is the rebuilding of generational boundaries so often weakened during the painful postdivorce period.[2]

A final task unique to the reconstituted family is the delineation of a relationship with the divorced biological parent. When the former spouse maintains a role with the children, all members of the reconstituted family are required to sort through feelings of loyalty, anger, jealousy, abandonment, and guilt in order to accept the former spouse's role in relation to the new family.

A Set for Scapegoating

As is the case with any family, reconstituted families are quite likely to reach the attention of mental health professionals through the presentation of a symptomatic child. The concept of scapegoating centers about the projection of family problems, especially parental conflict, onto the person of one child who exhibits disturbed functioning. This child is identified as the patient, while the family preserves its image of otherwise healthy functioning.[8]

Goldstein[4] has applied the notion of *pseudomutuality* to the reconstituted family, which has a vested interest in denying the expression of hostility lest anyone acknowledge marital conflict or the specter of disintegration of yet another family. Conflict is seen as the possible precursor to failure of the marriage, and the fear of this eventuality is frequently sufficient to cause the spouses to thrust the burden of dysfunction upon a child. The child, fearful of abandonment, angry about the loss of the biological parent, and angry at having to share this parent with the stepparent, is often all too willing to join in denying marital discord and to accept responsibility for causing the family problems. The child may eagerly assume the role of creating havoc, and become the symptom bearer, thus "permitting the family to maintain its solidarity."[8] The reconstituted family's need for pseudomutuality sets the stage for diverting family problems to a child predisposed to obstruct the integration of the new family.

Case Report

Two single parents, each of whom had referred a child to our clinic, courted and married each other while they were seen in treatment by two of the authors. Contact was maintained with the family several months after the marriage. Their passage from single-parent families to reconstituted family illustrates the developmental stages of the "combination family." Case material for this family is presented in the context of our treatment of one adolescent daughter, Susan, who serves as the family's symptomatic child.

Susan was 13 years old when her father, Bob, brought her to the clinic at the urging of Nancy, his soon-to-be fiancee. The precipitant to the referral was an angry altercation between Susan and Nancy's oldest daughter, the latest in a series of conflicts between Susan and Nancy's three children. The result of this episode was a rift between Bob and Nancy, which both feared might lead to the end of their relationship. Susan's father reported her presenting problems as frequent, explosive tantrums; inability to retain friends due to bossy, domineering behavior; and marked unhappiness with her current family situation.

Susan's parents had been separated for approximately 1 year. Shortly after the family's move to a new community, her mother, Gladys, underwent a psychiatric hospitalization. Her father elected to terminate the marriage at that time. Susan and her two younger sisters remained in their father's care and visited with their mother several times a week after her discharge from the hospital.

Bob, age 35, held a managerial position with a local business firm. His parents divorced when he was 4, and after living in several relatives' homes, he and his siblings were reunited with their mother when he was entering adolescence. His marriage to Gladys had occurred as a result of Susan's conception. Bob had always felt protective of Susan, and it was he, rather than Gladys, who stayed with Susan during an early hospitalization. Following the separation of Susan's parents, Bob and Nancy, who were neighbors, were brought together by their children's friendship. Nancy, age 38, had been divorced for 2 years from a psychotic husband. Her early years were spent with a passive, loving father and an "angry, unpredictable" mother who made repeated suicide threats during Nancy's adolescence. She was currently establishing herself in a gratifying career. Four months prior to Susan's referral, Nancy had sought help from the clinic for her youngest daughter, age 6, whose tantrums and uncontrollable behavior aroused

Nancy's concern about the adequacy of her mothering. This child's function-
ing was markedly improved after several months of play therapy and parent
counseling. Her behavior, unlike Susan's, did not appear to significantly
reflect the new family's course of development.

Since our involvement in this situation commenced as the
parents were starting to consider marriage, we were not present
to observe the first phase in the formation of this family: recovery
from loss and entering the new relationship. Nonetheless, our
initial work with the father and Susan brought to light their continuing preoccupation with a first-stage task—mourning the loss
of the first wife and mother:

Susan's kinetic family drawings depicted family scenes of several years
before. She drew a "happy picture" of the family clustered about a Christmas
tree; her "sad picture" portrayed mother and father throwing lamps at each
other while the children cried. Susan told the therapist she shared half the
blame for her parents' separation because she had argued with her mother
"at least half the time." She angrily described her father as "dumb" and
"stupid" because he divorced her mother. The father mirrored some of
Susan's feelings of sadness, guilt, and anger as he stated that he had not
wanted a divorce, but he and his children could no longer withstand the
emotional turmoil created by Gladys's histrionics and recurrent suicide
attempts.

Our early contacts revealed Susan and the two adults to be
deeply involved in the second stage of family formation: conceptualization and planning of the new marriage. In the course of
Nancy's therapy, she actively grappled with the first task of this
stage, resolving fears and doubts regarding a second entry into
marriage.

Nancy wondered if she and Bob could meet each other's needs, and worried
about possible similarities between Bob and her first husband. She asked
herself, "Is it right for my children for us to marry?", and she indicated her
concern about the ebb and flow of hostility between Susan and herself.
Nancy and Bob's ambivalence about the impending marriage brought about
a temporary "breakup" after a serious disagreement around buying a house.
Nancy acknowledged, regarding the marriage: "It's a bigger step this time."

Unlike the situation with many reconstituted families, Bob,

rather than the biological mother, provided the home for his children after his separation. Because of this arrangement, we felt the father moved readily into a relationship that could provide his children, especially his 2½-year-old daughter, with maternal care. This reality-based motivation appeared to counter his fear of failure and his guilt at abandoning his first wife. Bob nonetheless exhibited concerns about the marriage, fearing that Nancy was too lenient with his children, and questioning whether the marriage would be "right for Susan."

All three persons found it difficult to accomplish the task of investing in new family members as primary sources of gratification. As so often happens, we perceived a breakdown of generational boundaries, in this case between father and daughter:

> *Susan, appearing at least 3 years older in poise and mannerisms, described the responsibilities she had assumed in filling the void left by her mother's absence from the family. Father indicated that Susan had been a "little Mama" for the past 2 years. He spoke of Susan as having "a very special place" and of her being "number one with me."*

An impediment to the development of a primary relationship between Bob and Nancy was both Susan and Bob's reluctance to give up their overly close relationship:

> *Bob told the therapist that he felt Susan was telling him by her behavior that "we don't need Nancy." We saw father's ambivalence about his tie to Nancy as he spoke in double messages, expressing concern about Susan's belligerence toward her future stepmother and at the same time showing great pride in her "being a real fighter." Susan indicated her reaction to her father's growing closeness to Nancy by referring to Nancy as "the lady next door" or "the baby-sitter."*
>
> *Just prior to the marriage, we saw Susan yearning for a close relationship with Nancy, sitting next to her in the waiting room and seeking approval for her artwork. During one interview, Susan was asked to draw herself on a TV program. She chose, appropriately enough, "All in the Family." In the drawing, she and her younger sister were at home with their father. Nancy was depicted coming through the door bringing food to her father. At this point, Susan began referring to her future stepmother as "Aunt Nancy." As "aunt," Nancy becomes a part of the family but is not yet allowed a maternal role.*

Bob and Susan never appeared able to accomplish the third task of this stage—final resolution of the loss of the original family system:

> Bob maintained his anger at Gladys, and continued to identify Susan's depressed moods and excessive need for love and attention as "just like her mother." Susan's longing for the reunion of her original family persisted, and she suggested that her mother, rather than Nancy, join the family therapy sessions. In contrast, Nancy appeared to have resolved to a greater extent her feelings about her first husband. She told her therapist, "I feel sorry about his [mentally ill] condition, but not so sorry that I have to go back and take care of him."

The marriage signified entry into the third phase of family development, the actual reconstitution of the family. Susan was the focal point of difficulties in restructuring of family roles, a first task essential to melding of the two families. Issues of discipline reflected the state of Susan's acceptance of Nancy:

> Shortly following the marriage, Susan declared to her father, "No lady married to you by law is allowed to hit us unless there is a father's permission." Discipline issues also served to separate the marital pair, exemplified by Susan's drawing depicting father emerging from the parental bedroom in order to discipline his own two daughters for fighting. Susan's 7-year-old sister told Nancy, "I don't want you and Daddy to ever get a divorce." Susan, however, rejected Nancy in a nurturing role by comparing Nancy's cooking unfavorably with her mother's, and by spreading about the neighborhood tales that Nancy burdened her with all the household chores.

The family's state of integration was reflected in the new stepsibling relationships:

> Susan diagrammed the relative "brattiness" of her stepsiblings, and she was reported to incite continual battles with Nancy's daughter, resulting in conflict between Bob and Nancy.

An important problem in reconstitution of this family was the continued pressure exerted by Susan's biological mother, Gladys. Throughout our therapy, Gladys's contacts with Bob and Susan served to express her anger, to seduce her daughter into returning to her, and to gain emotional support when she found herself in difficulties. As Bob and Nancy's marriage approached, crises involving Gladys and her current suitor appeared to increase in frequency and intensity:

> *Susan related fearful dreams to her therapist in response to actual threats on the part of her mother's boyfriend against her father. Susan's fears of separation from her father, together with her own hostility toward him, caused these threats to arouse much anxiety and Susan sought refuge in closeness to Nancy.*

In the context of this situation, it was extremely difficult for the family to resolve the task of defining a role for the divorced biological parent:

> *Susan saw herself as caught between her biological and reconstituted families, graphically portrayed in her drawing of a courtroom scene. In this scene, Susan stands before the judge, choosing between her father and stepmother and her mother and the latter's boyfriend. In actuality, the family was involved in court proceedings at that time related to the biological mother's visiting rights.*

A further barrier to the integration of the family was Bob's hesitation to seek satisfactory legal resolution of a vague and ill-defined custody situation. Fearful that Gladys might contrive to gain custody of the children, he did not push for legal sanction of his own right to care for and raise the children. While the children's legal status continued in limbo, Gladys's role remained that of a potential threat to the integrity of the new family.

Discussion

Susan and her family's passage through the stages of step-family formation revealed the presence of opposing forces for integration and for disruption of the new family. These countervailing pressures were apparent in the family's attempts to cope with the tasks of each developmental phase.

Integrative forces were fueled primarily by the adults who wished to establish a marital union. Although Bob displayed much ambivalence about the marriage, his stronger drive was to marry Nancy and to forge a new family out of their separate households. Nancy experienced inevitable qualms about contracting a second marriage, but she, too, was impelled to enter the new marriage and family relationship. Susan's ambivalent need for a caring, supportive relationship with her stepmother was another integrative force.

Disruptive forces complicated resolution of the tasks at each stage of development. These forces were exemplified in Susan's continuing exclusive loyalty to her biological mother, and her persistent yearning for reunion of the original family. A further deterrent to integration of the new family was Susan and her father's reluctance to establish generational barriers and to relinquish the closeness of their relationship. Susan feared loss of her father to stepmother and stepsiblings, and resisted Nancy's acceptance as a significant member of the new family. A further disruptive force was the actual and potential threat to family stability posed by the biological mother.

In this situation as well as in other remarriages, we were impressed with the importance of the role played by a symptomatic child. The role is a complex one embodying the ambivalence of the entire system regarding the formation of a new family. Susan's behavior reflected the feelings and fears of other family members; her conflict with her stepmother served as a safety valve for negative feelings unexpressed between the parents. Open conflict between stepchild and stepparent is more easily tolerated by the new fragile family system than is conflict between the two adults. Parental anger symbolizes the danger of dissolution of the new family, and the system conspires to quell the threat of reexperiencing painful losses. Susan's disruptive behavior was less disturbing to the new system's equilibrium than was parental discord.

In our discussion of the stages of the reconstituting family's development, we have somewhat arbitrarily separated tasks into specific time frames. In reality, many of these tasks are taking place simultaneously, and some of them will remain forever short of resolution. We do not wish to imply that, once reconstitution is accomplished, the stepfamily will be indistinguishable from a biological family. We emphasize that the varying histories and loyalties of these families will continue to render the reconstituted family different from a biological family.

Conclusion

The increasing divorce and remarriage rates indicate a growing need for the development among mental health clinicians of skills to facilitate the evolution of new family systems that adequately serve all the members of a reconstituted family. We have found the concept of developmental phases and their tasks to be useful in our work with remarriage. In addition, we have found that taking a broad interactional view of a symptomatic child in a reconstituting family is essential if we are to be of adequate help to the child, the parent, and the stepparent. Regardless of whether family therapy *per se* is utilized, an appreciation of and an attempt to work with the family system is essential. With this developmental approach to remarriage, we can enhance our understanding of the nature of the problems faced by these families. In sharing with families the idea that many of their problems are developmental rather than arcanely pathological in nature, we invite them to look upon their difficulties as understandable and amenable to resolution.

References

1. Anthony, E. Children at risk from divorce: A review. In E. Anthony & C. Koupernik, (Eds.), *The child and his family* (Vol. 3). New York, Wiley, 1974.
2. Derdeyn, A. Children in divorce: Intervention in the phase of separation. *Pediatrics*, 1977, *60*, 20–27.
3. Fast, I., & Cain, A. The stepparent role: Potential for disturbances in family functioning. *American Journal of Orthopsychiatry*, 1966, *36*, 485–491.
4. Goldstein, H. Reconstituted families: The second marriage and its children. *Psychiatric Quarterly*, 1974, *48*, 433–440.
5. McDermott, J. Divorce and its psychiatric sequelae in children. *Archives of General Psychiatry*, 1970, *23*, 421–427.
6. Schulman, G. Myths that intrude on the adaptation of the stepfamily. *Social Casework*, 1972, March, 131–139.
7. Solomon, M. A developmental, conceptual premise for family therapy. *Family Processes*, 1973, *12*(2), 179–188.
8. Vogel, E., & Bell, N. The emotionally disturbed child as the family scapegoat. In E. Vogel & N. Bell (Eds.), *A modern introduction to the family*. NewYork: Free Press, 1960.

9. Wallerstein, J., & Kelly, J. Divorce counseling: A community service for families in the midst of divorce. *American Journal of Orthopsychiatry*, 1977, *47*(1), 4–22.
10. Wylie, H., & Delgado, R. A pattern of mother–son relationship involving the absence of the father. *American Journal of Orthopsychiatry*, 1959, *29*, 644–649.

VI

Developmental Life Transitions
Middle Age and Retirement

Middle age is a time to take stock of one's life. Having reached the halfway point in their lives, middle-aged individuals reappraise their career and marriage, contemplate the future, and try to come to grips with their mortality. Men and women who are established in a career may question the value of continuing their present work or profession. In a quest for greater satisfaction and self-definition, some individuals embark on a new career. Samuel Osherson[9] describes midlife as a time when a man may confront a crisis of loss of self, that is, he must come to terms with his failure to reach his boyhood ideals. Because most of today's middle-aged women did not have high career expectations as young women, many find that they are quite satisfied with their career achievements, and unlike men do not experience the crisis of failing to meet career goals.[1]

Middle-aged men and women share the tasks of making decisions about their future and facing old age and death, but each also confronts unique issues. In the first article, Lois Tamir describes the changes and psychological tasks that men experience during the transition to middle age. As a man enters middle age, a decline in physical functioning and the realization that he has lived half his life may trigger thoughts about death. His task is to gradually accept his mortality. In self-assessment, another integral task of middle age, a man examines his life and his place in the world and tries to accept life's contradictions. He may reflect on the cost of maintaining an overly masculine self-image and develop the more nurturant side of his personality. Finally, a middle-aged man wants to be remembered with affection. By serving as a mentor and offering guidance to younger persons, he can impart his knowledge and skills and ensure his personal legacy.

Work, family, and social relationships change as a middle-aged man reorganizes his life. If a man has reached the peak of his career, he must decide what to do next. If he has failed to attain his career goals, he needs to come to grips with his disappointment. Some men cope by overinvolvement in work, whereas others express less interest in advancement and instead come to appreciate the collegial aspects of work. Among middle-aged men, well-being is not linked primarily to the world of work but rather to marital contentment and the quality of social relationships. As child-care tasks decrease, middle-aged couples focus more on their relationship. Some marriages are strengthened as couples have more opportunities to be together, but long-standing marital problems also may resurface. In general, socially active men enjoy greater self-esteem and well-being.

Middle-aged women also experience mutliple changes. Increasing numbers of middle-aged women are single due to divorce or widowhood. Unlike the middle-aged man who worries that time is running out, these women may be concerned about all the years they have left before retirement with no husband or children at home and possibly no way of supporting themselves. Lack of job skills may limit their chances of finding a job. Women who have devoted themselves to being homemakers may face a substantial adjustment when their children leave home. However, the empty nest is not necessarily a painful crisis. Most midlife women look forward to freedom from motherhood responsibilities and the chance to pursue their own interests. In contrast to the middle-aged man whose interests shift from work to interpersonal relationships, the midlife woman may focus her energies on extrafamily activities such as going back to school or starting a career.[8]

As more people live to old age, middle-aged women and men are increasingly faced with the task of providing care and emotional support to elderly parents. Women may find themselves caught between competing demands from their family and elderly parents.[3] As middle-aged children face their filial responsibilities, they need to understand their parents' idiosyncracies and weaknesses as well as their strengths. Caregivers must handle feelings of impatience, frustration, and entrapment if the family member becomes physically ill and increasingly dependent. They often must cope with fatigue and guilt about not doing enough for their elderly parent. Marjorie Cantor[4] found that caregivers experienced more strain when they felt a close bond with the person who was receiving care. Thus, middle-aged children who care for elderly parents are at high risk of experiencing emotional tension. They must set aside personal desires, and give up their free time, opportunities for a vacation, and chances to socialize with friends.

In the second article, Betsy Robinson and Majda Thurnher describe adult children's experiences in caring for aged parents. Adult children frequently set aside 1 day a week to spend with their parents and to help them with everyday tasks such as shopping and banking. Adults with active, self-sufficient parents who coped successfully with aging spoke positively of their parents. But those whose parents required care or had symptoms of mental deterioration often described their parents in negative terms. They expressed irritation and frustration with them and resented their demands. Women felt particularly constrained by their aged parents, especially when they were responsible for helping with everyday activities and could not leave the parent unattended. Men reported helping their elderly parents as often as women, but they were better able to separate themselves physically and emotionally from them.

Colleen Johnson and Donald Catalano[6] have described the adaptive strategies of caregivers. Some adult children cope by distancing themselves from their parents and relying on non-family alternatives to provide care. A few remain physically close to their elderly parents but distance themselves psychologically from the situation. Some try to include other family members in caregiving, whereas other adult children may turn to role entrenchment, that is, they allow the caregiving role to become a full-time job that gives meaning to their life. Spouses who care for a physically ill mate use many of the same coping strategies, although they are more likely to become increasingly interdependent, intensify their relationship, and exclude others from it.

The caregiving role can be valuable in that it provides adults the opportunity to anticipate and prepare for their own aging as they help their parents negotiate the tasks of old age and death. However, because the role often puts such a strain on middle-aged children, they may need to rely on community resources such as homemaker services and respite care. These "societal" solutions may help them keep their elderly parents at home rather than in a hospital or nursing home.

As middle age draws to an end and retirement approaches, individuals must master yet another set of tasks. Retirees face issues related to the meaning of work, aging, and leisure time. They usually need to disengage from, and mourn, the loss of their work role, and develop satisfying and meaningful activities to replace the structure work provided. In the final article, Leland Bradford recounts the problems he encountered on retirement. He describes the losses he and other retired individuals experience when they leave an organization that has met many of their needs. The organization he worked for provided Bradford with companionship, a sense of belonging, and the social contacts needed for psychological well-being. In retirement, he lost the self-esteem that came from achievement of work goals, the power and influence he had acquired, supportive relationships with colleagues, and the structure provided by the workday. Without the daily agenda of work, Bradford was forced to initiate his own daily routine, a task that entailed finding meaningful activities to fill the empty hours each day.

Retired couples may discover new problems in their marital relationship. After retirement, Bradford felt like an intruder in his own home. During his work years, his office represented his domain, whereas his wife's domain was their home. Like other retired couples, he and his wife had to recognize each other's rights and work out ways to be alone and preserve their privacy in the home. Marital difficulties may also be triggered when a man's identity is threatened because he no longer is the family provider. Bradford recalls that a retired friend reacted to his sense of loss of mastery by becoming more domineering toward his wife. Finally, couples may grow apart through the years. Their differences may become obvious once they find themselves continually in each other's company. Leland Bradford suggests that a "marital review" can help couples avoid some of the conflicts that may arise during retirement.

Family and friends have a strong impact on individuals' adaptation to retirement. The transition to retirement is smoother if retirees and their significant social network members share congruent views and expectations about retirement. Conflict is likely to flare up if one partner believes that retirement is a time to enjoy life and pursue new activities, whereas the other sees it as a chance to slow down and prepare for old age. Different expectations about what retirement will be like may also lead to conflict. For example, one wife expected her retired husband to spend much more time with her. But he continued to pursue his own interests. When she confronted him with her dissatisfaction, he suggested she join him in one of his favorite activities—chopping wood.[5]

Factors such as poor health, low income, and retirement at an age earlier than expected[2] have been associated with poor adjustment to retirement. However, retirement can be a satisfying time of life if retirees receive support from significant family members and friends, share a congruent perspective of retirement with them, try to be responsive to their needs, and develop satisfying alternative roles. One such role, grandparenthood, can provide a source of activity and identity as grandparents take on the role of "valued elder." Grandparenthood gives meaning to life and links individuals to their past as well as to the future.[7]

References

1. Baruch, G. K. The psychological well-being of women in the middle years. In G. Baruch & J. Brooks-Gunn (Eds.), *Women in midlife*. New York: Plenum Press, 1984.
2. Beck, S. H. Adjustment to and satisfaction with retirement. *Journal of Gerontology*, 1982, *37*, 616–624.
3. Brody, E. M. "Women in the middle." *The Gerontologist*, 1981, *21*, 471–480.
4. Cantor, M. H. Strain among caregivers: A study of experience in the United States. *The Gerontologist*, 1983, *23*, 597–604.
5. Hornstein, G. A., & Wapner, S. The experience of the retiree's social network during the transition to retirement. In C. S. Aanstoos (Ed.), *Exploring the lived world: Readings in phenomenological psychology*. Carrollton: West Georgia College Press, 1984.
6. Johnson, C. L., & Catalano, D. J. A longitudinal study of family supports of impaired elderly. *The Gerontologist*, 1983, *23*, 612–618.

7. Kivnick, H. Q. *The meaning of grandparenthood.* Ann Arbor, Mich.: UMI Research Press, 1982.

8. Long, J., & Porter, K. L. Multiple roles of midlife women: A case for new directions in theory, research, and policy. In C. Baruch & J. Brooks-Gunn (Eds.), *Women in midlife.* New York: Plenum Press, 1984.

9. Osherson, S. D. *Holding on or letting go: Men and career change at midlife.* New York: The Free Press, 1980.

13

Men at Middle Age
Developmental Transitions

LOIS M. TAMIR

Most of us, regardless of education or profession, would probably agree that the middle-aged adult is at the apex of life. The middle-aged adult generally operates at his optimum level as he interacts with others, is at his peak earning capacity, and executes projects at his greatest level of efficiency. Why, then, has so much attention been paid to the so-called *midlife crisis*, a term now well ingrained in our vocabularies? I think an answer lies in the fact that the peak of life often stimulates a period of self-assessment. One cannot remain at a peak forever but must prepare to face a downhill journey or perhaps a walk along a plateau. This chapter examines the tasks confronted by men at middle age by virtue of this psychological state of affairs, tasks that are part of a natural developmental progression. It also takes a look at how these tasks are handled in three central spheres of life: work, family, and social relationships.

This chapter appears in abridged form from *Annals of the American Academy of Political and Social Science*, 1982, November, *464*, 47–56. Copyright 1982 by The American Academy of Political and Social Science. Reprinted by permission of Sage Publications, Inc.

LOIS M. TAMIR • Department of Psychology, University of Texas Health Sciences Center, Dallas, Texas 75235.

Tasks of Transition

The period in which this developmental dilemma comes to the forefront of the man's life appears to be the time in which he makes his transition to middle-aged status. For most men, this transition occurs when they are in their 40s. Although scholars of life-span development are often loath to pinpoint even approximate ages for developmental phenomena, the literature suggests that men in their 40s experience significant personal transition, crisis, or simply a heightened awareness of themselves. On a more dramatic level, clinical studies reveal that this population has a significant increase in mental health problems, including depression, alcoholism, and suicide. Whether dramatic or subtle, however, most studies that range over the span of adulthood display something atypical among middle-aged men, whether a blip in a curve, a deviation from the norm, or a qualitative transformation.

The problems a man confronts as he enters middle age are many and varied, overt and covert. Overt changes include his children becoming teenagers and often leaving home soon after, his parents aging and possibly dying, and his job or profession becoming more limited in future options. Covertly, it seems that lack of change may depress the man at middle age. No longer is he the object of attention at momentous events, such as weddings, births, first homes, or outstanding promotions.

This peak of life is also plagued with insults to one's sense of well-being. My own research, which has examined the transition to middle age based on a recent national survey, has documented this slump in a man's sense of well-being during his 40s.[14] Of interest is the fact that educational background seems an important criterion as to how a man deals with his move to middle age. College-educated men were more depressed, displayed more symptoms of psychological immobilization, had more drinking problems, and more readily turned to drugs to relieve nervous tension, although, surprisingly, their self-esteem remained intact. In contrast, men with a high school education or less were more likely to plummet only in the area of self-esteem. It is important to note that all these symptoms were limited to a very small age range, namely, men aged 45 to 49, a startling result, considering that they were compared with men ranging the entire life span.

In light of the research to date, it appears that there is an air of discontent seeping into the lives of men at this time but a discontent that need not be indicative of a full-blown crisis. Instead, it is likely that a period of introspection has begun and has taken a different form in accord with educational background.

This sense of introspection appears to be firmly anchored in the psychological tasks specific to middle age and in particular to men at this time. These tasks fall under five major headings: health, mortality, self-assessment, sex role, and generativity.

Health

Middle-aged men do not suddenly experience ill health, but the symptoms of physical decline, which had begun perhaps a decade earlier, begin to reveal themselves. The body becomes less reliable and predictable as arteriosclerosis develops, fat deposits appear, arthritis threatens, and testosterone production diminishes, to name just a few physical alterations. Even if these symptoms are minor, it is at this point that men begin to react more emotionally to physical changes. Accordingly, their wives are known to monitor their husbands' bodies more closely than their own.

Mortality

Highly related to the issue of health is the issue of mortality, for at middle age the man becomes painfully aware that he has lived perhaps half his lifetime. Bernice Neugarten best describes this phenomenon as a switch in focus from "time since birth" to "time left to live."[11] Elliott Jaques[8] has written most explicitly of the middle-aged man's coming to grips with his mortality, and he believes that this struggle defines middle age. Mortality, however, is not the only issue of middle age—the tasks of self-assessment, sex roles, and generativity are also powerful stimuli to personal change at the midlife transition. Nevertheless, these three tasks are integrally related to the tasks of accepting mortality, because that in itself can force the individual to confront internal psychological issues. The middle-aged man must make peace with himself in order to comfortably survive the remaining future.

Self-Assessment

Self-assessment, in contrast to mortality, is possibly the most integral task of middle age. It involves a process of examining one's individual life and one's place in the wider social environment. Self-assessment also involves coming to terms with life's contradictions. During youth and young adulthood the individual, working toward specific goals, typically relies on principles outlined in black and white. By middle age, however, the wisdom of experience allows the individual to recognize shades of gray and the multiple factors that sway the decision-making process and goal attainment. It is at this point that contradictions are recognized, not with outrage, but with acceptance, and according to the research by Daniel Levinson,[9] life's polarities are reintegrated. The psychologist Klaus Riegel[12] has described this stage as the highest level of cognitive functioning: dialectical thought.

Sex Role

One of the great polarities is the masculine/feminine dichotomy. Much research has documented the reintegration of masculine and feminine traits at middle age. Although women become more assertive and independent, men become more sensitive and nurturant. There are many possible reasons for this reintegration, in addition to the internal reworking of polarities just discussed. It may be that at this point the man takes stock of all the sacrifices he has had to make in order to maintain a strong masculine image, including enduring the stress of his job, and sacrifices in his interpersonal life and his relationships with his children. He may attempt to remedy the situation by developing a more well-rounded personality. It has been suggested, in fact, that all personality traits either previously submerged or not allowed to develop now begin to make their appearance in the transition to middle age.

Generativity

The final psychological task of middle age involves taking responsibility for future generations, be they one's own offspring or proteges, or a less tangible, more abstract group of younger adults. This means offspring guidance and developing a personal legacy that will leave an imprint on the future cohorts. Erik Erikson[5,6] writes most cogently of this task, labeling it a crisis of "generativity versus stagnation or self-absorption." If the adult in transition can successfully work through the tasks of middle age, he is free to contribute to others. If not, he will tend to stagnate, being more absorbed in himself than in what he can do for others.

Work, Family, and Social Relationships

Given these basic psychological tasks faced by men in the transition to middle age, it is useful to examine their repercussions at work, in the family, and with social relationships—three spheres of living upon which personal quality of life is highly contingent.

Work

Perhaps no other role is more integral to the identity of the male than the work role. Not only is work a source of income and sustenance for the man and his family, but it is also the clock by which the man assesses life's achievements as to whether they are on time, successfully early, disappointingly late, or woefully not forthcoming. And it is in the work environment that the man becomes most aware when he has reached his peak: most typically at middle age.

Usually by middle age, the male worker, be he blue collar, white collar, or professional, has reached a plateau. At best, a lateral shift in occupational position will occur. This tangible work situation in itself may stimulate self-assessment at middle age, for the man must psychologically maneuver himself out of a difficult no-win situation: if he has not achieved the success he has worked toward all his life, he will be terribly disappointed; if he has achieved what he has set out to do, he must assess whether it is actually all that wonderful, and where he should go from that point.

Research on how middle-aged men deal with this situation is

mixed. Although some researchers imply a sense of resignation from the work environment and a distancing from the cutthroat race for promotion,[3] others suggest a period of overinvolvement with work in terms of time and quantity.[1,4] Part of this overinvolvement may actually be because retirement is nearing and financial security becomes a key to future survival, in particular for the lower-middle- and working-class populations. The national survey research referred to earlier indicates the former pattern of resignation during one's 40s. As in the results described earlier, the patterns differ somewhat for college- and noncollege-educated men. In assessing the relationship between work and well-being, it was found that only during the 40s did work bear no relationship to well-being. Men at this stage could be thriving on the job, yet dissatisfied with life or, on the opposite end, unhappy with the work situation but generally satisfied with their lives. At all other ages men's work satisfaction was highly and significantly related to their sense of well-being. This surprising result appears to be a key indicator of some sort of disengagement from the work environment by middle-aged men, for work had little bearing on their psychological well-being at this precarious time in life, especially in comparison with their earlier years.

These survey results are far from isolated. *The Wall Street Journal*[15] has reported that managers from AT&T who were followed for 20 years displayed a significant drop in desire for advancement when they reached their 40s. No longer was their happiness correlated with work success.

Of interest with regard to the work environment are concerns with interpersonal relationships on the job. For college-educated men, the national survey revealed that only at the middle-age transition, the 40s, was the opportunity to talk with others at work highly and significantly related to job satisfaction when compared with older and younger men. If, in fact, there is a degree of job disengagement at this time, the interpersonal aspect of work is considered an important feature of work satisfaction. Perhaps the interpersonal side of work involves the emergence of the mentor–protege relationship that Daniel Levinson found in his research of men at middle age. Becoming a mentor certainly provides an excellent vehicle for accomplishing the task of generativity so crucial to a successful middle-age transition.

Family

In light of the difficult psychological work confronted by middle-aged men, there are bound to be repercussions at home and in relationships with wives and children. Other family members, too, are likely to be in transition. Mothers are no longer nurturing small children and possibly are investigating new opportunities outside the home. Children are now teenagers, seeking independence and freedom from parents. This situation makes for a complex interplay of interpersonal needs that are fulfilled or suppressed in the multiple relationships of family life.

It appears that during this time of transition, new terms are established for the relationship between husband and wife. Middle-aged spouses must shift their focus from a mutual concern with child care to a mutual concern with their own relationship, from roles of father/mother to roles of husband/wife. This shift of focus, of course, can either arouse interpersonal tension, because members of a strained relationship do not have their children as an outlet to divert attention from themselves, or it can solidify a relationship, allowing husband and wife further time to explore, rediscover, and enjoy one another. Indeed, Marjorie Lowenthal's research has indicated a more intense focus on the man's role as husband than as father during the middle years.

It is not surprising to read in the clinical literature that marriages that dissolve in middle age often do so as a result of underlying interpersonal problems that have existed from the beginning of the marriage. The presence of children can deflect these problems for quite a while, only to have the problems reemerge when the nest is emptied and husband and wife must face one another as separate persons once again.

The national survey study also reveals a striking pattern of results concerning the family lives of men in their 40s. Only men in their 40s viewed their adequacy as a father and adequacy as a husband as separate. Unlike men younger or older, this middle-aged group felt a psychological split between the two roles, perhaps because men at this age tend to introspectively assess their lifetime roles more. In turn, this split brings with it an emphasis, or rather reemphasis, on the marital role.

This shift to the ever-increasing prominence of the marital

role is displayed in the national study most clearly for men with a college education. Compared with older and younger men, the marital happiness of men in the 40s was most highly and significantly related to their psychological well-being. General happiness, life satisfaction, self-esteem, and the presence or absence of depression and alcoholism were more strongly related to marital happiness in the 40s than at any other age. Similarly, the AT&T study revealed that managers began to replace the primacy of work with the primacy of family when they reached their 40s.

The finding that there is a strong interdependence between marital contentment and a sense of well-being is of particular interest in light of the fact that, for men in their 40s, a sense of well-being is no longer contingent on the workplace. Apparently, for the middle-aged man, well-being takes an interpersonal turn, and he becomes more firmly embedded in his role as husband than in his occupational role, no matter how prestigious the latter.

Social Relationships

The final major sphere likely to have an impact on the quality of life at middle age is that of social relationships. Little is known about the social relationships of middle-aged men, or even about the social relationships of men at any age. Most psychological researchers simply concede that women maintain more intimate friendships with one another than do men. How men's friendships change through the life span is also unknown. Friendships can be especially important during times of stress. It is an area of living that merits more intensive investigation, especially with regard to transitional periods within the adult life span.

The little work done to date concerning the social relationships of men at middle age is highly contradictory. Although some research indicates a renewed interest in friends and community,[2,7] other research indicates a lull in friendship relations and a shallowness of social ties at this time. Perhaps this mixed set of results is because men at middle age represent a mixed set of individuals, some more socially oriented, some more withdrawn. Additionally, it is possible that many of the social relationships of men at this time are highly ambivalent. During a period of self-assessment, comparisons of self with others can be discouraging and a blow to self-esteem, thus dampening what could otherwise be cohesive, supportive relationships with others.

A striking pattern of results concerning the social relationships of men in their 40s has emerged from the national survey study. The self-esteem of noncollege-educated men, presumed to be the more working-class segment of the population at large, seemed more highly related to their sense of social connectedness during their 40s. Social connectedness includes a sense of feeling cared for, needed, and liked by others. Only at this transitional period in life does social connectedness relate so directly and strongly to self-esteem, a fragile personal characteristic at this time.

The social side of life seems to be a major contributor to a man's sense of well-being when he reaches middle age. Researchers of middle age[10] have shown an enhanced statistical relationship between social fulfillment and stress: those most socially active are least stressed; those most isolated are more subject to stress. Similarly, the men at middle age who feel distant from others are low in self-esteem. Men whose social connections are thriving maintain greater self-esteem.

The Trade-Off at Transition

The findings relayed in this article fit together like puzzle pieces to form a clear and integrated pattern of the lives of men in transition to middle age. Foremost is the fact that men at this time are in the midst of reworking their lives. Well-being is altered as lives are evaluated at conscious and subconscious levels.

Work, family, and social relationships appear to be reshuffled in the process of transition. The trade-off is one between occupation and people, between objective accomplishment and interpersonal emotion. The workplace is no longer as emotionally central, no matter how hard working the man in his 40s appears. Instead, it is the social side of work that sparks the interest of the middle-aged man, who perhaps is nurturing a protege, or delegating responsibilities to others in the most efficient yet sensitive manner.

Differences emerge along educational lines in relation to the types of close ties men in their 40s hold with others. The well-educated man appears more reliant on his wife than are men of more working-class backgrounds, to whom other interpersonal ties become more central. Although these interpersonal ties are not as defined as the marital tie, the marriage may very well be an integral component of a more amorphous sense of social connectedness. Further research is needed to clarify this speculation, for working-class men in particular have difficulty discussing personal issues.[13] The point remains, however, that nonmonetary social security holds the key to happiness at middle age for men of all levels of income and class.

References

1. Bardwick, J. M. Middle age and a sense of future. In J. G. Howells (Ed.), *Modern perspectives in the psychiatry of middle age.* New York: Brunner/Mazel, 1981.
2. Campbell, A., Converse, P. E., & Rodgers, W. L. *The quality of American life.* New York: Russell Sage, 1976.
3. Clausen, J. A. Glimpses into the social world of middle age. *International Journal of Aging and Human Development,* 1976, 7, 99–106.
4. Cooper, C. L. Middle-aged men and the pressure of work. In J. G. Howells (Ed.), *Modern perspectives in the psychiatry of middle age.* New York: Brunner/Mazel, 1981.
5. Erikson, E. *Childhood and society.* New York: Norton, 1950.
6. Erikson, E. *Adulthood and world views.* Unpublished paper prepared for Conference on Love and Work in Adulthood, American Academy of Arts and Sciences, Palo Alto, Calif., May, 1977.
7. Gould, R. L. The phases of adult life: A study in developmental psychology. *American Journal of Psychiatry,* 1972, *129*, 521–531.
8. Jaques, E. Death and the mid-life crisis. *International Journal of Psychoanalysis,* 1965, *46*, 502–514.
9. Levinson, D. J. *The seasons of a man's life.* New York: Knopf, 1978.
10. Lowenthal, M. F., & Weiss, L. Intimacy and crises in adulthood. *The Counseling Psychologist,* 1976, *6*, 10–15.
11. Neugarten, B. L. The awareness of middle age. In B. L. Neugarten (Ed.), *Middle age and aging.* Chicago: University of Chicago Press, 1968.
12. Riegel, K. F. Dialectic operations: The final period of cognitive development. *Human Development,* 1973, *16*, 346–370.
13. Rubin, L. B. *Worlds of pain.* New York: Basic Books, 1976.
14. Tamir, L. M. *Men in their forties. The transition to middle age.* New York: Springer, 1982.
15. *Wall Street Journal.* Labor letter section, March 16, 1982.

14

Taking Care of Aged Parents
A Family Cycle Transition

BETSY ROBINSON and MAJDA THURNHER

Thirty years ago Robert Havighurst[11] noted that the last developmental task of middle age is adjusting to aged parents. He defined this task as meeting the needs of aging parents in such a way as to make life as satisfactory as possible for *both* the parent and middle-age generations. However, most research into late-life, parent–child relationships has tended to focus almost exclusively on data gathered from the aged parent and neglected the viewpoint of the adult child. Only recently has there been growing awareness (or rediscovery) that the nature of the relationship between adult children and their parents is critical for the well-being of both.

The importance of adult children in the lives of the elderly has been well documented by gerontological research. Though most old people wish to be independent of their families, it is primarily children to whom they turn when in need of general assistance and, particularly, in times of crisis.[5,17,21,25,31] A number of studies have also indicated that parents generally live in close geographic proximity to at least one child, maintain close contact

This chapter appears in abridged form from *The Gerontologist*/the *Journal of Gerontology*, 1979, *19*(6), 586–593. Reprinted by permission.

BETSY ROBINSON • Division of Family and Community Medicine, University of California, San Francisco, California 94134. MAJDA THURNHER • Human Development & Aging Program, University of California, San Francisco, California 94134.

195

with their adult children, and receive various kinds of assistance from them.[13,22–24,28] In terms of assistance, it has been suggested that women feel greater responsibility for helping parents than do men.[9,30] Men, unlike women, have not been socialized to feel responsible for the emotional well-being of others,[1] an aspect that is increasingly relevant because it has been suggested that assistance in the form of emotional support has replaced physical care.[29] Mothers are also more likely to seek out children for emotional support than are fathers.[10]

Both ill health and the death of one parent and subsequent concern for the emotional, physical, and financial dependencies of the surviving parent are conditions that increase assistance by children. Often this results in parent and child sharing a household.[24,26] Newman,[18] for example, has reported that when disability of the parent rises to the point that extended care is needed, only two alternatives are considered: moving the parent to the home of a relative (most often that of a child) or moving the parent to a nursing home. Shifts in the demographic structure suggest that it will be those persons who are already engaged in or approaching their own process of aging who will be increasingly faced with caring for their parents. Brody[3] suggests that if adult children are confronting their own problems of aging, this may precipitate the institutionalization of the parent. Professionals (usually physicians) to whom adult children ultimately turn when they can no longer cope with an aged parent tend to recommend institutionalization rather than to suggest alternatives for managing the burden more easily at home.[6]

The quality of the parent–child relationship varies by the health status and activity level of the parent that has consequences for the general life satisfaction of both generations.[12] As the dependencies of the aged parent increase, both older people and adult sons and daughters are aware of potential conflict situations.[24] Newman[19] reports that interpersonal conflict and restrictions on the adult child's privacy and freedom are major reasons for stress and declining satisfaction for the child. In this respect, family size may be important because several can share physical and psychological burdens that would be onerous to one. Excessive burdens on family members are more important than the parent's specific health problem in seeking the admission of a parent to long-term care institutions.[14]

Our interest in the problem of parental caretaking arose when it became evident in the review of longitudinal data from a psychosociological study of normative transitions of the adult life span that the caretaking functions many older respondents were performing for their parents were perceived as stressful in that they were having a major impact both on the respondents' present lives and their plans for the future. The research reported here focuses on the perspective of the child and examines perceptions and attitudes toward the parent, the ways children related to and met the needs of their parents and the stresses generated by the caretaking relationship.

The Study Sample

This study is based on 49 respondents who had living parents drawn from a larger sample ($N = 114$) that formed part of a large-scale study of social and psychological change across the adult life course.[15] The respondents consisted of 23 men ranging in age from 45 to 65 years ($x = 55$) and 26 women ranging in age from 39 to 62 ($x = 50$). The living parents of these respondents comprised 16 fathers, age range 67 to 97 ($x = 81$) and 44 mothers, age range 64 to 95 ($x = 78$). The parents themselves were not interviewed. Three-fifths of the respondents were undergoing the transition to the empty nest and two-fifths the transition to retirement; each life stage consisted of roughly equal proportion of men and women.

Methods

The respondents were studied intensively at baseline and were given abbreviated follow-up interviews 18 months and 5 years later. The baseline interview that averaged 8 hours was predominantly open-ended but included structured questions, checklists, and rating scales. The follow-up interviews averaged 2 to 3 hours and contained open-ended questions focusing on changes that had occurred in the respondent's life. Respondents were asked to discuss important events they had experienced to describe their present goals and activities and to indicate how these had changed since the previous contact and to report on any changes they had experienced in interpersonal relationships.

The impact of the aging parent on the respondents' present lives and goals had not been anticipated and, hence, specific questions relating to interaction with parents at the two follow-up interviews had not been built into the research design. The present investigation, therefore, takes the form of a secondary analysis. For this analysis, the three rounds of protocols of respondents with living parents were systematically analyzed for information on late-life parent–child relationships. Because a number of researchers have specified certain conditions that increase or decrease interaction between elderly parents and adult children, the baseline data were first coded for the following areas: (1) geographical proximity of parent to respondent and respondent's siblings; (2) frequency of contact; (3) living arrangements of parents; (4) marital status of parents; (5) physical and psychological status of parent as reported by respondents; and (6) types of helping arrangements, if any.

A further examination of the affective nature of the relationship and the impact of a caretaking role on the present life and goals of respondents, due to the fact that they were based on largely spontaneous narrative data, was essentially qualitative. The information was uneven in scope, its richness largely dependent on the parent's proximity and respondent's concerns and responsibilities. Content areas examined were (1) type of stresses reported in the helping relationship; (2) mentions of gratifications and sacrifices; (3) descriptions of elderly parents and of relationships with them, which were rated on a 3-point scale (predominantly positive, neutral, or ambivalent, and predominantly negative). The follow-up data served to examine change through time, and a case history approach was used to trace changes in the relationship to parents and the determinants and consequences of change.

Although the analysis centers on relationship to parents during the 5-year period of study, it was felt advisable to examine

TAKING CARE OF AGED PARENTS

briefly two further areas in order to get a broader picture of the potential stress engendered by aged family members. The protocols of respondents whose parents were deceased at baseline were examined for instances of elderly parents residing in the home of the respondent and for the institutionalization of the parent, and the protocols of the total sample were examined for references to aged parents-in-law.

Prior to the baseline interview, 26% of our respondents had had elderly parents or parents-in-law (almost all were mothers/mothers-in-law) move into their household with the adult child assuming complete responsibility for care. (Parenthetically, we might note that another five respondents had also shared their household with other relatives, such as an aunt.) Also prior to the baseline interview, five of our respondents had found themselves no longer able to cope in caring for aged parents or parents-in-law and consequently had placed them in an institution, whereas another five respondents had institutionalized parents or parents-in-law without first bringing them into their home. In sum, 36% of our respondents were currently or had at some time in their adult life coped with decisions regarding caring for an older parent or parent-in-law in their own home and/or institutionalizing them.

Demographic and Caretaking Characteristics

Nearly one-half (47%) of our 49 respondents with living parents had one or both parents living in the same city as themselves; another 12% of the respondents had parents within easy driving distance (3 hours or less). The parents of the remaining 41% of our respondents lived in more distant parts of California or out of state. Our study confirms findings cited earlier that most older parents have children within easy visiting distance. Examining the location of elderly parents, we found only eight cases (16%) where the parent did not reside in the same city as at least one of his or her children, and only three of these (all widowed) could be said to be geographically isolated from their children. Of the five married couples who did not reside in the same city as one of their children, four were remarriages, which suggests some attenuation of filial bonds and obligations upon a parent's marriage.

The living parents consisted of 33% married couples, 61% widows, 4% widowers, and 2% divorced women. In terms of living arrangements of parents, all married couples resided in their own household, 23% lived alone, 16% lived with another relative or friend, 12% resided in the homes of our adult-child respondents, 8% were in institutions, and for another 8% the living arrangements of the parents were unknown.

Forty-seven percent of our respondents saw their parents weekly or daily (this included those who had parents living with them); 13% saw them at least once a month; and 40% saw them less than once a month. In general, contact with parents showed consistent patterns based on distance: when parents lived out of state or beyond a day's excursion, the norm was to visit them at least once a year; with parents resident in neighboring communities, an attempt was made to see them at least once a month. All but 2 of the 23 respondents with parents living in the same city saw them at least weekly.

There was often indication in the narrative data that adult children believed their parents wished to see them more often than the children wished or had time for, a discrepancy that may be attributable to the parent's abundant free time, scantier social networks, or greater emotional needs. The data suggest that a weekly visit or special activity with parents formed an acceptable compromise that symbolized and assured both parties of the continued solidarity of the parent–child bond. It was a common pattern to set aside a day in the week for visiting the parent or doing something special with the parent who was living in the household.

Forty-five percent of our respondents mentioned assisting parents. As expected, it was generally parents with physical and/or psychological disabilities who received help from a child. The eight parents who had health problems but were not being assisted by our respondents did not live geographically nearby or were in nursing homes. Over the 5-year period none of our respondents was helping a parent or parents in another state. This may be explained by the fact that, as noted earlier, the majority of geographically distant parents were living in close proximity to their other children, to whom they could presumably turn for assistance, and that when a distant parent devoid of such resources could no longer manage for him- or herself, he or she tended to be relocated to the vicinity of the respondent, most often joining the respondent's household.

Within our sample, 29 respondents lived in close geographic proximity to parents, and three-fourths of those mentioned gave some kind of help to parents, primarily in the tasks of daily living. Help with personal finances consisted primarily of writing out checks; none of our respondents mentioned giving direct financial aid to a parent. In some contradiction to other reported research, men were just as likely to report helping a parent as were women. However, the three respondents who were giving complete help to a parent (all mothers) were women, and throughout the 5 years of the study, women were more often involved in providing complete care than were men. Given the greater longevity of women and the greater likelihood of aged men to have spouses who could share in caretaking activities, one would conclude that severe stresses in late-life parent–child relationships will overwhelmingly involve mothers, with extensive caretaking functions falling primarily on daughters.

At baseline, one-half of the men and women mentioned personal sacrifices associated with helping a parent. For the total sample of 49 respondents with living parents, helping a parent (vs. not mentioning help) was significantly related to lower morale ($p < .01$), as measured by the Bradburn Affective Balance Scale.[2] Given this evidence of potential stress in late-life parent–child relationships, we next turn our attention to the ways in which our respondents perceived their parents over the 5 years, to the conditions under which stress was generated, and the consequences of stress for the respondents and its implications for their parents.

Impact of the Caretaking Role

At the baseline interview, about equal proportions of our 49 respondents with living parents gave predominantly positive evaluations of parents and their relationships with them, conveyed neutrality, or showed ambivalence or resentment. Consistent with other findings, appraisals of parents varied by the health status and activity level of the parent. The one-third of the respondents who spoke positively of parents also perceived their parents to lead active and self-sufficient lives: "They have a terrific marriage, and they are having more fun than they ever had"; "He still exercises regularly, is very spry, goes out a great deal and sings in a group." On the whole, successful aging on the part of the parent in terms of active engagement or, to a lesser extent, quiet self-sufficiency was a source of comfort and reassurance to the child. A few respondents commented on their good fortune that their parents were still alive, and 7 spoke of increasing closeness to the parent, viewing the parent as a continuing and dependable source of support. The latter attitudes tended to be those of women whose marriage was precarious or emotionally unsatisfying or those who had recently been widowed. One woman, for example, found reassurance in the fact that should her husband desert her, she could move in with her 86-year-old father ("As long as he is alive, I have a house"). In the absence of a supportive marital relationship, these middle-aged women seemed to turn to their parents, rather than children, for emotional sustenance.

Another one-third of the respondents, consisting of equal numbers of men and women, described their parents in predominantly negative terms, at times coldly and uncharitably. Many of these parents (all mothers) were reported to have symptoms of mental deterioration and sensory impairment and some to display paranoid tendencies and erratic behavior. One woman, for example, complained that she had "had a bellyfull" of her mother because she was forgetful, disoriented, and demanding. This woman also expressed fear of becoming senile like her mother. A number of other descriptions dealt with difficult personality traits: "My mother's personality was always a problem"; "She was always antagonistic, aggressive, and cruel to my father." Often-mentioned traits were nervousness and self-indulgence; ("Mother was spoiled rotten"; "Never cared for anything but cards and games"); one man expressed impatience at his mother's "stupidity," whereas a woman described her mother as "dull and disinterested." In commenting on progressive deterioration, respondents almost invariably pointed to earlier manifestations of present personality traits and problems in relationships. Some validity must be granted to their observations because it has been reported that people become more like themselves as they grow

older,[16] and it would follow that individuals who had been difficult to relate to in earlier periods of life would also be trying in old
age. On the other hand, it is also conceivable that with change in
personality and the increasing stresses involved in interacting in
such situations, earlier positive perceptions become blurred and
distorted. Regardless, the appearances or exacerbation of mental
symptomatology was apt to stress the adult child.

The relationship with elderly parents was most critical for the
29 respondents who had parents living within the same city or in
adjacent communities. Again, gratifying relationships with parents seemed to depend largely on the relative independence of
the parent and the values and cherished life-style of the child. In
this respect, 17 respondents showed positive or neutral attitudes
toward their parent. As may be expected, negative appraisals
were most likely to occur in instances where caretaking functions
were reported as confining and stressful. Twelve repondents expressed feelings ranging from irritation to exasperation and desperation about the infringements or constraints upon their life-
style induced by the parents.

For these latter respondents, responsibilities for the care of
the aged parent were perceived to occur at an inopportune time.
Some women had looked forward to freedom from worries and to
the pursuit of favored activities after their children had been
established. Some men and women were planning for retirement
and looking forward to extensive travel. There was the general
awareness that the time to make up for missed gratifications was
limited and that enjoyment should not be delayed. Under these
circumstances any unanticipated constraints on one's preferred or
hoped-for life-style were bound to evoke frustration, sometimes
accompanied by unwilled resentment. "I think I've waited on people so much of my life, and I wonder why I still have to do it," said
one woman. A second woman remarked that "the middle-aged
are sandwiched between their aging parents and their children;
just as you have raised your family, you have to take care of your
parents." Another woman, who felt her retirement plans for travel thwarted, commented, "We're at a stage where we should be
enjoying our lives. For many years we have been building up to
the future, and now we feel constrained. I guess it is terribly
selfish of me . . . but you are never free."

With few exceptions, as for example the man who regarded

his weekly and largely administrative meeting with his mother merely "a drag," the constraints in caring for a parent were experienced as severe, particularly for women. Though men mentioned having to "stay home nights" or being "tied down on weekends," women were far more likely to perceive the situation as oppressive, perhaps partly due to their higher emotional involvement.

As noted previously, men were as likely as women to report helping a parent, but they also appeared to have greater ability in distancing themselves physically and emotionally from their parents, and they appeared to experience less guilt and more readily accept the fact that it was not within their power to make the parent much happier. When men did have a high degree of contact with dependent parents, however, our data suggest that they were more likely to have negative perceptions of parents than were women. Possibly, contact with an aged parent is less rewarding for men than for women and results in greater irritability and impatience. Over the 5 years men recognized economic responsibilities and instrumental tasks but, unlike women, seldom felt responsible for the emotional well-being of the parent. They were also likely, not always unselfishly, to counsel the wife not to become overly involved with her own mother. Physicians were found to play a similar role in advising women to lessen their contact with the emotionally harrowing mother.

It was not so much the actual instrumental activity involved in the care of the parent which was viewed as burdensome, but the routines and confinement that were brought about by the parent's need: "The busy part about my mother does not bother me; it's the tied-down part that gets me." Some respondents had not taken a vacation for years because they felt they should not move beyond the reach of the parent. Some had set strict daily schedules which provided a sense of order and control, and some reassurance that one was meeting obligations to both the parent and one's self. It was often the infringement on such an established routine that precipitated crises.

To the extent that changes in relationship with parents across the 5-year period of study were mentioned, they were more likely to be negative than positive: 13 respondents commented on increasing difficulties and conflicts, whereas only 6 reported improvement, usually a sense of increasing closeness prompted by the parent's bereavement or frailty. Of these respondents, those who lived in the same city were more likely to report negative changes than did those whose parents lived farther away (when parents lived in the same city, negative changes outnumbered positive ones in the ratio of 11:2; when parents lived in outlying areas or at a greater distance, the ratio was 2:4). In some instances the changes were dramatic. One woman who at first contact expressed pleasure in visiting and doing things for her mother whom she described as the person closest to her and "an angel," displayed only hostility and resentment 5 years later when her mother's dependencies had increased and her capacity to reciprocate emotionally had declined. One man living with his octagenarian mother used to reserve 2 days for her when first interviewed. Five years later he described retirement as hell. His mother had become more demanding, and he felt that he could neither marry, travel, or move elsewhere, and he was fearful and desperate that he might die before he had a chance to enjoy some of the things he had worked for. A woman about to retire was suddenly faced with the task of taking her estranged mother into her household and was determined to create an optimal setting for her mother though this involved adopting a life-style totally inimical to her own nature and interests. Preparing for and psychologically adjusting to the move preoccupied her throughout the 18-month period between the baseline and the first follow-up and was accompanied by weight loss and insomnia. The 5-year follow-up found her living in a suburban community, deprived of vital cultural and social activities, and performing the role of homemaker and caretaker which she admittedly disliked. She suffered from constant frustration, tension, and irritability which she never permitted herself to reveal to her mother. Unlike most respondents, she stated that her mother was quite undemanding, and she attributed the acuteness of the situation to her own obsessive-compulsive personality and ludicrously exaggerated high standard of filial duty.

During the 5-year period of study one respondent had moved the mother into her home and five respondents had placed a parent in a nursing home (in two instances the parent had been living with the respondent); five respondents were apprehensively anticipating having to provide the parents with more care in the near future. The process of taking care of an aged parent was shown to include a series of phases and to extend over 2 to 5 years, during which there was growing anxiety, tension, and sense of confinement. All in all, nine respondents could be described as preoccupied and overwhelmed with the dependencies of the parent to the extent that their day-to-day lives were actuely disrupted and their future plans immobilized.

Our data accord with Brody's[4] and Wershow's[32] findings that children strive to delay the parents' institutionalization at considerable cost to themselves. In the majority of instances in our study, the relocation of the parent—or parent-in-law—occurred not precipituously but after a lengthy period of the parent's steady mental and physical deterioration, which imposed severe psychic stress on the child and taxed his or her ability to cope with the situation.

Conclusions

In our study, stress resulted from late-life parent–child relationships in two primary ways. First, coping with perceived mental deterioration of the parent produced a stressful situation and generally resulted in negative portrayals of parents by children. While it can be argued that at some point institutionalization becomes the only solution, the deterioration in family relationships may begin in the early stages of the parent's mental impairment, and this may possibly be circumvented by providing children with better awareness of the processes of mental decline. In our sample, much of the ambivalence and antagonism which was felt toward the parent resulted from the child's failure to fully understand observed changes in the parent.

Consistent with other studies, stress also resulted when the caretaking relationship was experienced as confining. Confinement was less clearly linked to the physical or mental status of the parent than it was to infringements on the life-style or hoped-for life-style of the adult child. Along with attempting to meet the parent's emotional needs, which perhaps the child alone can provide, our adult respondents were mainly helping parents in the activities of daily living—taking them to the doctor, cleaning the house, preparing meals, and the like. As the child became more involved in performing services for the parent, and, particularly, when the child felt he always had to be available, the situation became problematic.

The one area in which our respondents were not giving help was in terms of financial assistance to parents. This is no doubt largely a consequence of elderly parents taking advantage of such programs as Social Security, Supplemental Security Income, Medicare, and Medicaid.[7,8,20] In light of the apparent success of those health and income programs, one solution for easing burdens that the caretaking relationship imposes might be found in expanding social support systems such as in-home meals, housekeeping services, transportation and escort services, and particularly respite services. Except for an occasional housekeeper and one full-time nurse, none of our respondents reported receiving or seeking outside family help in the care of a parent. While it has been reported that children often serve as mediating links between parents and social institutions,[27] our data suggest that adult children also have to be made more aware of the community resources available, which may ease their own caretaking responsibilities and sense of confinement. Unfortunately, because of eligibility requirements, even where these various supports are available for elderly people and their families, middle-income people may not have them as options.

The current trend toward earlier discharge from acute-care hospitals and an expected increase in home care may result in more adult children becoming involved in caring for physically dependent parents. We feel an awareness of the stresses evoked by a caretaking relationship and active involvement by health and social services professionals for reducing these stresses will be needed if life satisfaction is going to be maintained for both adult child and parent generations.

References

1. Adams, M. The compassion trap. In V. Gornick & B. K. Moran (Eds.), *Women in sexist society*. New York: New American Library, 1972.

2. Bradburn, N. M. *The structure of psychological well-being.* Chicago: Aldine, 1969.
3. Brody, E. M. The aging family. *Gerontologist,* 1966, *6,* 201–206.
4. Brody, E. M. Follow-up study of applicants and non-applicants to a home. *Gerontologist,* 1969, *9,* 187–196.
5. Brody, E. M. *Long-term care of older people: A practical guide.* New York: Human Sciences Press, 1977.
6. Calkins, K. Shouldering a burden. *Omega,* 1972, *3,* 23–36.
7. Cameron, P. Pre-medicare beliefs about the generations regarding medicine and health. *Journal of Gerontology,* 1972, *27,* 536–539.
8. Crouch, B. M. Age and institutional support: Perceptions of older Mexican Americans. *Journal of Gerontology,* 1972, *27,* 524–529.
9. Gray, R., & Smith, T. Effect of employment on sex differences in attitudes toward the parental family. *Marriage and Family Living,* 1960, *22,* 36–38.
10. Hagestad, G. O., & Snow, R. B. *Young adult offspring as interpersonal resources in middle age.* Paper presented at the annual meeting of the Gerontological Society, San Francisco, Nov., 1977.
11. Havighurst, R. J. *Developmental tasks and education.* Chicago: University of Chicago Press, 1948.
12. Johnson, E. S., & Bursk, B. J. Relationships between the elderly and their adult children. *Gerontologist,* 1977, *17,* 90–96.
13. Kerckhoff, A. C. Nuclear and extended family relationships. In E. Shanas & G. Streib (Eds.), *Social structure and family: Generational relations.* Englewood Cliffs, NJ: Prentice-Hall, 1965.
14. Kraus, A. S., Spasoff, R. A., Beattie, E. J., Holden, D. E. W., Lawson, J. S., Rodenburg, M., & Woodcock, G. M. Elderly applicants to long-term care institutions. II. The application process; placement and care needs. *Journal of the American Geriatrics Society,* 1976, *24,* 165–172.
15. Lowenthal, M. F., Thurnher, M., Chiriboga, D., & Associates. *Four stages of life: A comparative study of women and men facing transitions.* San Francisco: Jossey-Bass, 1975.
16. Neugarten, B. L. Personality and patterns of aging. *Gawein,* 1965, *13,* 249–256.
17. Neugarten, B. (Ed.). Aging in the year 2000: A look at the future. *Gerontologist,* 1975, *15,* 1–40.
18. Newman, S. *Housing adjustment of older people: A report of findings from the first phase,* Ann Arbor: Institute for Social Research, the University of Michigan, 1975.
19. Newman, S. *Housing adjustment of older people: A report of findings from the second phase.* Ann Arbor: Institute for Social Research, the University of Michigan, 1976.
20. Palmore, E. The future status of the aged. *Gerontologist,* 1976, *16,* 297–302.
21. Riley, M. W., & Foner, A. *Aging and society, Vol. 1: An inventory of research findings.* New York: Russell Sage Foundations, 1968.
22. Rosenberg, G. S. *The worker grows old.* San Francisco: Jossey-Bass, 1970.
23. Rosow, I. *Social integration of the aged.* New York: Free Press, 1967.

24. Shanas, E. *The health of older people.* Cambridge: Harvard University Press, 1962.
25. Shanas, E. Social myth as hypothesis: The care of the family relations of old people. *Gerontologist,* 1979, *19,* 3–9.
26. Stehouwer, J. The household and family relations of old people. In E. Shanas, P. Townsend, D. Wedderburn, H. Friis, P. Milhøj, & S. Stehouwer (Eds.), *Old people in three industrial societies.* New York: Atherton, 1968.
27. Sussman, M. B. The family life of old people. In R. Binstock, & E. Shanas (Eds.), *Handbook of aging and the social sciences.* New York: Van Nostrand Reinhold, 1976.
28. Sussman, M. B. Relationships of adult children with their parents in the U.S. In E. Shanas, & G. Streib (Eds.), *Social structure and family: Generational relations.* Englewood Cliffs, N.J.: Prentice-Hall, 1965.
29. Sussman, M. B., & Burchinal, L. Kin family network: Unheralded structure in current conceptualizations of family functioning. *Marriage and Family Living,* 1962, *24,* 231–240.
30. Townsend, P. Emergence of the four-generation family in industrial society. In B. L. Neugarten (Ed.), *Middle age and aging.* Chicago: University of Chicago Press, 1968.
31. Troll, L. E. The family of later life: A decade review. *Journal of Marriage and Family,* 1971, *33,* 263–290.
32. Wershow, H. J. The four percent fallacy: Some further evidence and political implications. *Gerontologist,* 1976, *16,* part 1, 52–55.

15

Can You Survive Your Retirement?

LELAND P. BRADFORD

I was the chief executive of an organization I had helped found, as well as a professional behavioral scientist, and I should have known better. But I didn't. After 25 years of working under the strain of building an organization, of interweaving the ideas and needs of the key staff with a multiplicity of outside forces, I was ready for the beautiful promised land of retirement. I persuaded my wife to leave our lovely Georgetown home and move to North Carolina, where I could golf to my heart's content and enjoy relief from the stress of having to make daily decisions. I thought it would be just wonderful.

How wrong I was! The first year was awful. The organization moved on without me. Important decisions I had made were reversed. No one called for advice. As far as I could see, no one

This chapter appears in abridged form from the *Harvard Business Review*. "Can You Survive Your Retirement" by Leland P. Bradford (November/December 1979). Copyright 1979 by the President and Fellows of Harvard College; all rights reserved. Reprinted by permission.

LELAND P. BRADFORD • Deceased, a founder and former director of the National Training Laboratory, Arlington, Virginia 22209.

cared. I even felt that my professional reputation had vanished. It hurt.

At times I thought with empathy of a friend who had been president of a large multinational company. He had told me, before he retired, that he had everything planned carefully. A year after his retirement, some of his former vice-presidents told me he came to the office at least twice a week seeking someone who was free to lunch with him.

I found that golf did not fill a day. The consultation and volunteer work I did was not satisfying. Other interests paled before the challenges I had faced. Life felt empty. I was not aged, just a little older. I had plenty of energy, and I felt just as competent as I had been.

When for the umpteenth time I complained to my wife about the emptiness of my life, Martha exploded, "I've heard enough of your complaining! You dragged me away from the city and home I loved best. Do you know why I don't like it here? Do you know why I've gone to the hospital twice this year for checkups, only to find nothing wrong? It was because I'm unhappy. Did you consider my life in retirement when you retired?" I hadn't, though I thought we had talked everything over. Maybe I had just talked about *my* retirement. What she said woke me up, and I listened.

Then we talked for days, for weeks, it seemed like months— at breakfast, teatime, the cocktail hour, during evenings when there were no parties. We came to know each other's feelings and problems better. We asked ourselves if we were the only ones to react this way, so we looked about us and talked to many others on the golf course and at small parties. We found we weren't alone, although people usually covered up at first before acknowledging the empty hours they dreaded and their sense of futility and uselessness. (We learned later of a census study showing that many persons die 4 to 5 years after retirement, seemingly out of a sense of uselessness. And according to a famous French physician, people can indeed die of boredom.)

Only after we had talked through our own difficulties to our satisfaction did we begin to question why this transition period was so very difficult and so different from others we had negotiated. Was it because it marked an ending, or were there other causes? Here are our conclusions.

What One Loses in Retirement

As we thought about what had happened to us and to others, we began to see how organizations inadvertently fulfill a number of basic psychological needs for people. The loss of these gratifications on retirement can be devastating unless effectively accommodated to or replaced.

Acceptance and Socialization

The organization, for almost all positions, provides colleagues, work groups, teams, committees, units, or departments. Members perforce feel a sense of belonging that they share with others, whether the cohesive factor is task completion or antagonism within groups or the company. Conflict adequately handled is energizing. Task accomplishment is a mutual gain. Work provides the contacts vital for psychological well-being. Otherwise, there are no correctives for perceptual distortion, no antidotes for loneliness.

I found all this out. I felt the alienation of no longer being a part of groups I had belonged to for 40 or more hours a week for more years than I cared to remember. Even in my childhood, when I had been temporarily ostracized by playmates, I had not felt so keenly excluded, bereft, outside, disposable.

I thought again of my friend who had returned hungrily to the office to seek the companionship of his past subordinates. What was different for him, and now for me, was the apparent lack of an arena offering equal challenges and companionship. I found it harder than I ever expected to say a permanent good-bye to a lifetime work career. It took time and suffering to find an adequate solution.

Goals, Achievement, and Affirmation

Organizations provide goals and tasks to be formulated and accomplished. During the middle years these are interwoven with personal financial aims and family responsibilities. Goals make achievement possible, sometimes with soul-warming results. Achievement brings affirmation from others and from one's self.

Without this periodic affirmation, self-esteem and self-worth diminish. They are intricately interdependent and, oh, how important!

To be without goals is to be purposeless, to have no reason to arise in the morning; for some, even to live. I teetered on the brink of goallessness, and it took Martha to awaken me. Also, a perceptive club member said to me, "Do you realize the purpose of our club is to keep useless people alive?" That helped wake me too.

Not long ago I had lunch with a man whom I had known for years. Highly successful in the positions he had held, he was generous, sensitive to others, and a good companion. He had been retired for a couple of years. During the 2 hours of lunch, I don't think I got in three sentences. He didn't tell me what he was doing, because he wasn't doing anything to talk about, but he did talk about the well-known people who sought him out and the artists and musicians who wanted his company. I left our luncheon saddened. He who had achieved so much was now reduced to seeking affirmation from others in superficial ways. How had retirement so drastically stripped him of his sense of achievement?

Power and Influence

Companies provide for most employees some degree of power and influence. For top executives, of course, the degree is great, though most would admit to various constraints. Power conveys importance to the person and aids the formation and perception of identity. Power increases the areas in which accomplishment can occur and leads to the gaining of more power.

For executives and others who have known considerable power, its sudden loss at retirement can be an acute deprivation. The shock for many is not only great but also bewildering. Events are less under one's control, and the importance in others' eyes that power gives has evaporated. Must the person who has lost power continue to vie for it, or can the individual find power and importance within himself?

On the board of directors of a local organization of not much significance sit some former executives of well-known companies.

The board meets periodically for a stated 2 hours each meeting. For 5 to 10 minutes real work is accomplished. These executives, before retirement, would have ended a meeting in no more than 15 minutes. Now they are content to spend the 2 hours. Why? One might guess that, since they have little else to do, 2 hours fill a portion of a day. One might also hazard a guess that for those 2 hours power and influence are again theirs.

Support Systems

Individuals need a variety of support systems for psychological and emotional health. Colleagues, friends, neighbors, clubs, community responsibilities, family, and others serve as support systems providing recognition, admiration, assurance of abilities, reality testing, feedback on behavior, and encouragement.

When retirement comes, and particularly if the couple moves away, many support systems disappear. I wish I had thought to list all my support systems before I retired, then crossed off those I would miss. I could then have gone on more than just intuitive feeling in deciding which ones were crucial to replace.

Routines and Time

The busy executive with wide-ranging interests and multi-faceted decisions to make seldom realizes the stabilizing force of set routines—regular staff meetings, daily agendas on the desk each morning, planned luncheon engagements, organized trips, prearranged social events.

When retirement comes, most of these routines stop. At first it seems heavenly: no clock ruling you, no secretary reminding you of your luncheon appointment, no hurried breakfast, no train to catch. So I found it; but not for long, because habit is strong. Besides, inasmuch as my day no longer had its ready-made structure, I was left with the aggravating necessity of making many small decisions. Therefore, routines need to be set; else why should one get out of bed at all? This is a small but significant change in the transition to retirement.

Where we now live there is no postal delivery. Sometime during the morning, everyone goes to the post office to meet friends, exchange gossip, make golf dates, and sometimes arrange parties. Gradually routines like this become established, but only if the person deliberately develops them; no longer does the organization create them.

Before retirement, the expenditure of time, like routine, is primarily under the control of the organization, and time spent on nonwork activities is fitted into the slots remaining. During the driving, challenging, responsible work years, time becomes a scarce and precious commodity: it is the duty of secretaries and assistants to ensure that this precious resource is effectively used.

In retirement the reverse is too frequently true. Time must be filled, somehow, to pass the day. Time can lead people into the dangerous wasteland of empty time, where no purpose is present to stir any interest or desire. If empty time recurs each day, the will and motivation to seek new interests dwindle. Boredom joins with apathy to reduce the joy of living and speed psychological if not physical deterioration.

In my early days of retirement I would become irritated on the links if a slow foursome in front held up our play. My partners, longer retired, would say, "What's your hurry? What else do you have to do today?"

For many of us, golf was followed by time at the bar, perhaps some bridge, more cocktails at home or at a party, followed by a dull evening. The intense preoccupation with work and community responsibilities had precluded leisurely reading in former years. Interests and new skills not developed before retirement were difficult to cultivate after retirement.

So the challenging hours of yesterday become empty hours today, often with disastrous consequences.

Problems of the Retired

The very different conditions of retirement create new problems stemming from existing situations. One is sufficiently common and serious to be critical in a misery-free transition to retirement.

Marital Difficulties

Marriage, as a dynamic process, alters of course with changing conditions. The abrupt passage from work to retirement should require consideration of possible marital adjustments. There are a number of factors leading to this necessity.

The Rights of Each. I never realized that my work career, title, status, job responsibilities, office, secretary, even desk represented my turf, or territory, and thus largely defined my identity to others and to myself. When I thought of turf I thought of the way animals fight to secure or defend a bit of space. It was only at retirement, when all aspects of my turf were given to another, that the dreadful realization of being turfless struck home. For an awful moment, I became uncertain of my identity. I knew who I had been, but I was not certain who I was. The sudden movement from "I am" to "I was" was difficult to adjust to.

I had always thought of the home as mine as well as Martha's. But now I found that it was her turf. It had been her territory to manage, where she had made and implemented decisions and dealt with a host of people. I had never thought of the time and knowledge she had put into managing the home.

It was not long before it occurred to me that I was intruding on her turf. I managed to be in the wrong place at the wrong time—for example, we kept bumping into each other in the kitchen. It was her domain, and I was obviously curtailing her freedom of action. We talked it through and worked out accommodations that gave me some turf without depriving her and allowed us time alone as well as shared time.

We observed how "turf loss" and intrusion problems beset other retired couples. Once we were looking at clothes in the downstairs section of a store. Sitting on the steps leading downstairs was a gray-haired man. A woman standing near us saw us glance at him, and she felt impelled to speak. "Since he's retired he goes wherever I go. I can no longer shop in peace," she said, with a hostile look toward the stairs. "It's like having a child with you all day long. I don't know how long I can stand it!"

Then there is the extreme where intrusion means control. An acquaintance of ours had always been restless, but his nervous energy had fit well with the demands of his high-level corporate position. He did not slow up even in retirement. No sooner did he and his wife return from one cruise or plane trip, with stops at various cities, than he was planning another. His wife grew more weary with each trip.

Finally she spoke up, saying she couldn't take it any longer.

He brushed her feelings aside. "Nonsense," he said. "Travel is broadening. It's good for you." That silenced her; she couldn't stand up to his strong (and insensitive) personality. But finally, for the first time, she complained openly and bitterly to her friends.

Unless the couple can undertake a conciliatory review of their "turf loss" and intrusion problem and make adjustments to it, irritations will grow, bitterness will mount, and conflicts will continue. But such a marital review is not easy to make. Talking through the problem requires a sense of self-worth on the part of each so that feedback can be openly given and nondefensively received. It requires respect of each by the other and sufficient self-understanding so that each feels secure.

The turf-intrusion problem is typical of the mutually affecting strains that become especially stressful in retirement, when husband and wife find themselves spending much more time together. The turmoil that one of them experiences upsets the other. Unless each can share the problems and can accept help and support from the other, relations that before were calm become potentially explosive.

Sex Role Questions.   Particularly for the man who has lost his turf, the fear of losing a masculine image is bothersome. He has had an identity as the family provider, the family head, the ultimate judge on major issues. Title and position in the eyes of others bolster one's self-image, and a man tries to project himself to others as a strong and competent person worthy of their respect.

Because a man cannot overtly assert his macho drives, he directs them into various innocent and socially acceptable channels. The individual may only be dimly aware of these drives, but they are strong.

Not long ago Martha and I attended a small dinner party with four other couples, all friends or acquaintances. The host had always appeared to us to be a quiet, unobtrusive man. That night, however, he was assertive and extremely aggressive toward his wife. If she broke in on his conversation, he told her to wait until he was finished talking. He corrected her and instructed her not to talk unless she knew what she was saying. She made no protest, out of good manners or perhaps for other reasons. The other guests looked as embarrassed as we were.

Martha and I talked the matter over when we arrived home. What we had seen was not the couple's normal pattern of relationship. One hypothesis stood out in our thinking: the husband, without realizing it, was endeavoring to show the other men at the party that, though long since retired, he was still a man and master of his home.

Growing Apart. Over the years sharp differences in work responsibilities may have brought first imperceptible and then palpable differences in the levels of growth of the partners. Because so much of the day was spent apart, these differences may not have been important. But with the closer living of retirement, they become almost unbearable.

One man we know rose far in his company through sheer ability. His frequent new contacts, coupled with his absorbing mind, brought continual expansion of his interests. His wife stayed home and socialized with a tight circle of friends. Then he retired, and he suddenly found they had little in common and even less to communicate about. It seemed they had come out of different worlds, and there was nothing they could do but to live out their lives as best they could. My wife and I agreed that both were to blame—he because he had done nothing to help her grow, and she because she had insulated herself and had made no effort to develop.

So at retirement, couples need to undertake a marital review. Those who have negotiated this transition successfully probably made sensitive adjustments as needs arose without waiting for problems to become serious. But those who think that their relationship will remain the same and make no accommodations are in for trouble.

VII

Developmental Life Transitions
Death and Bereavement

Our acquaintance with loss and death spans a lifetime. Partial losses throughout our lives prepare us for the death of close family members and for the ultimate loss—the loss of ourself. But even a lifetime of preparation cannot blunt the pain of grief—the initial shock and numbness, followed by the agonizing yearning, and later the waves of sadness aroused by memories of the loved one. During the slow, arduous process of adjustment to bereavement, grieving persons need to let go of the dead person, give up their grief, and build other relationships to fill the void left by the loved one. Parkes and Weiss[5] note that bereaved persons must be able to understand their loss intellectually and explain how it happened. Emotionally, they must confront every aspect of the loss until the distress associated with thoughts of the loved person diminishes, and they are able to recall memories of the dead person without pain. Finally, bereaved persons must change their self-image to match the new reality. For example, widows need to accept their new identity as a single head of household.

Sometimes a lengthy illness provides family members with time to assimilate painful changes and begin anticipatory grieving. In the first article, Dorothy Paulay recounts how she coped with her husband's critical injury following a car accident and his slow decline and eventual death after 5 years. As her husband, Jean, lay in a coma suffering from brain damage, Dorothy kept a vigil at the hospital, waiting for her husband to awaken so she could begin to help him recover. She vented her anger at the doctor who gave a pessimistic prognosis and limited the awareness of her loss by minimizing the seriousness of his illness.

Eventually, Jean emerged from the coma. With the help of his wife and son, he relearned how to walk and talk but remained in a sanitarium. During the lengthy period of her husband's gradual decline, Dorothy managed by focusing on the present and limiting interactions with the outside world to people and things directly related to her situation. She and her son involved themselves intensively in Jean's care and rehabilitation. However, after 4 years, Dorothy and her son finally acknowledged that Jean might never recover. Once she gave up her struggle to help him recover, Dorothy was able to invest her energy in rebuilding her family life. Because her long ordeal provided time for anticipatory mourning, Dorothy was able to cry and let Jean go when she saw that the end was near. With time, she successfully made the transition from wife to survivor and came to see her experience as a source of strength and her life as having been enriched by it.

When the initial outpouring of support fades, widows face tasks of overcoming loneliness and forging a new identity, issues that are similar to those of divorced persons (see Chapters 10 and 11). Widows can cope effectively with loneliness by keeping busy, developing new roles, or focusing on existing roles such as that of grandparent. Judith Saunders describes widows as having to forge an "uncoupled identity."[9] In the transition to such an uncoupled identity, the widow must decide whether to dispose of her husband's belongings and whether or not she will wear her wedding band. Giving away her husband's possessions and removing her ring are concrete signs that she is breaking the bonds she had with him. Changes in social patterns such as seeking new friendships, engaging in new social activities, and dating also signal movement toward a new identity.

The anguish of a widow or widower is surpassed only by that of parents whose child dies. Linda Edelstein found that bereaved mothers experienced several losses—loss of their maternal identity, loss of future hopes and expectations, and loss of the illusion that their family is safe from tragedy and that they can prevent their child from dying. Bereaved mothers sometimes cope with their losses by reaching out in a maternal way to someone in need of help. Parents also try to keep the child's memory alive.[2] Some parents may temporarily make their child's room a shrine and keep it just as it was when the child died, or they may commemorate the child in pictures. One mother kept memories of her dead child alive by creating a "cry box" that contained her child's special possessions—kindergarten pictures, smelly old sneakers, and the like. The child's siblings spent hours telling stories about the child's possessions and in this way worked through their grief.[1] Other parents may create a memorial, establish scholarships, or give money to the child's favorite sports facility.[2]

People often cope with tragedy by finding meaning in it. In the second chapter, Margaret Shandor Miles and Eva K. Brown Crandall explore the varied resolutions of grief by parents whose child has died. Some parents saw life as meaningless and thought they would never get over the loss of their child. But many of the parents found some meaning in their loss by establishing memorials to their child, identifying the uniqueness of him or her, helping others, and developing deeper religious beliefs. Such parents became more compassionate and caring, lived life more fully, and were more aware of the preciousness of each moment. Parents who are able to find meaning in their bereavement may experience growth rather than despair.

The course of adjustment to the loss of a child or a spouse may depend on personal factors and on circumstances surrounding the death. For example, Therese Rando[7] studied parents whose child had died of cancer and found that parents of children with long-sustained illnesses fared more poorly than those whose child had a shorter illness. Prior loss was also associated with poorer bereavement outcomes, whereas anticipatory grief was related to better adjustment. Similar issues affect adaptation to the death of a spouse. Good conjugal bereavement outcome is associated with some aspects of the event itself, such as having forewarning of the death as well as with marital cohesion and independence, the absence of concurrent life crises, and the presence of adequate social support.[5,8]

Aspects of the social environment—our values, beliefs, customs, and the support available from family, friends, and neighbors—have a significant impact on how we see death and cope with it. In the third article, Kathleen B. Bryer discusses death from the perspective of the traditional society of the Amish.

She explores the family and group structure of the Amish, their funeral customs and mourning rituals, and their personal experiences and feelings about death. The Amish society provides many conditions that facilitate coping with death and bereavement. Death is seen as an integral part of life. Religious beliefs make death less frightening and help the Amish accept it. Most Amish people die at home with family members in attendance. In the process of caring for the dying person, family members can begin anticipatory grieving. They also have a chance to take care of unfinished business and to talk with the dying person about death. (For a discussion of the specific tasks faced by dying persons, see Sylvia Poss.[6])

When a death occurs, Amish neighbors take responsibility for notifying others about it, making funeral arrangements, digging the grave, and preparing the food for the meal after the funeral. After the body is embalmed, it is returned to the home. Family members dress the body in white clothing that has been sewn and set aside especially for the funeral. Customs such as these help members of the community prepare for death. Family, friends, and neighbors gather at the home to view the body and participate in the funeral service. After the funeral, the community continues to be sensitive to the emotional needs of the bereaved family. Support is offered for at least a year after the death. For example, a widower's sister helped care for his children until he remarried.

Our modern society often fails to provide the kind of help that is available to members of the Amish community. Prevention programs for bereaved persons that offer reassurance and guidance can facilitate adjustment to loss of a loved one. For example, a counseling program for persons at high risk of poor adjustment following bereavement resulted in their experiencing less tension and anxiety and using less medication, alcohol, and tobacco.[4] New widows who obtain emotional support and practical assistance from widows who have resolved their grief tend to manage bereavement tasks better and to readjust more quickly than those who do not receive such support.[11]

Successful adaptation to grief can leave the bereaved person wiser and better able to experience life fully. John Schneider[10] describes the final phase of the grief process as one of transforming the loss into a growth experience. Grief can be transmuted into creative energy, as was the case for Mary Jane Moffat,[3] a writer who worked through her widow's grief by writing poetry and reading literature that captured the painful emotions she struggled to master. She compiled her poetry and readings into a powerful book on mourning in the hope that it would enable other persons to make peace with their grief.

References

1. Arnold, J. H., & Gemma, P. B. *A child dies: A portrait of family grief.* Rockville, Md.: Aspen Systems, 1983.
2. Edelstein, L. *Maternal bereavement: Coping with the unexpected death of a child.* New York: Praeger, 1984.
3. Moffat, M. J. (Ed.). *In the midst of winter: Selections from the literature of mourning.* New York: Random House, 1982.
4. Parkes, C. M. Evaluation of a bereavement service. *Journal of Preventive Psychiatry,* 1981, *1,* 179–188.
5. Parkes, C. M., & Weiss, R. S. *Recovery from bereavement.* New York: Basic Books, 1983.
6. Poss, S. How the terminal patient accepts dying. *Patient Counseling and Health Education,* 1980, *2,* 72–77.
7. Rando, T. A. An investigation of grief and adaptation in parents whose children have died from cancer. *Journal of Pediatric Psychology,* 1983, *8,* 3–20.
8. Raphael, B. *The anatomy of bereavement.* New York: Basic Books, 1983.
9. Saunders, J. M. A process of bereavement resolution: Uncoupled identity. *Western Journal of Nursing Research,* 1981, *3,* 319–332.
10. Schneider, J. *Stress, loss, and grief: Understanding their origins and growth potential.* Baltimore: University Park Press, 1984.
11. Vachon, M. L., Lyall, W. A., Rogers, J., Freedman-Letofsky, K., & Freeman, S. J. A controlled study of self-help intervention for widows. *American Journal of Psychiatry,* 1980, *137,* 1380–1384.

16

Slow Death
One Survivor's Experience

DOROTHY PAULAY

Each of us is destined to be a survivor. Death awaits all of us, of course, but for practically everyone death will be experienced first as a survivor, as someone near or known to us dies. Our reactions to these deaths, along with the culture, race, mores, customs, and ethics of our times, will help to shape our feelings toward our own death. While much has been written recently about the problem in our death-denying culture of coming to terms with the fact of death, for the most part discussion has been in terms of adjusting to the death of a loved one which has just occurred or to one's own death which is imminent.

But there are many kinds of survivors, just as there are many kinds of deaths. Research has shown that practically everyone desires a quick, clean death with minimal suffering and no or very short illness. The individual prefers that for his loved ones, too, although not so suddenly that there is no warning, no preparation time to adjust to unanticipated loss. Sometimes, however, there is no choice. The death is not quick and painless. Instead, there is the slow, inexorable debilitation of a chronic illness or traumatic

This chapter appears in abridged form from *Omega*, 1977–1978, *8*(2), 173–179. Copyright 1977, Baywood Publishing Co., Inc. Reprinted by permission.

DOROTHY PAULAY • 10401 Wilshire Boulevard, Los Angeles, California 90024.

injury through which both patient and family must suffer. The
survivors of such a death go through a different qualitative experience of death and dying, especially if the process takes not days
or weeks but years. It is worsened by the process of being forced
to watch the disintegration and loss of the image of the loved one
as he slowly dies.

The following is one therapist's account of her own personal,
intimate experience with dying in confronting the lingering death
of her husband. I have written it in order to describe one survivor's working-through process and to offer whatever insights
were gained which might be useful in helping other survivors of
similar long-term illness and death of a loved one.

I suddenly became a member of our death-denying society,
when I learned that my husband, Jean, was in a car accident. It
was a head-on collision—both cars were completely demolished—
both drivers were alone—Jean was unconscious under the wheel.
The driver of the other car was found walking around. Both men
were taken to a hospital. The other patient was discharged within
3 days with slight bruises. Jean remained in a coma for a week.
Luck had chosen its victim in this encounter.

As a clinical social worker, I had often listened and helped
others cope with severe life stresses and with death. I know that a
patient goes through a series of stages in his struggle with his fatal
illness and that his family also goes through stages in accepting it.
But while I had been able to help others, I found that I couldn't
help myself. I couldn't accept the doctor's statement that Jean's
brain was partially damaged and that he could never again be as I
had known him. I denied the seriousness of Jean's illness, the
degree to which he had been injured. It is through this experience
that I really learned about my attitude toward life, death, and
dying.

I was filled with anger at what had happened, at luck which
had singled us out for its cruelest of blows, which had robbed a
man of all his abilities, and a family of its husband and father.

I directed my anger at the medical profession. I know doctors
are human. They get sick and sometimes even die. At the hospital,
the doctor in charge of emergencies said that Jean was terminal.
He didn't want me to see him. He felt the sight of the injury might
be too much to take. I insisted on seeing him. Reluctantly, the

doctor directed me to a small room where he was lying on a table. He had plunged from the height of agility and health to the depths of total paralysis. Normally slender, his swollen body looked large, heavy; his face was covered with cuts. I stayed with him a few minutes and left.

That day and the rest of the week I remained around the hospital, waiting for him to regain consciousness. I wanted to be there when he came back to life to start him immediately on the road to recovery. I was filled with resolve. No matter how badly hurt Jean was, I would help him as I had helped others. But this was more blind wish than understanding. With only part of his brain functioning, my husband was severely disabled for $5\frac{1}{2}$ years until his death from pneumonia.

Even in the face of the doctor's hopeless attitudes, our 13-year-old son Pete and I retained the belief that he would recover. We were determined to help him do so, and we were partially successful. For 4 years Pete and I devoted ourselves to caring for Jean. He relearned to walk and talk. At times he was rational, aware of his disability, sometimes grateful and appreciative of our attention, and sometimes angry, confused, and depressed. He was aware of how much he had lost and showed great courage in facing the loss of everything that had been meaningful. For some it takes the form of hopelessness; for others it can be used to discover untapped inner strengths.

As if to support our own need to deny, we received numerous phone calls and letters expressing shock, sorrow, and deep concern over Jean's condition. These wishes to be with us in spirit nourished and supported me. Letters reminded me that "Jean possesses the strength and will to get well." Another letter: "With his tremendous vitality and zest, if anyone has the spirit or will to accomplish the impossible, Jean will do it." From a rabbi: "I have seldom asked the God I serve to counter the laws of nature, but I would gladly forgive and praise Him for any miracle that might restore Jean to his charming, ebullient, capable, thoughtful self."

My efforts to cope with the situation were mostly denial—a "splitting off" of emotions. My personal life shrank. I limited my interest in the outside world to only those people or things that had a direct bearing on my immediate situation. I lived in the present only—concern about the future came later. I also became aware of my reaction to the way others acted toward me and toward Jean. I got a great lift from people's interest in Jean and their hope for him. When they seemed to give up, I was angry that he no longer merited their hope. I felt some people were uncomfortable in my presence, and their distress created discomfort in me. The more anxious they became, the more I felt their wish to avoid me. My ability to reach out or to receive expressions of human feelings decreased.

At the time of the accident, three doctors stated that Jean could not last the day. One doctor, trying to be objective, decided the unvarnished facts were best for me. He said, "He won't live. If he does he will be blind and totally paralyzed—a vegetable." As I look back now, I realize I wanted to be told the truth in spite of my denial, my inability to face possible death. But I also desperately needed some spark of hope. Miracles sometimes happen. Truth can be cold, brutal, cruel. It should be tempered with gentleness and empathy.

Sometimes the denial in the family is its only defense to help it get through the crises, to give it time to integrate an unhappy truth. I didn't want to talk about Jean's impending death. I didn't want to admit he was dying. I couldn't. I preferred denial. Some of the doctors didn't understand and therefore didn't allow it.

As Jean slowly regained consciousness, his doctor asked me what language he was speaking. I didn't know. I consulted his brother and learned that he was reciting the atonement prayer in Hebrew. Jean's background was that of an orthodox Jew. At age 13 he had rebelled against religious rituals which had no apparent meaning to him and against the Hebrew language which he didn't understand. But he returned to partial life by traveling the tortured pathways of ingrained ancient customs with the Hebrew prayer of atonement.

When Jean was semiconscious, I could at times reach him. This gave me hope that through our relationship I could help him get well, a hope I needed desperately. A sick person seldom gets well alone—he is helped by a give-and-take relationship. Unless there is some shred of hope, the survivor is hard put to be helpful. As Jean was regaining consciousness he suddenly would ask, "Why are you here?" And I would say, "Because I love you." One day he asked the question and I, feeling tired and discouraged, said, "Because I am here." To my surprise he corrected me with, "Say, because I love you." I thus became aware of how much he needed my love and support.

When he was moved from the hospital to a sanitarium and tube feeding was discontinued, he reached Nirvana—"This is heaven, who found this place—excellent food." Then, thoughtfully, "Hope it doesn't cost too much." I admired his drive and determination to get well. My own hope was reinforced by his warmth, his humor, his optimism, his thoughtful self. "I will get well," he would say. "Some day we will see the world together." At other times he asked, "What makes you feel so sure that I will get well, and when I do, how will I feel?" He would say, "Tell me from the beginning what happened. Tell me all you know and that way I too will know." He would ask questions in an attempt to orient himself to the present, past, and future. He would then say, "Be patient with me and my questions. I ask so I have someone to blame if it doesn't come out right." When I looked and felt low he was kind. When I acted strong he was hostile and angry.

As the months wore on, his personality became moody, alternating between elation and sadness. Sometimes he was frustrated, agitated, angry. I found notes he had written expressing his confusion and depression.

> *I love life and love it dearly, but today I am a lost man. Get better, for what? Why is life cruel? I am not cruel—why make life so? I am good—why isn't life equally so?"*

He would say:

> *The only thing I know is what I don't know. I cannot fill the void. I feel so uncertain. Strange to lose one's memory. I am human—I am not getting better—I am getting worse. Tell me, who was the man I talked with? Strange that a mind can't make itself understood. I feel alone and lost. I am not concerned over not walking, but I am concerned about the confusion of my mind. People can see that I can't walk; they can't see my confused mind.*

Jean felt himself an unworthy burden and was ashamed of his inability to function. Sometimes he viewed his illness as a punishment for real or imagined misdeeds. He was terrified at being abandoned now that he was sick. He felt alone and unlovable. He would say:

Life to me is very troublesome because I am a burden to you. I always have been independent. I don't want my life to be dependent on you. I must gain strength so I don't tire so quickly, so I can walk and use my right hand.

When the feeling in his hand returned he was overjoyed. "I feel like a new man—no longer a cripple."

Our son Pete was excellent with Jean. He helped him regain his physical strength and emotional worth. Jean was so proud of him as expressed by his notes: "Pete, I am fortunate to have you as my son." Another note; "Pete was like a breath of spring. The young man has an air of maturity that gives me a feeling of proudness. I can only give him my love and tell him he is wanted and loved by his mother and father."

Pete would try to help Jean by allowing him to do whatever he thought he could do himself; to recover feelings of self-worth; to feel accepted and wanted. We were honest and direct. We pulled for him and with him. We tried to be tolerant and understanding of his inconsistent behavior, his frustrations, his helplessness.

We helped him recover from his aphasic period, a complicated condition affecting the ability to use or understand speech. In this aphasic period he had an intense need to repeat over and over a certain word. Being a good speller, he spelled out words. He was aware of words coming out wrong, but with only part of his brain working he had no control over the words. There were reverses, opposites of what he meant. Sometimes he did not want to reveal how mixed up he was. He asked for sugar; given sugar, he had meant butter, so he sprinkled sugar over bread. Match for cigarette—napkin for blanket. He would say, "cold hot air," "dark sunshine outside," "election results are bad for the winner." "When you exhaust your sleep, you're well slept out." "I wouldn't wish this on my worst enemy that I like." We frequently laughed with him, when he realized what actually had come out instead of what he meant.

Jean's behavior reflected his inconsistent and often poor judgment. He set fires, tore magazines. At times he was noisy and belligerent. He had poor control over his anger and anxiety. He might start with a good idea but would end up applying it inappropriately. This behavior did not make him popular in sanitariums. They would request that he be removed, and I would have to start another search for a new sanitarium. Several times I found a new one where he would be the first patient and could remain until the sanitarium was filled. Then again I would be asked to move him.

In the fourth year of Jean's illness, Pete started a conversation with "When Daddy gets well . . ." I suddenly heard myself, "Daddy may never get well," and Pete said, "That's what I have been thinking." It was the first time that we could say aloud this fear of permanent disability—death—that we had denied, pushed aside for over 4 years.

It was the turning point in my life. I lost hope for my husband's recovery, then redirected it to rebuilding our family life. I redistributed my time and my energy and started to cope at last with the reality of Jean's illness. I continued to care for him, to arrange satisfactions to fill his limited life, but my hopes and goals were directed in rebuilding my own life and in separating myself from the impossible struggle to overcome by sheer will power his disabling illness. Having experienced Jean's struggle with life, I have learned that death is not always an "enemy"—sometimes it is a friend. It can be an end to a long life; it can sometimes be regarded as a privilege earned by intense suffering. I found comfort in Freud's attitude toward the person who had died: "admiration for someone who has accomplished a very difficult task." "Death," he said, "was a friendly idea."

I learned that fear of dying is not only human, a feeling I need not be ashamed of, but something I can learn to handle. Fear of death may be more a problem for the living than for the dying.

I have learned the hard way that my way of feeling is not the universal way. There is no one way of coping with dying. There is no "ought to feel" or "ought to be." Each person looks at life and death with a different set of values. There is gratifying richness in the variety of individual differences.

Late one night, Jean's doctor, who had proved most helpful to me, phoned. The sanitarium had called him to visit Jean. The doctor reported Jean had pneumonia with a 105° fever and that I should be prepared for the ending. Doctors on three previous occasions had prepared me for his death. I had not been ready to separate from him those times, and I didn't. This time I let him go—freed him. I cried the rest of the night.

Early next morning I was at the sanitarium. To my amazement I found Jean up walking around the room in an angry, complaining, demanding mood—fever normal. I remained with him that morning, questioning my sanity. Was last night's phone call from the doctor a dream? The following night Jean died.

I gathered my strength—isolated my feelings—phoned Pete at an out-of-state camp. In the mortuary, being with the body which had been Jean's, I experienced a different separation, a different turning point. I felt relief for him, a void for me. He was part of me and he was gone. I made the necessary arrangements for the funeral. But this was not for me. This was to carry out the beliefs and practices of society. I talked with the mortuary representative, chose a casket, talked with the rabbi. During the funeral I was there in body, my feelings in control. I was aware of the many people who had come—I talked with them. Pete was my greatest emotional support. With him I shared the loss.

After the funeral I withdrew, needing to allow myself to feel the pain of my loneliness, to experience the void. I was sad for the loss of the healthy Jean; a small part of me was still clutching at the sick Jean.

I find myself doing what he did, saying what he said, enjoying what he had enjoyed. The spirit of the delightful, capable Jean has remained with me.

I have examined my attitude toward life, death, and dying. I have learned that the energy used in concern over the nature and meaning of death may be made available to cope with life's crises. Only by coming to terms with death, by accepting it as a companion, and knowing that it will eventually possess me, can I possess my life and make it richer and more meaningful.

My experience now became a source of strength. It is part of me and belongs to me. It has heightened my awareness of the shortness of life by emphasizing its quality and beauty. We tend to die the way we live. Now I feel freer, more comfortable to listen sensitively to others and help them deal with theirs.

17

The Search for Meaning and Its Potential for Affecting Growth in Bereaved Parents

MARGARET SHANDOR MILES and
EVA K. BROWN CRANDALL

The loss of a loved one through death is virtually a universal human experience. Few individuals who live a normal life span can escape the experience of losing a close relative or friend. The grief process that characteristically follows such loss is considered one of life's most profound and unique human experiences.[1]

In the past two decades, this process of grief has been examined, studied, and conceptualized by numerous authors from a wide variety of disciplines. The major focus of many of these publications has been on describing the cognitive, behavioral, emotional, and physical manifestations of grief[2-6] and on the evaluation of the outcomes of the grief experience on bereaved individuals.[7-11] For the most part, the grief-outcome studies have examined problematic, negative outcomes in an attempt to isolate variables that may be predictive of negative sequelae of grief, such

Reprinted by permission from *Health Values: Achieving High Level Wellness*, 1983, 7(1), 19–23. Copyright 1983 by Charles B. Slack, Inc.

MARGARET SHANDOR MILES • School of Nursing, University of North Carolina, Chapel Hill, North Carolina 27514. **EVA K. BROWN CRANDALL** • School of Nursing, Washburn University, Topeka, Kansas 66621.

as severe emotional problems, ill health, or early death. Less attention has been paid to the study of potentially positive outcomes that may occur in the bereaved. A number of authors, however, have mentioned the idea that grief, although very painful and difficult to endure, can potentially lead the sufferer to grow and mature as a human being.[1,6,12–17] Koestenbaum, in particular, has noted:

> You do not know what it means to be human, you do not know the essence of your humanity, unless you have opened the window to your nature. And this window is opened only by suffering: pain, death and all the negative experiences of life. This is an ancient truth. . . . Suffering leads to insight, to knowledge about what it really means to *be*.[14] (p. 54)

Because of the unique relationship between parent and child, the death of a child has been identified as one of the most profound human losses. To parents, children represent a part of their own being and their immortality. In addition, the parental role carries with it a deep feeling of responsibility for the physical and emotional well-being of the child. The death of a child, then, sends the bereaved parents into a deep and painful existential "search for meaning."[18–20] This search has been articulated clearly by Frances Gunther in the epilogue to the book *Death Be Not Proud:*

> Death always brings one suddenly face to face with life. Nothing, not even the birth of one's child, brings one so close to life as his death. . . . The impending death of one's child raises many questions in one's mind and heart and soul. It raises all the infinite questions, each answer ending in another question. What is the meaning of life? What are the relations between things: life and death? the individual and the family? the family and society? marriage and divorce? the politics and religion? man, men and God?[21] (p. 250)

In the conceptual model depicting the process of parental grief, developed by one of the authors (Miles),[19,20] this "search for meaning" has been identified as an extremely important aspect of the grief process. Ultimately it may be a key factor in a positive "growth" versus a negative "despair" resolution of the grief experience. To learn more about this search for meaning and the subsequent impact on one's views about life, open-ended data from bereaved parents collected in three separate studies were examined in order to assess both the positive "growth" resolutions and negative "despair" resolutions following the profound experience of losing a child through death. Specifically, the data were examined to determine how the death of a child affected the parents' views about themselves, about others, and about life in general.

Related Literature

Hill, a family systems theorist, in his theoretical treatise about factors affecting families under stress, points out the great importance of the interpretation made by the family about a crisis event. This interpretation, which he defines as "meaning," is based on the family's value system and its previous experiences with crisis. In his view, families with adequate resources may still fail to deal adequately with a crisis because they interpret it negatively rather than positively.[22,23]

Coming from an existential theoretical base, Koestenbaum notes that all individuals must make a fundamental decision regarding the overall view they impose on life. Two choices are apparent: a joyful/optimistic or a despairing/pessimistic view of life. According to Koestenbaum, confronting death, grief, and suffering particularly in one's own life can contribute to a meaning of life that is optimistic.[14] One of the greatest contributors to the existential concept of meaning is Victor Frankl, founder of the movement called *Logotherapy*. In his theoretical framework, emphasis is placed on how an experience of great pain can help us find our deepest meaning and conquer negative attitudes. On the other hand, despair is caused by suffering in which the sufferer sees no meaning. Frankl is not suggesting that one settle back and adjust to a painful loss but that one get in touch with the feelings of outrage and anger and direct them into finding the meaning of one's own existence.[13]

Several authors writing specifically about grief have noted the importance of meaning in the resolution of grief. Marris considers bereavement a process of change that can lead the bereaved into a new sense of purpose about life; he believes that the context of meaning, which helps the bereaved to develop new purposes, must be based on the fundamental structure of meaning developed in childhood. It is through the struggle between one's past identity and conceptualizations about life and the present conflicts engendered by the loss that new viable interpretations about life and its meaning are reformulated.[16] Cassem notes that loss and grief are indispensable to growth. He views bereavement as a continual process experienced throughout life. Cassem sees the ability to integrate misfortune into one's life in a positive, growth-producing manner as a mark of maturity. Thus, prior maturity is probably the best predictor of who can negotiate the bereavement process and grow.[12] Simos in her book on grief, indicates that suffering can be a force in providing life with meaning; however, for life to be tolerable after a loss, there must be an active search for the restoration of this meaning. This is first sought by addressing questions about the cause of death. Later, questions are addressed that attempt to find answers to the existential problem: "Why me? Why him?" Since the answers to these "why" questions may never be adequately answered, the bereaved are faced with the existential choice of how to deal with the resultant suffering.[6] In his studies of survivors of holocaust and disaster, Lifton has noted two patterns of response. One pattern is that of numbing, in which one's personal identity becomes constricted. The other, more positive response, is the struggle for rebirth/transformation, in which new modes of being are sought through a complex process of personal change. This process may involve exploration, experimentation, and risk that is facilitated by support from others and by prior personal strengths.[15]

Schneider has postulated a holistic model of grief that attempts to integrate motivation for growth into the resolution of grief. The last phase, called "transcending the loss," represents the growth of the individual no longer to be bound by the power of what was lost or by attempts to rectify areas of personal vulnerability. Its purpose is to develop the capacity of the individual to extend beyond grief, to new commitments, balance, and wholeness in life.[17] Like Schneider's model, Mile's conceptual model of parental grief includes a phase called the "search for meaning." The search at first involves an attempt to determine why the death occurred. Later, the search becomes deeper and more existential and involves deep profound questions about religion, self, life, and others. "Why me? Why my child? Where was God? How can life go on? What is my life all about?" Meaning may be found in:

1. adherence to religious and philosophical beliefs
2. identification of the uniqueness of the child's life and death
3. memorialization of the child's memory
4. becoming involved in activities that can help individuals and society

The search for meaning is hypothesized to ultimately affect the type of resolution made to the child's death.[19,20] The importance of this search for meaning in bereaved parents is supported by Craig, who suggests that an essential part of the grief work of bereaved parents is the resolution of the meaninglessness of the crisis.[18]

Methods

Since the concept of meaning and its ultimate impact on personal growth, especially within the framework of grief, is still under development, it is difficult to know how it can be measured and studied. Perhaps one method for beginning to evaluate the potential development of meaning and personal growth in the lives of the bereaved is to look at statements made by them about their experience. Information from open-ended questions which asked bereaved parents in various ways to describe themselves were examined in this descriptive analysis seeking clues regarding both positive "growth" resolutions and negative "despair" resolutions to the death of a child. The data were collected in three separate studies, which are part of an ongoing research program on parental bereavement.

Findings

In the first study, 61 bereaved fathers responded to a mailed questionnaire in which they were asked to respond to six open-ended questions about their loss experience. In the last question they were asked to list/discuss anything else about their grief which they wished to share. Twenty-four fathers discussed their changed views about life or their present perspective about how the loss affected them overall. Of these 24 comments, 9 indicated a positive resolution, 9 evidenced a more negative view of life, while the remainer indicated that the father was still attempting to understand his loss or indicated some neutral statement. The positive responses included: learning to prioritize and reorganize my goals; becoming more sensitive and helpful to people who hurt; losing my fear of death; learning to appreciate young people; and realizing the importance of spending more time with my family. Negative responses tended to reflect the ideas that life had stopped; that one will never get over it; and that no good will ever come from the death.

In the second study, completed by Crandall and Miles,[24] 8 bereaved fathers and 30 bereaved mothers were asked to complete a 20-statement questionnaire responding to the phrase "A Bereaved Mother is . . ." or "A Bereaved Father is . . ." In content analysis of the data, one of the major categories that emerged was "bereavement outcomes" which included 29% of the mothers' 457 responses and 26% of the fathers' 105 total responses. The data were further analyzed into subcategories which included both positive and negative outcomes. Positive outcome subcategories included: "cherishing memories"; "feeling more positive about life"; "being more compassionate and more caring of others"; "being more spiritual"; and "feeling stronger." The positive outlook statements accounted for 40% of the responses of mothers and 33% of the responses of fathers that were coded into the "bereavement outcome" category. The negative outcome subcategories included: "not being able to forget or recover" and "being unable to resolve the loss." These accounted for 19% of the responses of the mothers and 22% of the responses of the fathers coded into the "bereavement outcome" category, a substantially smaller percentage of responses than in the positive subcategories. The remainder of the subcategories included statements that indicated that the parent was still seeking answers and working toward recovery.

Specific comments of both mothers and fathers that were coded into the positive subcategory of "changed attitude about

life" included some of the following: grateful, more compassionate, more appreciative, more serious about life, more aware of the
importance of other loved ones, aware of the fragility of life, and
having a greater understanding of life and death. In another
ongoing study of bereaved parents whose children died of chronic disease or sudden accidents, subjects were specifically asked to
comment about their "changed views about life." Of the numerous comments made by the 36 parents, 40 responses indicated a
positive outlook, whereas only 13 responses were negative.
Positive responses included learning to live each day to the fullest;
being more understanding of others who have experienced loss;
feeling more loving toward others; having a stronger faith; being
aware of the preciousness of life; being a better person in general.
Negative responses included having a negative meaningless view
of life; just existing; feeling suicidal and lacking trust.

Discussion

The data presented here must be considered with caution
because of the imprecise, indirect method of measuring meaning
and growth. The parents studied were not directly asked about
their search for meaning or about their potential growth as a
result of their child's death. It was felt that directly asking parents
these questions would bias their responses toward the negative
pole, since bereaved parents are sensitive about the idea that
growth could occur because of their child's death. In addition, the
small convenience sample of parents who agreed to participate in
these studies were, for the most part, members of a self-help
group for bereaved parents. Parents who attend such groups may
be a special group of individuals who differ in important ways
from the general population of bereaved parents. For one thing,
they are parents who are seeking help in their grief, and because
of their attendance at a self-help group they may be more apt to
find meaning and to grow. It should also be pointed out that the
period of time since death was not considered in data analysis and
may be an important factor in the evolution of the "search for
meaning."

Nevertheless, it is interesting to note that so many of the

comments given by these parents indicated that they had found some meaning and had grown in some important ways following the deaths of their children. The most commonly reported growth responses included being more compassionate and caring of others, especially the bereaved; having a stronger faith; and being aware of the preciousness and fragility of life which helped them live each day more fully. Additional clues about the potential for finding "meaning" in life following a child's death can be found in numerous newspaper clippings and magazine articles about bereaved parents who have started self-help groups, such as Compassionate Friends, and community action groups such as Mothers Against Drunken Drivers. Through such activities, these parents are making major contributions to society.

Focusing on the potential for "growth" resolution when a child has died is meant in no way to minimize the deep and long-lasting pain of grief which is experienced when a child has died. Rather, it is meant to point out the importance, as described by Frankl, of channeling the pain and rage into meaningful endeavors which can contribute to recovery and can assist society as well.[13] Finally, research needs to focus more on this process of searching for meaning after the death of a loved one and on its potential for affecting the ultimate outcomes of grief in the bereaved. In addition, clinicians who are counseling the bereaved need to be aware of the importance of helping grieving clients deal with the existential search for meaning in their loss.

References

1. Shneidman, E. *Voices of Death.* New York: Harper & Row, 1980.
2. Balkwell, C. Transition to widowhood: A review of the literature. *Family Relations,* 1981, *30,* 117–127.
3. Clayton, P. J., Halikes, J. A., & Maurice, W. L. The bereavement of the widowed. *Diseases of the Nervous System,* 1971, *32*(9), 597–604.
4. Parkes, C. M. *Bereavement: Studies of grief in adult life.* London: International Universities Press, 1972.
5. Sanders, C. M. Comparison of young and older spouses in bereavement outcomes. *Omega.* 1980–1981, *11*(3), 217–232.
6. Simos, B. G. *A time to grieve: Loss as a universal human experience.* New York: Family Service Association of America, 1979.

7. Clayton, P. J. Mortality and morbidity in the first year of widowhood. *Archives of General Psychiatry*, 1974, *30*, 749–750.
8. Kraus, A. L., & Lilienfield, A. M. Some epidemiological aspects of the high mortality rate in the young widowed group. *Journal of Chronic Diseases*, 1959, *10*, 207–217.
9. Maddison, D., & Walker, W. L. Factors affecting the outcome of conjugal bereavement. *British Journal of Psychiatry*, 1967, *113*, 1057–1067.
10. Parkes, C. M. Determinants of outcome following bereavement. *Omega*, 1975, *6*, 303–323.
11. Young, M., Benjamin, B., & Walis, C. Mortality of widowers. *Lancet*, 1963, *2*, 454–456.
12. Cassem, N. H. Bereavement as indispensable for growth. In B. Schoenberg, I. Gerber, A. Weiner *et al.* (Eds.), *Bereavement: Its psychosocial aspects*. New York: Columbia University Press, 1975.
13. Frankl, V. E. *Man's search for meaning*. New York: Simon & Schuster, 1963.
14. Koestenbaum, P. *Is there an answer to death?* Englewood Cliffs, N.J.: Prentice-Hall, 1976.
15. Lifton, R. J., & Olson, E. *Living and dying*. New York: Praeger Publishers, 1974.
16. Marris, P. *Loss and change*. New York: Pantheon Books, 1974.
17. Frears, L. H., & Schneider, J. M. Exploring grief and loss in a wholistic framework. *Personnel and Guidance Journal*, 1981, *59*(6), 341–345.
18. Craig, Y. The bereavement of parents and their search for meaning. *British Journal of Social Work*, 1977, *7*(1), 41–54.
19. Miles, M. S. *The grief of parents: A model for assessment and intervention*. Paper presented at the Annual Conference, Forum for Death Education and Counseling, Orlando, Florida, 1979.
20. Miles, M. S. Helping adults mourn the death of a child. In H. Wass & C. Corr (Eds.), *Childhood and death*. New York: Hemisphere Publishing Corporation, 1984.
21. Gunther, J. *Death be not proud*. New York: Harper & Row, 1949.
22. Hill, R. Generic features of families under stress. In H. J. Parad (Ed.), *Crisis intervention: Selected readings*. New York: Family Service Association of America, 1965.
23. McCubbin, H. I., Joy, C. B., Cauble, A. E., Comeau, J. K., Patterson, J. M., & Needle, R. H. Family stress and coping: A decade review. *Journal of Marriage and the Family*, 1980, *42*(4), 855–871.
24. Crandall, E. K. B. *Grieving fathers and mothers: Their self-concepts*. Unpublished master's thesis, University of Kansas, 1982.

18

The Amish Way of Death

A Study of Family Support Systems

KATHLEEN B. BRYER

The meaning of death has been a central human concern since the beginning of time. Societal issues change, and with these changes come demands for new approaches to the problems associated with a rapidly changing world. But the basic concern of people throughout history has been the concept of their own mortality. Becker[2] stated that "the fear of death is natural and present in everyone, that it is the basic fear that influences all others, a fear from which no one is immune, no matter how disguised it may be" (p. 15).

To face death is to begin to master life. Familiarity with the face of death brings with it a reordering of the priorities of life, thus granting to death the position of ultimate importance it deserves. Kastenbaum[9] wrote:

> Death is one of the central themes in human development throughout the life span. Death is not just our destination; it is part of our "getting there" as well. Death-relevant thoughts, experiences, and circumstances always accompany us. (p. 43)

This chapter appears in abridged form from *American Psychologist*, 1979, *34*(3), 255–261. Copyright 1979 by the American Psychological Association. Reprinted by permission of the publisher and author.

KATHLEEN B. BRYER • West End Medical Center, Lancaster, Pennsylvania 17603.

The lessening sense of permanence in modern society, exacerbated by the specter of mass annihilation and the pressing problems of the nuclear family, requires new thinking about the meaning of life and death. The crisis caused by the death of a loved one has many parallels with other life crises such as divorce, separation, abandonment, abortion, mobility, and unemployment. In these instances a disruption has occurred in interpersonal relationships, and no longer is there the particular person or situation that has gratified the individual in a special way.

A study of the way of life and death within the traditional society of the Amish presents a rare opportunity for examining their centuries-old method for coping with death. The Amish people see death as a part of the natural rhythm of life, within a religious belief system based on the teachings of the New Testament, which sees the person's relationship to death as one of human temporality and divine eternity. This concept of the transcendental nature of life can take much of the fear out of death and dying. The relational systems within their traditional society provide the Amish people with a sense of *Gemeinschaft*, of community.

Attitudes toward death as found in the Amish society can result in an easier acceptance of death than is often found in the American culture, where contemporary belief systems tend more toward the secular than the transcendental. Uncertainty about a hereafter can produce great anxiety and dread:

> When a society's values and institutions are seriously questioned, life transitions become anxious and traumatic. . . . What does it mean to grow old when old people are isolated . . . apart from family and ongoing community? What does it mean to die when science has challenged sacred religious beliefs and in the place of spiritual comfort has left only the "scientific method"? (p. 26)[12]

Coping with death is becoming increasingly difficult. Steele[14] proposed that in Western society we as individuals and as a culture are left with science to provide the support and guidance on issues of death that ritual and belief once provided. And death, which once occurred mostly in the home, in the presence of the family, now occurs more often in an institutional setting. Kastenbaum[10] saw death interpreted as an event, with the implication that death happens at a particular place. He stated that our response to the time–space dimensions of the death event includes the tendency to contain it within a limited, specifiable framework so that we can feel relatively free of death at other times and in other places.

Today the doctor and the hospital provide the framework for the death event. The orientation of the individual to his or her own death is often left to the individual alone, without the extensive social network on which his or her ancestors could rely. Death has lost the important position that custom had given it. The manner of dying in modern society has become solitary and hidden, one that can put individuals into a frightening isolation that cuts them off from family and friends. As American psychologist Dael Wolfle stated, "We have the curious situation that medical progress has made death more stressful for relatives, more expensive for the family, and more troublesome for society" (quoted by Troup & Greene,[16] p. 4).

According to Aries[1]:

> Common attitudes toward death, such as are being discovered today by sociologists, psychologists and doctors, seem so unprecedented, so bewildering, that as yet it has been impossible for observers to take them out of their modern context and put them into historical perspective. (p. 136)

The Amish Way of Life

The Amish are direct descendants of the Swiss Anabaptists whose members suffered severe persecution for their stand against incorporation into the state churches of Europe during the 1500s. The Amish, named for their leader, Jakob Ammann, are a conservative group who broke away from the Swiss Anabaptists because of doctrinal differences between 1693 and 1697. They accepted William Penn's offer of religious liberty and settled in Pennsylvania at least as early as 1727. At present there are approximately 80,000 Amish living in 20 states in the United States, in Ontario, and in several small settlements in South and Central America (Hostetler, personal communication, January 27, 1977).

The Amish live in a familistic society in which family and community integrity are essential for survival. Because of their commitment to preserving their unique way of life, the Amish people have not had the melting-pot experience in America. Their major cultural patterns include a strong religious orientation, an agrarian life-style, patriarchal authority, distinctive dress and language, separation from the world, and mutual assistance given freely in all times of need. The Amish people take care of their mentally or physically impaired, their aged, their children and adults in need. There is no marital separation or divorce. In some families, there are as many as four generations living in the same household.

Closely aligned with their closeness to the earth is their time orientation:

> Within the bounds of nature they can feel secure. They work with the seasons, not by the hour. The difference between an Amish buggy and a car is not just the horse in front; it can also be seen on the dashboard. In an Amish buggy you may find a calendar; in the car, a clock with the seconds ticking away. (p. 14)[17]

Today they live at the same unhurried pace as that of their ancestors, using horses instead of automobiles, windmills instead of electricity, Pennsylvania-German dialect instead of English, and facing death with the religious tenets and steadfast faith of their forebears.

The function of the Amish family today is little changed from that of centuries ago. The *ars moriendi* of the 15th century specified that people must know of their coming deaths so that they will be able to die well, in a manner that gave death the important position it deserved.[1] The Amish people have retained this emphasis on the importance of death. Hostetler[7] viewed every death in Amish society as a sober occasion of great importance. It is a time for reinforcement, not only of family support systems, but also of the ability of the society to hold itself together.

The Amish Way of Death

The importance that the Amish place on their funeral ceremonies is reflected not only in the familiarity with death but also in an intensified awareness of community. As an Amish man reported in a family interview, "The funeral is not for the one who died, you know; it is for the family."

At the time of death, close neighbors assume the responsibility for notifying others of the death. The bereaved family has only two tasks: first, the appointment of two or three families to take full charge of the funeral arrangements; second, the drawing up of a list of the families who are to be invited to the funeral.

The Amish community takes care of all aspects of the funeral occasion with the exception of the embalming procedure, the coffin, and the horse-drawn wagon. These matters are taken care of by a non-Amish funeral director who provides the type of service that the Amish desire.

The embalmed body is returned to the home within a day of the death. Family members dress the body in white garments in accordance with the Biblical injunction found in Revelation 3:5. For a man, this consists of white trousers, a white shirt, and a white vest. For a woman, the usual clothing is a white cape and apron that were worn by her at both her baptism and her marriage. At baptism a black dress is worn with the white cape and apron; at marriage a purple or blue dress is worn with the white cape and apron. It is only at her death that an Amish woman wears a white dress with the cape and apron that she put away for the occasion of her death. This is an example of the lifelong preparation for death, as sanctioned by Amish society. The wearing of white clothes signifies the high ceremonial emphasis on the death event as the final rite of passage into a new and better life.

Several Amish women stated that making their parents', husbands', or children's funeral garments was a labor of love that represented the last thing they could do for their loved ones. One Amish woman related that each month her aged grandmother carefully washed, starched, and ironed her own funeral clothing so that it would be in readiness for her death. This act appears to have reinforced for herself and her family her lifelong acceptance of death and to have contributed to laying the foundation for effective grief work for herself and her family. This can be seen as an example of the technique of preventive intervention called "anticipatory guidance" (p. 84),[3] which focuses on helping individuals to cope with impending loss through open discussion and problem solving before the actual death.

After the body is dressed, it is placed in a plain wooden coffin that is made to specifications handed down through the centuries. The coffin is placed in a room that has been emptied of all furnishings in order to accommodate the several hundred relatives, friends, and neighbors who will begin arriving as soon as the body is prepared for viewing. The coffin is placed in a central position in the house, both for practical considerations of seating and to underscore the importance of the death ceremonials in Amish society.

The funeral service is held in the barn in the warmer months and in the house during the colder seasons. The service is conducted in German and lasts 1½ hours, with the same order of service for every funeral. The guests view the body when they arrive and again when they leave to take their places in the single-file procession of their carriages to the burial place.

Viewing the coffin again at the cemetery entrance, the guests gather at the grave dug by neighbors the previous day. As all watch silently, the grave is filled with earth. After scripture reading and prayer, followed by a hymn and the Lord's Prayer, the mourners bow their heads in silent prayer. Following the interment, the family and close neighbors return to the home, where a meal has been prepared by the families in charge of arrangements.

Calm acceptance of death, undergirded by a deep religious faith, is an integral part of Amish culture. The anticipation of death lies at the core of much religious activity:

> The inevitable fact of death needs to be reckoned with and accounted for; it has to be explained and included in a wider scheme of representations, a belief system, a religion. . . . J. Bowker argues that religion has failed to disappear because of the great "constraint" of death; the role of religion is to find a way through this limitation to human existence. (p. 1)[6]

In research conducted by Templer[15] on death anxiety, results indicated that those who have a strong attachment to their religious belief system, who are certain of life after death, and who believe in a literal interpretation of the Bible apparently have lower death anxiety. Ray and Najman[13] found that people can accept death and be anxious about it at the same time: "They appear to be simply people who can take a realistic view of death and even see positive aspects of it" (p. 314).

In Amish society, reactions to death are given expression in culturally sanctioned behaviors that are firmly rooted in a belief in life after death for those who remain loyal to the faith. The high visibility and close proximity of the dead are important aspects of the Amish death system; death is real and exerts a powerful influence in this society.

Relational Support Systems

Before Death

The Amish family system, rooted in accountability, operates as an in-house, extended-network system. It is usual to share the care of a family member who is physically or mentally impaired. Going from one household to another for monthly visits within the family, the needy individual can benefit from the fresh supply of interest and patience that is available and freely given.

Experience with death is common in Amish families, with most deaths occurring in the home, in the presence of family members, regardless of length of time needed for care. Most of the families interviewed for this study had experienced taking care of a terminally ill family member, with length of care ranging from several days to 20 years. One Amish woman responded to the question of whether she or her husband had ever taken care of a dying family member by saying, "Oh yes, we had the chance to take care of all four of our old parents before they died. We are both so thankful for this." In their intensive caring they had the opportunity to work through their grief in the anticipation of the death of each parent. In the process, they were moving toward the personal reorganization that is needed in order to return to the tasks of living that follow the death of a loved one.

Kalish[8] cited the British study conducted by Cartwright, Hockey, and Anderson in 1973 regarding family members' care of the dying person. It was found that even though the primary caretakers often became physically and psychologically exhausted during the terminal period, they probably had the least guilt and the fewest feelings of having unfinished business of anyone in the family.

Feifel[4] reported that the terminally ill emphasized the importance of the family more than did a control group of healthy normals; the closer the former individuals felt to personal death, the more important those people and places became that represented psychological security. Lerner[11] stated that three-quarters of the deaths in the United States take place in institutions, despite the fact that most people say they would rather die at home.

In all but three Amish families in the present study, death occurred at home, with ample opportunity to communicate with the dying person about the feelings associated with the impending death, instructions for putting personal affairs in order, and suggestions by the dying person to surviving family members about the importance of preparation for one's own death. An aged widow related that her husband told her as he was dying, "It is better this way; you could better take care of yourself if I die first than I could if you would die first."

Some of the dying persons spoke of death with some distress, according to the interviewed family members: one man stated that his father cried a lot during his last days; another said his sister had difficulty accepting the fact of her death but then began to accept it quietly and calmly within the circle of her family. Those who did not speak directly with dying family members reported that there was generally a quiet acceptance of the coming death that was felt by the family; all stated that this sense of acceptance was a strong factor in their own grief work following the death. In the process of being with their dying loved ones, there was opportunity for emotional expression and working through the anticipatory grief reaction.

At Death

The Amish face death with realism and acceptance; it is seen as an expectable part of a life that is rooted in a primary, face-to-face community. Their customs and rituals of death provide two critical functions: first, they ameliorate the frightening aspects of death by viewing it through a belief in immortality; second, they summon the support of the extended family and the community to provide resources and nurturance for the bereaved.

Even though the Amish emphasize death as a spiritual victory over temporal life, they do not ignore the fact that death is also the separation from loved ones; they are familiar with the profound sense of loss and sadness. Massive support, both physical and psychological, is immediately available. One bereaved father said:

> The thing that meant so much to me was people's caring and wanting to help and support. And the spiritual side, the call on God makes it easier to accept. My upbringing gave me help to straighten myself out; I had nine children to raise.

Another widower, who had four young children at the time of his wife's sudden death, related that his sister came to his house to care for the children until his subsequent marriage to a woman with whom he had five additional children.

When a death occurs under tragic circumstances, it is not unusual for other Amish families who have lost family members under similar circumstances to travel to the home of the grieving family, sometimes from considerable distances. Previously unknown to one another, these families meet to share the same experience with death. Their words of sympathy and support and their presence at the funeral provide a same-experience therapy that can be of great help for the bereaved family and community.

Childhood responses to death affect personality development; conversations with older people about death can make a decided difference in the way a child absorbs experiences with death.[12] Kastenbaum[9] stated that the reality of early insights and the process through which the child moves toward a network of death conceptions have a definite impact on the overall pattern of cognitive and personality development:

> Should death take on the aura of overwhelming catastrophe (something that even big, strong adults cannot cope with or even talk about), then the child may be en route to long-standing problems in thinking about the future in general. (p. 30)

A conversation with two young Amish girls illustrates this concept: two sisters, aged 11 and 13, related in detail their experience 2 years earlier with the death of their beloved grandfather who lived with them in a three-generational household. The girls spoke of their treasured early childhood memories of their grandfather. As he became more feeble and unable to move about the farm, the sisters looked after him and entertained him each day with word games and reading aloud to him. One day the care of the aged man was left to the sisters while the parents visited distant friends. The old man died that morning. The sisters' calm recital of the death experience and their feelings at that time demonstrated their ability to deal with the fact of a loved one's death, in spite of the unusual conditions of the situation.

Lifton and Olson[12] stated:

> A child's concept of death is likely to be charged with fear when earlier death imagery has overwhelmed imagery of life and continuity. Experiences that reinforce imagery of life's connection, movement, and integrity will encourage an attitude of trust and hope. . . . This is very different from having the reality of death kept from him [sic]. (p. 50)

The real power in the Amish way of death is that they do not ignore it, thereby allaying the anxieties created by events they cannot fully understand or control. The reality of the death of the body is firmly impressed on the mind and emotions; this makes it difficult for fantasies to develop in the bereaved. The presence of the body in the home, the repeated viewing, the continuing community support, and the family participation in the actual disposition of the body all serve as constant reminders of the fact of death.

After Death

The role of the extended relational system of the Amish is one of accountability for the needs of the bereaved individual and the family during the long period of psychosocial transition after the funeral. The rate of remarriage following death of a spouse is reported to be one of the highest in any culture, according to Hostetler (personal communication, January 27, 1977). This fact illustrates the strong commitment to repairing the rupture in the family unit at time of death and to responding to the emotional needs of each member of the family.

The high level of support shown the bereaved family is maintained for at least a year following the death. Support is given through increased correspondence, evening and Sunday visiting throughout the year, special scrapbooks and handmade items for the family, new work projects started for a widow, and quilting days that combine fellowship and productivity.

A widow reported that she and 15 other widows maintained a circle letter that made its rounds every 4 months throughout several states. She found this communication a great source of help to her in sharing the special problems of the widow. She also told of an occasion when 60 Amish widows met to discuss common experiences and problems; she said it was one of the best days she had had in recent years, and she looked forward to another occasion like it in the near future.

According to Feifel,[5] normal mourning lasts for at least 1 year after death; he believed that it is essential that community support be available for at least that first year:

> It is plain that we not truncate the grief and mourning process. The dead must die before we are able to redefine and reintegrate ourselves into life. And the greatest gift we can offer to the bereaved is to be with, not treat, them. (p. 9)

Conclusions and Implications

The Amish families interviewed in this study all listed the following conditions as the most helpful aspects of coping with death in their society: (a) the continued presence of the family, both during the course of the illness and at the moment of death; (b) open communication about the process of dying and its impact on the family; (c) the maintenance of a normal life-style by the family during the course of the illness; (d) commitment to as much independence of the dying person as possible; (e) the opportunity to plan and organize one's own death; (f) continued support for the bereaved for at least a year following the funeral, with long-term support given to those who do not remarry.

In Amish society, most individuals can face death confidently, with the assurance that they will be able to live out their days at home, surrounded by loved ones who will help them to plan and organize their own deaths. Their strong religious belief system provides a framework for calm acceptance of the impending death. And in keeping with their concept of death as a natural part of the rhythm of life, the Amish people have a deep sense of continuity across the generations; they know that their families will receive massive support from the community when they die.

References

1. Aries, P. The reversal of death: Changes in attitudes toward death in western societies. In D. Stannard (Ed.), *Death in America*. Philadelphia: University of Pennsylvania Press, 1975.
2. Becker, E. *The denial of death*. New York: Free Press, 1973.
3. Caplan, G. *Principles of preventive psychiatry*. New York: Basic Books, 1964.
4. Feifel, H. Perception of death. *Annals of the New York Academy of Sciences,* 1969, *164,* 669–677.
5. Feifel, H. *New meanings of death*. New York: McGraw-Hill, 1977.
6. Goody, J. Death and the interpretation of culture: A bibliographic overview. In D. Stannard (Ed.), *Death in America*. Philadelphia: University of Pennsylvania Press, 1975.
7. Hostetler, J. A. *Amish society*. Baltimore, Md.: Johns Hopkins Press, 1963.
8. Kalish, R. A. Dying and preparing for death: A view of families. In H. Feifel (Ed.), *New meanings of death*. New York: McGraw-Hill, 1977.
9. Kastenbaum, R. Death and development through the lifespan. In H. Feifel (Ed.), *New meanings of death*. New York: McGraw-Hill, 1977.
10. Kastenbaum, R. *Death, society, and human experience*. St. Louis, Mo.: Mosby, 1977.
11. Lerner, M. When, why and where people die. In O. Brim (Ed.), *The dying patient*. New York: Russell Sage Foundation, 1970.
12. Lifton, R. J., & Olson, E. *Living and dying*. New York: Praeger, 1974.
13. Ray, J. J., & Najman, J. Death anxiety and death acceptance: A preliminary approach. *Omega,* 1974, *5,* 311–315.
14. Steele, R. L. Dying, death, and bereavement among the Maya Indians of Mesoamerica: A study in anthropological psychology. *American Psychologist,* 1977, *32,* 1060–1068.
15. Templer, D. I. Death anxiety in religiously very involved persons. In *Death anxiety*. New York: Mss Information Corporation, 1973.
16. Troup, S. B., & Greene, W. A. (Eds.). *The patient, death, and the family*. New York: Scribner's, 1974.
17. Zielinski, J. *The Amish: A pioneer heritage*. Des Moines, Iowa: Wallace-Homestead, 1975.

VIII

Coping with Unusual Crises
Special Family Stressors

Many ordinary families face extraordinary problems, such as the physical or mental illness of a family member, family violence or incest, legal troubles, or forced migration to another country. These special challenges magnify the issues raised by normally expected life transitions. Families who experience such stressors face the tasks of maintaining open communication in emotion-laden situations, developing ways of meeting the competing needs of different family members, coping with role changes, handling the stigma associated with many of these situations, and seeking support to supplement limited family resources.

One common family stressor is the serious physical illness or injury of a spouse or child, such as the sudden quadriplegia that may follow a severe car accident or the gradual decline that occurs among children with muscular dystrophy or older adults with a chronic brain disease. The family members of these patients face several complex tasks. They must help their loved ones control their symptoms and try to prevent new medical crises, assist in carrying out special treatment procedures (such as home dialysis for end-stage kidney failure), and form adequate relationships with health-care professionals. They need to maintain a sense of inner mastery of their divergent feelings and try to preserve a satisfactory self-image, for example, by helping their ill spouse or child as much as possible but not feeling overwhelmed by guilt when they cannot do everything he or she asks. Moreover, they must conserve family resources and their relationship with the ill family member and try to sustain hope in the face of an often uncertain prognosis. (For an extended discussion of these issues, see the companion volume on coping with physical illness.[7])

The interdependence and powerful emotional ties that bind family members together make it especially hard to cope with behavioral problems such as battering, incest, or the presence of an alcoholic or mentally ill spouse. In comparison to a physical illness, these behavioral problems may be more encompassing and raise more difficult issues, such as the extent to which the individual is to blame for his or her aberrant behavior, how much other family members are at fault, and the need to take sides in situations where supporting one person may risk irretrievable harm to another. When a wife learns of an incestuous relationship between her husband and daughter she may be torn by "divided loyalty," wanting to support her daughter and yet fearing the loss of her husband. In turn, the sexually abused girl may keep her torment secret out of fear of punishment or in order to protect her father and maintain family unity. Years later, victims may try to make sense of their experience, examine the character and motives of their father, or consider such family circumstances as the death of their mother or lack of sexual relations between their parents.[9]

Often family members keep problems "within the family" and seek their own solutions. Alcoholism is a problem that family members frequently try to handle on their own. In the first article, Jacqueline Wiseman describes strategies wives use to "treat" their husband's problem drinking. Initially, wives believe their husbands' drinking is voluntary, and so they use logical arguments to persuade them to drink less. When gentle urging to cut down on drinking fails, a wife may intensify her efforts and try to convince her husband that drinking will ruin his health or cause him to lose his job. When this strategy does not work, disappointed wives step up their efforts and nag their husbands. Next, wives may resort to pleading and threaten to leave, but their husbands often respond angrily to such pressure and do not take the threat of separation seriously.

When these approaches fail, wives shift to indirect strategies that involve manipulating the environment so their husbands will have less desire or opportunity to drink. One strategy is acting "normal." A wife may pretend her husband has no drinking problem and converse with him or cook and clean as if he is not drunk. Some wives also engage in a "taking-over" strategy. They manage demanding tasks that might upset their husbands and try to be better wives in the hope that this will free their husbands of burdens and cause them to drink less. Wives also choose nondrinking companions for their husbands, limit the money available to them, and keep their husbands busy so they will not have time to drink. These coping strategies may be effective in some situations, but they did not work for the women Wiseman studied. Many of these women gave up the "home treatment" and sought professional help. (For an account of an alcoholic woman's struggle to recover, see Meryman.[6])

The personal and social resources of family members have a significant impact on their ability to cope with family problems. Spouses of alcoholics tend to function more effectively when they experience fewer life stressors, are located in more cohesive and expressive families, and are less likely to use avoidance coping strategies.[8] Abused wives with an education, employment skills, and helpful relatives manage to get out of their marriage quickly—an option that may not be available to women who have few resources and are dependent on their husbands. (For some illuminating interviews with battered women, see Giles-Sims.[3]) Also, women whose husbands are imprisoned cope more successfully with this long-term stressor if they are better educated, enjoy higher social status, come from cohesive families with an egalitarian division of labor, and have more family and personal resources.[5]

Relocation is another common stressor for modern families. Whether families move because of a job transfer or in search of a better life, all face a loss of their familiar environment and a disruption in their social relationships. However, if individuals are able to cope successfully with these losses, relocation can ultimately be a positive experience. For example, Jeanne Brett[1] found that although mobile husbands and wives are less satisfied with their social relationships, perhaps reflecting the loss of old friends and the problem of finding new ones, they are more satisfied with their marriages and family life than stable couples. She notes that the challenge of moving and setting up a new household may increase feelings of competence and bring families closer together because they must rely on each other for support until they can find new friends.

The adjustments required of immigrants and refugees are much more dramatic than those experienced by families who relocate within a country. Immigrant and refugee families need to relinquish their attachment to their country of origin, invest emotionally in their new country, and build a "psychological bridge" between their present life and the past. In the early postmigration period, immigrants must mourn the loss of friends, language, social norms, and culture. In addition, they face the practical tasks of finding a house, transportation, and a job—tasks that may be especially hard for certain groups such as rural Vietnamese refugees who do not have the skills to cope with modern Western society.[4] Immigrants also need to overcome the problems associated with not knowing the language of their host country. The inability to clearly express their thoughts and communicate their needs makes it hard for immigrants to develop close relationships with people in the host country and contributes to their sense of isolation and low self-esteem.

In the second article, Carlos Sluzki describes five stages of family migration, different types of family coping mechanisms, and the conflicts and symptoms that may occur when families relocate. The first step in the migration process is the preparatory stage—when the family makes a commitment to migrate. There may be euphoria after the decision is made but also a sense of feeling overloaded and dismayed at the prospect of the move. Step 2 is the act of migration. Step 3, the period of overcompensation, occurs in the early weeks and months after the move when the family focuses primarily on meeting its basic needs. Many immigrants try to block out the dissonance in their new culture and make little or no effort to acculturate. The fourth step, decompensation and crisis, occurs after about 6 months. Conflicts and symptoms arise as the family tries to adjust to the new country. The family needs to strike a balance between maintaining traditional values and beliefs that are necessary to their identity and modifying those that conflict with the new culture. Conflicts can flare up when children adapt more readily to the new culture's language and perspectives than their parents or when family structure and roles are challenged, such as when a wife finds a job before her husband. Step 5, the transgenerational impact, concerns the conflict of values that may occur when issues that were not dealt with by the first generation arise in the second. This is especially likely when immigrant parents live in an ethnically homogeneous area that shelters them from the new culture, whereas their children are exposed to divergent values in school and the media.

Coping strategies of specific groups of immigrants reflect their unique problems. A major problem for Latin American women is worry about children who have been left behind in the care of maternal kin until they can bring them to the United States. Parents may cope with concerns about their absent children by "not thinking too much" about the problems of family members who have remained behind. Latinos' beliefs in self-sacrifice for their children and loved ones help them face demanding work conditions.[2]

Refugees who are forced from their country by poverty, oppression, and war often experience multiple losses, and unlike other immigrants are unable to plan ahead. For example, many Vietnamese had only a few days to prepare before fleeing their country. They faced the sudden loss of family members, property, careers, businesses, social attachments, social status, and their culture. Once in this country, single men formed pseudofamilies as support systems to substitute for the families they left behind. Work provided a way of avoiding homesickness and tension and enabled the refugees to improve their social and economic status. Another strategy involved placing hope in the future generation. Refugees took pride in their children's educational accomplishments. Finally, the refugees coped by taking a fatalistic approach to life. The best adapted Vietnamese refugees came from well-functioning families, experienced the fewest social and economic losses, were somewhat familiar with modern Western culture, and were able to find social support.[4]

Adaptation to relocation is a gradual, long-term process. This process may be facilitated if, as Carlos E. Sluzki suggests, immigrant families are able to learn their new country's language and get information about its customs before they move and if they can maintain contact with people from their country of origin and have brought with them meaningful objects from their country to make them feel at home in their new life.

References

1. Brett, J. M. Job transfer and well-being. *Journal of Applied Psychology*, 1982, *67*, 450–463.
2. Cohen, L. M. Stress and coping among Latin American women immigrants. In G. V. Coelho & P. I. Ahmed (Eds.), *Uprooting and development: Dilemmas of coping with modernization.* New York: Plenum Press, 1980.
3. Giles-Sims, J. *Wife battering: A systems theory approach.* New York: Guilford Press, 1983.
4. Lin, K., Masuda, M., & Tazuma, L. Adaptational problems of Vietnamese refugees. Part III. Case studies in clinic and field: Adaptive and maladaptive. *Psychiatric Journal of the University of Ottawa*, 1982, *7*, 73–183.
5. Lowenstein, A. Coping with stress: The case of prisoners' wives. *Journal of Marriage and the Family*, 1984, *46*, 699–708.
6. Meryman, R. *Broken promises, mended dreams.* Boston: Little, Brown, 1984.
7. Moos, R. (Ed.). *Coping with physical illness: New perspectives.* New York: Plenum Press, 1984.
8. Moos, R., Finney, J., & Gamble, W. The process of recovery from alcoholism. II. Comparing spouses of alcoholic patients and matched community controls. *Journal of Studies on Alcohol*, 1982, *43*, 888–909.
9. Silver, R., Boon, C., & Stones, M. Searching for meaning in misfortune: Making sense of incest. *Journal of Social Issues*, 1980, *42*, 855–871.

19

The 'Home Treatment'

The First Steps in Trying to Cope with an Alcoholic Husband

JACQUELINE P. WISEMAN

It is now recognized that alcohol addiction generates problems that extend beyond the heavy drinker to the family and particularly the spouse. Yet for several decades, when the spouse (and especially the wife) was the focus of research, primary emphasis was on her as an unwitting causal agent in her husband's problem drinking, due to the presumed presence of "pathological" personality traits such as dominance, dependency, or sadomasochism. More recently, Steinglass and others[11,16–18] have taken a functionalist, systems approach and attempted to show that the wife is a part of a family "system" that may help maintain the husband's problem drinking. Where the focus has been on the coping behavior of wives of alcoholics, investigators have been concerned with their management of the problem over a considerable time span of their husband's drinking career and do not detail early attempts to get their husbands to stop or cut down.[4–8,10] This

This chapter appears in abridged form from *Family Relations*, 1980, *29*, 541–549. Copyright 1980 by the National Council of Family Relations, Fairview Community School Center, 1901 West County Road B, Suite 147, St. Paul, Minnesota 55113. Reprinted by permission.

JACQUELINE P. WISEMAN • Department of Sociology, University of California-San Diego, La Jolla, California 92093.

effort to fit the wife into the etiology of alcoholism, or condense her attempts to cope with a husband's long drinking career into major stages, has resulted in ignoring what might be the first line of defense in the battle with a man's compulsive drinking behavior—the wife's early intervention efforts.

This chapter contains a delineation of the many aspects of what will be referred to as the "home treatment" attempted by wives of alcoholic men as they try to handle their husbands' problem drinking in the privacy of their homes when they first become aware that he may be an alcoholic. Like the proverbial iceberg below the surface, there exists a career of amateur therapy by the wife of an alcoholic which is enacted long before her drinking husband comes to the attention of professionals in the field.

Shibutani[15] has pointed out that all acts, even coping ones, depend on how the individual actor defines the situation and how he or she defines and symbolizes the meaning of any attempt at amelioration and the counterreactions these inspire. In the course of such definitions, the social actor takes into account how others feel about the action, and then moves tentatively toward it, "building it up" piece by piece, checking and rechecking the usefulness of the decision. Reports on the hidden drama of the home treatment indicate that maneuvers by the wife reflect her understanding of the nature of alcoholism, her adjustments to the reactions of her husband to reform attempts, and her changing perception of their relationship and her subordinate status vis-à-vis her spouse. Furthermore, there appears to be an *approximate* time order to the methods that are tried.

Wives of alcoholics who attempt to cope alone with the heavy drinking of their spouses find themselves in dual and somewhat contradictory roles: both therapist and close kin. Like the professional therapist, the wife searches for ways to help her husband with what she perceives to be a serious problem affecting both him and the entire family. Like many cases that therapists handle, the husband–client seldom admits he drinks too much. Again, like the professional, the wife gropes for ways of helping her "patient" in the face of his denial and even hostility to her efforts.

However, unlike the professional, the wife usually has an established and close relationship with the patient that existed *prior* to her attempts to help him stop his drinking. This has both advantages and disadvantages. Although this relationship may give the wife an edge over the professional in empathetic understanding, she is often, unlike the professional, the person with the *least power* in the dyad. This is quite the opposite from the professional relationship, where the therapist is seen to be of higher (or dominant) status in the role relationship with his client due to his acknowledged expertise.

Without this advantage, the wife of the alcoholic is forced to use approaches to her husband's problem drinking that do not depend on role power based on authority of knowledge and training. Thus, the stage is set for strategic interaction, since it is lack of power that is usually the genesis of inferior role position strategies. Yet, as will be seen, the approaches wives develop through trial and error bear a striking resemblance to some professional therapeutic stances.

Methodology

Seventy-six wives of alcoholics were interviewed in depth and also answered a five-page structured questionnaire concerned with pertinent background data. Wives were asked to discuss how they decided their husbands were alcoholics, what they did after they decided this, what persuaded them to try to get their husbands into professional treatment, how they handled this matter, their experiences (and their husbands') with professional treatment, and what effects the alcoholism of the husband had on their marital relationship and their lives in general.

Wives were recruited through an advertisement placed in newspapers in the city selected for the study. This approach is preferred over recruiting through Al-Anon because the latter offers a distinct philosophy of life to wives of problem drinkers, a fact which could confound the findings. Thus, Al-Anon members were interviewed only as they surfaced through advertisements.

The wife's word that her husband is an alcoholic was accepted because there was no way to check back with the husband inasmuch as many women came in secret to be interviewed. However, there were reassuring indicators that the husbands who were discussed by their wives were indeed alcoholics: first, all had undergone some sort of treatment for their alcohol problem at least twice; additionally, the consistencies in the behavior of the husbands, as described by the wives, lend credence to the belief that a uniform population (in terms of the existence of problem drinking) was being tapped.

The Home Treatment

Wives of alcoholics were asked, "When you first decided that your husband was an alcoholic, what did you do? What did you do next? What did you do after that? Then, what did you do?" The aggregate behaviors reported had a time order—that is, almost all wives tried the same first approach to the problem of their husbands' alcoholism, and almost all adjusted their approaches to a series of failures in the same ways. However, many of these wives were offering retrospective data that span 10 to 25 years of marriage. Some have said that they tried one thing and then another, and then they would go back and try the entire repertoire again. Thus, the exact order of home treatment attempts cannot be known, although it would appear that the time order presented here is at least indicative of the general progression of events.

The Direct Approach

At the outset, the wife saw her task as providing logical reasons to her husband for quitting his heavy drinking—arguments so persuasive that they outweigh any motives her husband may have for continuing. Although the wife probably had been told that alcoholism is a "disease," at this point she still believed her husband's drinking was voluntary. Thus, she initially proceeded on the theory that the use of alcohol can be halted or reduced if the drinker is persuaded of the necessity to do so.

Logical Persuasion and Its Fate.   When wives tried to "talk things over" with their husbands, most started out rather low key, affecting a casual attitude while still making their concern clear.

Usually, when we are alone, I tell him, "You gonna start to drink again, you better be careful." But I would not nag him. I'd say, "You're drinking

*again; you better be careful or you'll end up in trouble." Usually he says,
"No, I won't, Babe."*
   *[I'd say] "John, do you have to drink that much? Now is it really
necessary?"*

As can be seen, the early approach centers on suggestions for
more moderate drinking, rather than stopping altogether. The
responses by the men were, however, primarily defensive.

*I'm taking care of myself. I'm not drinking so much now. Don't worry.
I'm not drinking too much. It's your imagination.*

When convinced that a gentle nudge toward cutting down on
alcohol intake is not going to work, wives escalated to "presenting
a case." Their arguments usually had three major foci:

1. The husband had better start realizing that he has a real
   drinking problem, and his drinking has gotten out-of-
   hand.
2. His drinking is adversely affecting other areas of his life
   and relationships with others.
3. His drinking, if continued, will ruin his health.

Sample comments from wife-respondents were:

I told him that if he kept drinking, he'd be out of a job.
   *I tried to show him what was bothering me. The fact that we didn't have
any money; the car; he has ulcers also . . . the fact that he was always
complaining about a headache, his stomach and everything.*

Wives reported that the reaction of some husbands to these
stronger arguments remain mild, and even become conciliatory as
they offer agreement and promises to cut down their drinking.
However, these promises rarely were kept for long.

*He was very intelligent, and he would always agree. Then he would really
get drunk and get a big hangover and say, "That is it. You are right, honey,
no more." I live in hope until the next time (he starts drinking again).*

Nagging—Wives Escalate Their Campaign. If social bonds,
especially those in the marriage relationship, are based on shared
meanings, reciprocity, and trust, then it is not surprising that a

great deal of strain was felt by the wife as she experienced the
disappointment of a succession of such broken promises and that
she moved from logical discussion to nagging.

> *I felt let down, you know. Somebody didn't keep their end of the bargain.*
> *Now I just don't believe him, and tell him so.*
> *I'd be a screaming, nagging bitch, that's what I've become.*

Husbands did not react to a wife's nagging and quarreling
with the same equanimity they showed when she attempted logical persuasion. A frequent reaction was to suggest to the wife that
she was driving him to drink by her continual complaining.

> *Well, he said I was nasty when he drank, so this is why he drank. Who wants*
> *to come home to a nasty woman? I admit I did start to get nasty.*

It is at this juncture that men used countercriticism to end the
nagging *and* to explain their drinking.

> *Once he said, "You're too fat. Stop eating and I'll stop drinking."*

The preceding strategy placed the wife in a no-win position.
Logical discussion and sweet reasonableness do not result in any
long-term reform. When she became more forceful, he began to
blame her for his excessive drinking. In despair and desperation,
these women turned to a persuasive strategy used by many wom-
en in other situations—emotional pleading and threatening.[13]

Emotional Pleading and Threats to Leave.   Wives' descriptions of how they acted when they became too emotional to continue to discuss their husbands' drinking dispassionately indicated
they still believed that their spouses could stop drinking if they
wished. Wives also hoped their husbands' love would cause these
men to cease their excessive alcohol intake in order to end her
unhappiness.

> *I begged him. I pleaded, I cried. I was very emotional and I cried and said*
> *that if [he] loved me, he wouldn't do this to me and the children.*

Husbands who were constrained when their wives raised the
subject of their heavy drinking calmly and who limited themselves

to countercharges when wives made accusations produced some defensive escalation[14] and exhibited anger when approached by an emotion-wrought wife.

He said, "Well, you go your way and I'll go mine. I am not an alcoholic."

With talk on all levels failing, but still holding to the belief that their husbands could voluntarily stop their drinking, wives of alcoholics often turned next to threats of separation or divorce. The purpose, however, was to hasten reform and ultimately to salvage the marriage. These women hoped *not* to have to carry through on their threat.

At that time, I threatened: "You either stop or I will leave." I guess that when I said I would leave him, I hoped that it would sort of, you know, make him realize.

Husbands responded to these threats primarily with cavalier disinterest, although remorseful promises (such as they made in response to tearful pleas) were sometimes forthcoming. These drinking husbands appeared to be guessing that there was a lack of real seriousness in the threat. They may have known that it is economically very difficult for the average wife to manage such a move on her own—especially if small children are involved. They also may have counted on their wives lacking the courage for such a drastic action. Women, themselves, admitted these problems. They said:

The threats I used to use on him would roll off his back and he would say, "Well, maybe you're right, maybe we should give up and quit and get a divorce."

James and Goldman[8] and Estes[2] have noted that wives of alcoholics often develop an entire repertoire of coping styles for living with an alcoholic. As one fails to produce the desired results, another is tried. The findings of this study—more narrowly focused on the early period of trying to get alcoholic husbands to stop drinking excessively—substantiate these two reports. Starting with the direct approach, wives passed through logical discussion, emotional pleading, nagging, and threats, and then often go back to some one of these methods in the hope that they would yet be effective. It is at this juncture of failing several times at various direct approaches that wives began to develop indirect moves— strategies they hoped would help the husband cut down on his drinking *without his being aware of the fact the wife was trying to change his behavior.*

The Indirect Approach

The development of hidden antidrinking strategies signals a turning point in the wife's view of alcoholism and her power to do anything about it. She no longer sees excessive drinking as so completely voluntary and is beginning to consider the possibility that his drinking is a compulsion.

Her assessment of their relationship changes as well. She has learned that he will not stop drinking just for her sake, nor does he show concern at the ritual threat of separation. Because of this, she often feels a loss of closeness with her husband. At the same time, she may also experience feelings of being more aware than her husband of the danger he is in. Using a type of reasoning that is startlingly like that of professional therapists, wives try out a range of behind-the-scenes manipulative approaches to managing the husband's environment in such a way that he either has less desire or less opportunity to drink.

Acting "Normal" or "Natural". One indirect approach is not unlike the so-called therapeutic milieu that enjoyed popularity in treating mental illness in the 1960s.[12] The essence of the method is that professional therapists construct the environment of the alcoholic in such a way that he will experience less stress and have a reduced desire to drink. The wife, lacking the resources of an institution, must therefore create the nonstressful environment within her limited sphere of power and competence.

The wifely version of the therapeutic milieu is what wives referred to as acting "normal" or "natural." The wife stopped trying to persuade her husband to stop his heavy drinking. Instead, she pretended the drinking or the drunken behavior was not occurring. Often the wife will try this method after deciding that the daily hassle of the direct confrontation was useless, as well as being hard on her emotions. It should be stressed, however, that "acting normal or natural" was more than just resignation. It was a mode of "reasonable" behavior that wives assumed in reaction to their husbands' drinking; it was intended to elicit the same type of "reasonable" behavior in return.

I acted a lot of ways when he was drunk. Inside, I acted like, "Let's pretend it is not happening." Now, I try to act like a normal person (like he thought I was abnormal) because I thought if I acted normal in some way, that he would act normal.

A major setting for these attempts to act natural was the home at the end of the day when the husband returned quite obviously drunk. The wife then tried to act like she thought she would act if her spouse were sober.

[When he came home] I just talked to him like I'm talking to you. I just pretend like nothing is wrong. Sometimes it would work, and other times he would keep at me 'til I got mad.

In an effort to reduce such strain, wives of alcoholics used props and activities to aid in acting natural. Often they went on a self-conscious and feverish round of cleaning and cooking activities when their husbands came home drunk, for it is easier to play-act at "naturalness" if one has some concrete routine involving behavior that will take up excess nervous energy.

[I act normal by] being in the garage washing, in the den, or finding something to do—nervous energy. I am so busy with things that I don't even pass the kitchen to see what he is doing.

Goffman[3] discussed the strains that develop in the family of a deviant (in this case, a mentally ill member) when loved ones try to help him, and keep him from harming himself, while at the same time working hard at appearing "normal" so that such surveillance is not noticed. The problematic person also notices the forced normalcy but pretends to be unaware of being watched. Thus, the interaction becomes stilted, and the home becomes "an insane place."

Taking Over. A touching extension to acting natural is added by the wives who actively attempted to make all facets of the home and marriage better for their husbands by taking over anything that might put demands on their mates or upset them. In addition to trying to be better wives and housekeepers, such women took care of more details of running the house and other areas of life. Their hope was that an extremely pleasant, burden-free atmosphere would reduce their husband's need for liquor. It is quite possible that this coping approach is the foundation for the traits of "dominance" and "desiring a dependent marriage partner" that were earlier ascribed to the wife of an alcoholic by psychiatrists and social workers.

> *I do all the shopping. I take him to work and bring him home, pick him up from work, and I pay the bills and, you know, things like that. Well, I thought it would help him, that I could, you know, help with some of the responsibilities. I thought maybe he could have been tired—they need a drink to relax. I thought that might be the problem.*

Another indirect strategy involved selecting "safe," nondrinking companions or visitors for social occasions.

> *I tried getting us involved with people that didn't drink as much as we did, but he found them very dull.*
> *If he would say, "I am going to go out for a little while," I'd say, "Take Mike with you." He is 5 years old. I figure if he [the husband] has the child with him, he would not go to the pub.*

Wives also tried to manipulate the money available to their husbands for alcohol. Those wives who had direct access to the family money and got the paycheck first hid the checkbook or hid extra money. Wives who found it difficult to physically withhold or hide money, however, took a more indirect course and often attempted to spend so much that there was little or no money left for alcohol.

Neither approach was successful in preventing most husbands from getting money to buy alcohol. Desperation finally drove the wife of an alcoholic at one time or another to try and curtail the supply of liquor available in the home. They poured out liquor, smashed bottles wherever they found them, or hid the liquor supply from their husbands. This direct and time-worn strategy is more histrionic than really helpful to finding a solution for the problem.

Industrial Therapy.   Quite often part of the therapeutic milieu in the mental hospital or institutional setting is what has been termed "industrial therapy."[1,19] This "I.T." refers to routine work around the ward, which is assigned to patients in an attempt to keep them out of trouble, taking up free time with a "useful pursuit." A variation of this approach has been invented by wives of alcoholics, who exhibit great versatility in the creation of tasks and a subtlety of task management. Because their rather special form of industrial therapy grew out of their subordinate position in the marriage dyad, however, wives attempted to increase the number of activities where their husbands usually and voluntarily drink less. By this strategy, women reduced their spouses' intake without creating an awareness of manipulation.

> *I try to keep him busy. I bought paintings for him . . . You know, those paint-by-the-numbers things.*
>
> *I tried to interest him in reading, but that didn't work. [I tried] gardening. . . . We did a lot of gardening together. We planned out our landscaping and, of course, the house which I thought was the final, ultimate. . . . Eventually, I had to subcontract practically everything, because he just could not grasp hold of it . . . it didn't work.*

Drinking Along with Him.   With some vague intent of forcing him to "share the supply," or "showing him," or "letting him see what it is like to be living with an alcoholic," or forcing him to "cut down in order to be a better example to her," some wives turned to a dangerous and dramatic strategy—they tried to drink as much as the men did. Most wives found this an impossible task; they usually were unable to match their alcoholic spouses drink for drink. Either they became ill and passed out, or they retreated from the approach upon becoming frightened that they themselves might be developing a serious drinking problem.

Other wives reasoned that if a husband's drinking could be restricted to the home, he would drink less. To get him to drink at home, they start drinking with him, trying to create a party atmosphere that would be competitive with the inviting social milieu of the bars he frequented. But, as with "use-the-supply" and "fighting-fire-with-fire" approaches, most wives found the "home party" strategy failed because they couldn't match their husband's intake stamina.

It was great [drinking with him at home], but then after two or three drinks, I had enough and I was ready to go to bed. By then he was so happy . . . he'd want me to sit with him 'till three o'clock, and if I refused, and say, "I have to go to work, I don't want to drink more," then, well, he'd go out. So you see, there was no way of stopping him.

Miscellaneous Indirect Strategies. In their desperation to turn back the tide of their husbands' increasingly heavy drinking, wives also tried a variety of other strategies—all covert in nature and some reflecting what stress can do to a person's powers of reasoning.

I tried behavior modification. The biggest behavior mod I've done is definitely withhold sex.

I remembered he loved his boots, and I thought somehow, if I do something to these boots so he can't wear them to go out drinking, then he won't go; [so] I hid them.

The "Hands-Off" Approach

After extensive efforts at various aspects of home treatment, wives began to feel (sometimes through counseling or at Al-Anon) that they personally could do little about their husbands' drinking. McNamara[9] has pointed out that for many wives, this is a relief.

I figure after trying everything out, I figure let me leave him alone. It will either kill him or cure him, or something, but let him do it on his own. I cannot fight him. I fight, I get less results, so I figure let me let it be.

After allowing the problem to lie fallow for a time, however, the wife finally turned to professional help for her husband. She realized at last her inability to do anything to help him. This awareness signals a greater acceptance of the illness theory of problem drinking, as well as a definite end to any hope of handling the problem within the family. The home treatment was terminated. Coping began to focus on how to adjust to an alcoholic in the family. Parenthetically, contact with alcoholism treatment professionals, initially on behalf of her husband, may eventually result in the wife arranging for counseling for herself.

References

1. Belknap, L. *Human problems in a state mental hospital.* New York: McGraw-Hill, 1956.
2. Estes, N. J. Counseling the wife of an alcoholic spouse. *American Journal of Nursing,* 1974, *74,* 1251–1255.
3. Goffman, E. Insanity of place. *Psychiatry,* 1968, *32,* 357–388.
4. Jackson, J. K. The adjustment of the family to the crisis of alcoholism. *Quarterly Journal of Studies on Alcohol,* 1954, *4,* 562–586.
5. Jackson, J. K. The adjustment of the family to alcoholism. *Journal of Marriage and the Family,* 1956, *18,* 361–369.
6. Jackson, J. K. Family structure and alcoholism. *Mental Hygiene,* 1959, *43,* 403–406.
7. Jackson, J. K. Alcoholism and the family. In D. J. Pittman & C. R. Snyder (Eds.), *Society, culture, and drinking patterns.* New York: Wiley, 1962.
8. James, J. E., & Goldman, M. Behavior trends of wives of alcoholics. *Quarterly Journal of Studies on Alcohol,* 1971, *32,* 373–381.
9. McNamara, J. H. The disease conception of alcoholism: Its therapeutic value for the alcoholic and his wife. *Social Casework,* 1960, *41,* 460–465.
10. Orford, J. F., & Guthrie, S. Coping behavior used by wives of alcoholics: A preliminary investigation. *International Congress of Alcohol and Alcoholism, Proceedings,* 1968, *1,* 97.
11. Paredes, A. Marital-sexual factors in alcoholism. *Medical Aspects of Human Sexuality,* 1973, *7,* 98–115.
12. Rapoport, R. N. *Community as doctor: New perspectives on a therapeutic community.* London: Tavistock, 1959.
13. Safilios-Rothschild, C. Patterns of familial power and influence. *Sociological Focus,* 1969, *2,* 7–19.
14. Schelling, T. C. *The strategy of conflict.* New York: Oxford University Press, 1963.
15. Shibutani, T. *Society and personality.* Englewood Cliffs, N.J.: Prentice-Hall, 1961.
16. Steinglass, P. Experimenting with family treatment approaches to alcoholism, 1950–1975: A review. *Family Process,* 1976, *15,* 97–123.
17. Steinglass, P., & Moyer, J. K. Assessing alcohol use in family life: A necessary but neglected area for clinical research. *The Family Coordinator,* 1977, *26,* 53–60.
18. Steinglass, P., Weiner, S., & Mendelson, J. H. A systems approach to alcoholism: A model and its clinical application. *Archives of General Psychiatry,* 1971, *24,* 401–408.
19. Wiseman, J. P. *Stations of the lost: The treatment of skid row alcoholics.* Englewood Cliffs, N.J.: Prentice-Hall, 1970.

20

Migration and Family Conflict

CARLOS E. SLUZKI

Millions of people migrate each year. They do it alone or in organized aggregates, by their own decision or forced by decisions of
others or by natural cataclysms, carrying with them truckloads of
household items or a bundle of essentials. They travel on a luxury
ocean liner or crammed in the *bodega* of a *sampan,* are received
with press conferences, or sneak in under barbed-wire borders by
night. They look forward with hope or backward with fear. They
belong to a culture in which high geographic mobility is the rule
and count on skills to deal with the process of migration, or they
have been raised in a highly sedentary culture in which uprooting
means near catastrophe. They are thoroughly familiar with, or
completely ignorant of, their situation on arrival, the language
and customs of the new place, the people, the dwelling situation,
the work they are going to have. One way or another, countless
numbers of people manage to break away from their basic support networks, sever ties with places and people, and transplant
their home base, their nest, their life projects, their dreams, their
ghosts.

There is a unique drama that characterizes migration in each

This chapter appears in abridged form from *Family Process,* 1979, *18,* 379–388.
Copyright 1979 by Family Process, Inc. Reprinted by permission.

CARLOS E. SLUZKI • Department of Psychiatry, Berkshire Medical Center, Pittsfield,
Massachusetts 01201.

case. In fact, this drama often becomes a part of the treasured heritage of each family. The concrete anecdote covers the widest spectrum. It may consist of the sheltered move from coast to coast of an executive's family for reasons of promotion in his work or the precarious move of the family of a political refugee who is given asylum in another country as an option to continued jail and torture. It may be the hopeful move of a family to a medical center where an offspring may receive continuous treatment for a chronic disease or the doomed move of a Puerto Rican from a low-paying job in San Juan to a low-paying job in the Bronx. It may be the move forced by racial and religious persecution in Nazi Germany or present-day Uganda or Southeast Asia, and so on, in an endless variety.

However, despite this array of anecdotes and scripts that derive from the culture and the circumstances of each family, the process of migration—both across cultures and across regions within cultures—presents outstanding regularities. In fact, if we focus our attention on patterns, rather than content (as we shall do in this discussion), we may develop a model of the migratory process that has a reasonable degree of cross-cultural validity, a model that is, so to speak, "culture free," regardless of how culture specific the styles of coping and the prevalent themes may be.

Stages of Migration Process

The continuum of the process of migration can be broken down into the following discrete steps: (a) *preparatory stage;* (b) *act of migration;* (c) *period of overcompensation;* (d) *period of decompensation;* and (e) *transgenerational phenomena.* Each step has distinctive characteristics, triggers different types of family coping mechanisms, and unchains different types of conflicts and symptoms. Each of these basic phases of the migratory process will be described in detail in this chapter, with emphasis on specific types of urgencies, conflicts, and crises. This will be followed by some general guidelines for preventive interventions that are relevant when dealing with families presenting conflicts related to the migratory process.

Preparatory Stage

This prologue to migration begins when the first concrete moves are made by family members toward a commitment to migrate. These moves can be an exchange of letters, a request of an application for visas, or any other act that substantiates the intent to migrate. The time span of this stage obviously varies with the circumstances but in most cases is also contingent upon the family style (from an "explosive" decision to a lengthy rumination).

In the course of the preparatory stage, a first "up-and-down" curve will frequently appear, expressed as a short period of euphoria and an also short period of overload, dismay, and poor performance that habitually does not acquire major proportions and tends to be explained away as the natural result of efforts, tensions, and emotions. In the course of those ups and downs, however, new family rules about roles and functions in relation to migration begin to be negotiated among members. These rules, explored during the preliminary stage, will be fully incorporated once migration takes place.

Migration is described by migrants as an act loaded either with negative motivations and connotations (such as "to escape political oppression") or with positive connotations (such as "to make a better living"). It is important to realize that the choice of one given connotation over the other is sometimes reasonable but on other occasions quite arbitrary, although not random. So, "to make a better living" (positive) may imply "to escape from a bad living situation" (negative). The choice of one given emphasis as reason for migration—with the value judgment attached to it— may provide us with valuable clues about the family's coping styles, including rules about which roles are to be played by each member.

In spite of the fact that it is usually the result of a collective decision, some people tend to be labeled as "responsible" or motivator of the migration. Did they move because it was beneficial for the job situation or the career of one member of the family— more frequently the husband—while the other one—more frequently the wife—was dragged behind? Did they move because one of the kids was chronically ill, and they needed to locate near an adequate medical facility? If so, who insisted on the move, and was it useful in terms of the care of the illness? Was somebody rescued by the move? Who experienced the greatest loss in the move? The anecdotes that consolidate roles of heroes and villains, victims and oppressors, remain frequently as family myths and appear repeatedly as themes of family feuds or as the unmentioned "skeletons in the closet."

Another important issue in this regard stems from the frequent assumption that, if the move had a positive motivation or even far exceeded the family's expectations in terms of advantages, there is no reason to mourn what has been left behind; any sadness or mourning is immediately labeled as pathological or an act of ill will. In fact, those family members "in charge" of mourning have the greatest chance of being scapegoated by the rest (thus isolating those members in charge of the painful task of coming to terms with the past).

The opposite situation can also be found. Families who have escaped from extreme situations such as total annihilation may remain anchored to their past, in a state of permanent collective remembrance, mourning, and involvement with those dreaded circumstances from which they—and not others—escaped. In these cases, the member of the family who breaks away first from the collective family mourning is frequently scapegoated as a traitor (to the family, to those who stayed behind, etc.). The confrontation notwithstanding, this role accomplishes a collective need: that of testing the new reality (done by the "traitor") while appeasing the guilt (done by the "accusers").

The Act of Migration

Migration is a transition with little or no prescribed rituals. In most cultures and circumstances, migrants are left to deal with the painful act of migration with only their private rituals. The most noticeable exception takes place in Israel, where the Ulpan—an initial residential program and intensive teaching of Hebrew to new immigrants—entails a whole complex ritual of initiation. There are also minor exceptions in other cultures, such as the "welcome wagon" ritual performed by neighbors to newly moved families in middle-class America.

It must be kept in mind that, although the very act of migration may constitute a brief transition (a 3-hour leap by plane), in many other cases the act proper may take a considerable time. Such is frequently the case with people displaced by wars and with people who migrated with intermediary stays in countries of transition or in internment camps. This protracted process may lead to the establishment of strong allegiances among people exposed to the same vicissitudes, to the point of becoming a primary net as strong as the one left in the country of origin. Such has been the case, for instance, with European Jews escaping the Holocaust who shared long pilgrimages on board ships before reaching a country that would accept them (leading to surrogate-family names such as *schiffbrudern* and *schiffschwestern*—ship brothers and ship sisters). The same occurs at present with the "boat people" from Vietnam.

The mode or *style of the migratory act* varies considerably. Some families "burn bridges," and the act of migration has the character of something final and unchangeable. Contrariwise, others affirm that they migrate "only for a while," regardless of the unlikelihood of a return. Some families decide *a priori* that the country they have chosen will be it, whereas other families explicitly include trial periods in their plans in order to decide among countries. Some families migrate in block and blindly, without any previous exploration of the field. Others organize the move cautiously, sending some members as "scouts" to prepare the terrain, secure jobs and dwelling, and the like. Some families migrate legally and can have access to institutions of the country of adoption, whereas others migrate illegally, thus enhancing their (adaptive) mistrust and alienation from mainstream institutions. Finally, some families choose to migrate, and some are forced to do so.

Period of Overcompensation

Migratory stress does not take its heaviest toll in the weeks or even months immediately following migration. On the contrary, the participants are frequently unaware of the stressful nature of the experience and of its cumulative impact. In fact, it is a period in which a heightened task-oriented efficiency can be noted, aided by a strong increase in the split between "instrumental" and "affective" roles within the family, in the service of the basic need for survival and adaptation in an environment and a culture that is, to a greater or lesser extent, alien.

Ethnicity can be defined in terms of the orientation it provides to individuals by delineating norms, values, interactional modalities, rituals, meanings, and collective goals. That orientation—that *weltanschauung*—does not operate in a vacuum but is dialectically supported by regularities of the environment that generate the experience of *consonance*. A person walking in the street with a baguette under his arm is consonant—for a perceptual set tuned up for Paris, not Boston. To be surrounded mainly by blond people is consonant—for Stockholm, not San Juan. For men to go arm in arm is consonant—for Rome, not Omaha. A 1:00 to 4:00 siesta break is consonant—for New Orleans in the summer or for Jamaica, not Brooklyn. In fact, each individual subscribes to a certain organization of reality and, hence, makes constant predictions about how things are going to be and how people are going to act and react. Each unpredicted variation on any of those features shatters that person's premises about reality and calls for a complex calibration of either the perceptions ("are my senses reliable?") or the prediction ("are my values, or is my common sense, reliable?"). These calibrating, adaptive mechanisms are mobilized by the *dissonance* resulting from any mismatch between expectations and environment.

In the period immediately following migration, the first priority of the family is sheer survival, that is, the satisfaction of its basic needs. Given those priorities, the process of cancellation of dissonance or the denial of its subjective impact is maximal precisely at the period in which the bombardment by dissonant experiences is also maximal. As a result of this mechanism, it is not infrequent to observe that recent immigrants show a clear focus of attention—of consciousness—while the overall field of consciousness is blurred or clouded (similar to certain patients with concussion who appear overall stunned and confused but maintain a narrow focus of clear consciousness).

A concurrence of extreme circumstances and lack of coping skills can trigger massive crises in this period, with family disorganization or multiple symptoms. But that is not the rule. In fact, the majority of migrating families manage to establish and maintain for months a relative moratorium on the process of accultura-tion and accommodation. During this period immediately follow-ing migration, therefore, conflicts and symptoms tend to remain dormant. The only observable feature is that previous family rules and styles tend to appear slightly exaggerated. For instance, if the members were mutually close, physically or emotionally, they will seem even closer, if they were mutually distant, they will increase their autonomy further, in spite of the fact that the lack of an extended social network may force them to spend more time together.

A moratorium technique developed occasionally is the collec-tive myth that "they will return to the country of origin after some time." Families cling to the old country's norms and refuse to engage with the new environment. Needless to say, that coping strategy can last for only so long, and eventually the fantasy will collapse under the pressure of the new reality, triggering a major crisis.

One way or another, the period of apparent calm and over-compensation gives way, some 6 months after it started, to an era of major crisis, one in which the long-range responses to migra-tion take place.

Period of Decompensation or Crisis

This is a stormy period, plagued with conflicts, symptoms, and difficulties. In fact, the majority of the migrated families that are brought to the attention of family therapists can be placed at one point or another of this phase of decompensation. In it, the main task of the recently migrated family takes place: that of reshaping its new reality, maximizing both the family's continuity in terms of identity and its compatibility with the environment. These two facets of the task sometimes compete and require a reasonable compromise for their accomplishment. It is indeed a frequent and necessary adaptation to retain certain family habits, even though they differ from those of the new context, while getting rid of other traits because they go too much against the grain of the culture of adoption or because they would require an extended family no longer available. The balance is delicate and difficult to reach. The whole collective task is complex, painful, and unavoidable. Frequently, the crisis creeps into the family through the offspring: children tend to catch up with the new culture and the new language (verbal and nonverbal) much more rapidly than their parents do, unleashing a clash of values and styles that strikes at the core of the family.

Many family rules and values that were effective in the country of origin may prove to be less adaptive in the culture and circumstances of the country of adoption. But for a family to change its styles and rules (some of which may have been pivotal ones) requires that the group activate delicate and complex *rules about changes of rules*. In many cases, families have not previously established these rules about rules and embark on the still more difficult task of developing them *de novo*. For instance, how may parents reach an agreement on ways of discussing contraception with their adolescent daughters raised in the United States when the norms of their culture—and therefore their present rules— preclude the explicit discussion of issues about sexuality in general even within the parental couple?

The effect of the strengths and weaknesses of the family coping mechanisms in the context of the new culture is cumulative and will express itself in the course of the months, sometimes years, after the migration. Many family functioning rules will prove to be adaptive in both cultures and will not show any change. Many others will have undergone changes affecting the distribution of roles and norms that may involve every member of the family. Finally, many other patterns will be retained at the expense of a certain degree of alienation from the extrafamilial world. Some of these patterns are maintained because they become central to the family identity, as a sort of cohesive ritual. Others are kept simply because the family has not been able to develop ways to cope with the changes in role entailed by the change of rules.

As mentioned before, in order to cope with the immediacy of migration, families frequently develop a split between instrumental and affective roles: one member—usually the male—deals with (present and future-oriented) instrumental activities that entail a connection with the current environment, and the other— usually the female—centers on present and past-oriented affective activities that entail a sustained connection with the previous environment (including maintenance tasks such as letters, phone calls, etc., and mourning of what has been left behind). This rule about distribution of roles, that may be adaptive during the first few months, has the potential of a catastrophic runaway in the system if rigidly maintained. The outward-oriented member will develop autonomous adaptive traits and establish a new satisfactory network of his (her) own, and the inward-oriented one will maintain a relative isolation that becomes more marked by comparison. The autonomous member will experience the other one, relatively ignorant of the norms and customs of the new environment and with fewer new acquaintances and friends, as interfering with the instrumental need and reacts to that experience with still more autonomy. This further fences off and enhances the experience of solitude of the already isolated, past-oriented member, who will respond either by clinging more to the past or by clinging more to the other member, who, in turn, will feel dragged down by that situation and increase his (her) disengagement. The whole process escalates progressively into a major crisis of the relationship.

It is interesting to notice the power of this rule about polarization of roles. In those families in which this split of roles escalates into a divorce, it can be seen that the past-oriented member frees herself (himself) from the fixed role *only after the separation*; forced at first by the need to cope, she (he) soon "discovers" her (his) previously untapped abilities to deal with the present environment and to plan the future.

An inverse case, not infrequent in migrant families of rural origin, is that the woman will find an unskilled job in the city more easily than the man, thus challenging drastically their previous family structure and roles. In these circumstances, even though on occasion a switch of roles may take place uneventfully, much more frequently the man will become symptomatic (depressive, alcoholic, or with somatic complaints), or a major crisis of family disorganization will ensue.

Some families manage to mourn what has been left behind and integrate it constructively into a blend of old and new rules, models, and habits that constitute their new reality. For them, the positive side of the experience outweighs the disruptive nature of the stress, and they emerge from the process—some 3 years after migration—with new individual and collective strengths. In other families, whatever has been left behind in the country of origin, may become increasingly idealized (making adaptation more difficult) or denigrated (making mourning and working through of the loss more difficult). High levels of intrafamilial confrontations may cause the family to consult a therapist, with some members representing the values of the country of origin, and some, those of the new society. The factionalization will appear as tension and overt conflict between spouses, with the additional tug-of-war of offspring factions—or across generations, with the tightening of intragenerational coalitions. These tendencies build into a major interpersonal crisis or crystallize into a medical or psychiatric complaint. In fact, in order to deal with, or express, accumulated stress, tension, pain, and conflict, family members will frequently activate the socially acceptable and interactionally powerful pattern of the "somatic complaint" or the "psychiatric problem" and occasionally the socially less acceptable pattern of "social deviant" (e.g., as a juvenile delinquent).

Transgenerational Impact

Families, in their function as main socializing agents, convey not only the norms and mores of their culture at large but also the specific styles, modes, values, and myths that constitute an ad hoc, family-specific view of the world and of their own history. It comes as no surprise then to discover that any long-term delay in the family's adaptive process will tend to become apparent when a second generation is raised in the country of adoption. Whatever has been avoided by a first generation will appear in the second one, generally expressed as a *clash between generations.*

This clash is maximally apparent in families belonging to cultural groups that have been ghettoized by choice or by force in their country of adoption. A neighborhood that mimics the country of origin constitutes an environment that buffers the cross-cultural exposure and slows any adaptive change. If the second generation becomes socialized in that same secluded environment, the process will repeat itself with no apparent consequences. However, if the process of socialization takes place in a milieu that reflects the norms and values of the new country, what has been delayed by the first generation will take the form of an intergenerational conflict of values.

Such is the case, for instance, with families of Chinese origin living in American Chinatowns. Offspring of immigrant parents, who are raised in the United States and who interacted actively with the larger society through schools, mass media, and informal and formal contacts of various sources, tend to clash dramatically with their parents in terms of values, norms, and mores. In a more or less subtle way, this intergenerational clash takes place in almost any immigrant family with an intensity that shows an inverse correlation with its previous capacity to thoroughly work through the complex process of migration.

In many cases, however, the clash is intercultural rather than intergenerational. The conflict between the child's dominant style of coping—congruent with the family culture—and the differently defined rules and boundaries within large sectors of the extrafamilial world results in a label of "delinquency" for the child's behavior and its consequences (see Minuchin *et al.*, pp. 351–352[1]).

Preventive Implications of the Model

As may have been observed throughout this description of the migratory process, each step presents its own phenomenology, its own specific types of conflicts, and its own available coping modalities. Each step implies a normal level of conflict for the family, and each has the potential of triggering family crisis. The nature of the crisis depends on the family's own style and resources, or lack of them, and the presence of environmental support, or added strain.

Several *preventive implications* can be derived, centered either in the preparatory stages or in those that immediately follow migration. It would be important to convey to families who contemplate migration the convenience of (a) forseeing and anticipating periods of loneliness and rootlessness (in order to legitimize that experience and avoid any negative labeling); (b) ensuring the maintenance of contact with people from the "old place," resisting the temptation to deal "surgically" with those ties; (c) learning the language of the new country before the move (if applicable); (d) acquiring prior information about practicalities of the new reality (e.g., how does one get a doctor?) as well as the more subtle area of social rules (e.g., do people shake hands or not when greeting?); (e) ensuring some level of continuity in their own physical environment by carrying with them those meaningful objects— framed pictures, decorative objects—that were markers of their private space and placing them in the new dwelling immediately in order to generate a sense of familiarity and continuity.

With the possible exception of the first one, the middle-class bias of the points just mentioned is obvious. Most of them require the luxury of time and money as well as a strong future orientation. Solutions that cut across social classes and deal especially with the less protected families of lower socioeconomic levels should be built into standard health protection procedures. For instance, the impact of migration could be buffered substantially by ad hoc community organizations or equivalent collective projects aimed at providing interim networks of reference in the countries of destination for families in the process of immigrating. These surrogate extended families could help immensely in terms of providing both practical expertise and emotional support during the tough first period of insertion. It should be noted, however, that the middle-class, individualistic orientation of public health policies in most countries of the Western hemisphere define these problems and policy issues as the responsibility of those who are affected by them rather than the responsibility of the society at large.

References

1. Minuchin, S., Montalvo, B., Guerney, B. G., Rosman, B. L., & Schumer, F. *Families of the slums*. New York: Basic Books, 1967.

IX

Coping with Unusual Crises
Man-Made and Natural Disasters

Disasters strike indiscriminately, leaving victims stunned by multiple losses and feeling vulnerable in an environment they once considered safe. Initially, disaster victims confront dramatic unexpected changes as they experience losses of family, home, personal property, and possibly even their community. Following a disaster, families face the tasks of uniting and supporting each other, seeking help from relatives, friends, and relief agencies, and reestablishing a home life and some semblance of normality. Later, victims may face a "second disaster" as they encounter difficulties in replacing lost possessions, finding out who is responsible if the disaster is man-made, and obtaining compensation. Moreover, families who have lost their home face the problem of moving and adjusting to a new environment.

Disasters vary greatly in their nature and magnitude. Goldine Gleser and her associates[4] have suggested that most floods should produce relatively little lasting psychological impairment because there is minimal threat to life, warnings usually allow time for evacuation, and only part of the community is affected. Tornadoes, cyclones, and severe earthquakes are likely to be much more stressful due to their suddenness and great destructive potential. Technological catastrophes such as the nuclear accident at Three Mile Island and the toxic chemical leak in Bhopal, India, also may be especially stressful due to the victims' sense of loss of control over the technology, the assumption that such disasters are potentially preventable, and the lack of a "low point" after

289

which the situation can be expected to improve. Victims may be unable to resume normal lives because they are plagued by the suspicion that even worse consequences are yet to occur.

In the first article, Michael R. Berren, Allan Beigel, and Stuart Ghertner describe a model for classifying disasters. The authors categorize disasters according to type (man-made versus natural or a combination of the two), duration (a fire may be over in just a few minutes, whereas a famine may last months or even years), and the extent of personal impact on the victims, as when one earthquake does relatively little damage whereas another destroys an entire city. The potential for occurrence or recurrence is also important. Natural disasters such as tornadoes and hurricanes are regular seasonal events in certain parts of the country. In contrast, airplane crashes are rare and unlikely to recur for a given individual. Finally, although little can be done to prevent most natural disasters, many man-made disasters can be averted or their consequences forestalled. These characteristics can be used to contrast different disasters and to help plan appropriate interventions.[2]

Although the characteristics of disasters vary widely, disaster victims show many common reactions. During the impact phase, they confront the threat of injury and death. In the immediate postimpact phase, shock may be juxtaposed with the euphoria of having survived. In general, disaster victims quickly direct their energy toward rescue activities and try to deal with the effects of the disaster. Grief may be delayed while they are intensely involved in these pursuits. Later, however, some victims experience chronic stress and lingering grief. (For a discussion of survivor reactions prior to and immediately after a disastrous fire, see Valent.[8])

In the second article, Robert Jay Lifton and Eric Olson discuss five main survivor reaction patterns and the long-term psychological effects of the Buffalo Creek flood. The first pattern is the death imprint and death anxiety. The death imprint includes the vivid memories of death and massive destruction that may plague survivors for many years after a disaster. Death anxiety was reflected in terrifying dreams in which survivors were threatened by disaster-related forms of death and had to struggle to remain alive. A second pattern of survivor reactions is death guilt that is related to having survived. Survivors felt guilty about not being able to save relatives or thought that if they had died another person might have lived. A third reaction, psychic numbing, helped survivors minimize their emotional pain. Survivors were apathetic, depressed, withdrawn, and suffered from memory difficulties. Fourth, survivors experienced impairment of human relationships. Although they needed nurturing and support, survivors had difficulty accepting it when it was offered. Moreover, family members often were unable to help each other because they were overcome by their own grief. The final response pattern involved the survivors' attempt to find an acceptable explanation for the disaster in order to resolve their anger and discover new meaning in their life.

Successful coping strategies tend to vary with the type of disaster. Following the Buffalo Creek flood, men who began cleaning and restoring their homes were less anxious and impaired in the long run than those who were unable to do so. These men may have fared better because their self-confidence was bolstered by their involvement in constructive activity.[4] Yet victims at Three Mile Island who used problem-focused coping strategies tended to report more stress than those who relied on emotion-focused strategies. Because it was impossible for individuals to control the continuing radiation danger at the power plant, those who favored problem-focused strategies were destined to fail, and thus their stress levels remained high.[1]

Victims may also band together and cope as a group. For example, victims of the Love Canal disaster formed a homeowners association[3] that served as a self-help group that provided information and support and voiced community concerns (see Chapter 1). In communities that experience natural disasters with some regularity, citizen groups may prepare for future disasters. Thus, previously organized groups can help to make and lay sandbags if a flood threatens or provide first aid and rescue services to victims of a tornado. These active coping strategies help members of the community gain a sense of control even though they are quite powerless to influence the event itself.

Demographic and personal factors, such as age, can influence adjustment following a disaster. Although greater maturity and more extensive coping experience may provide middle-aged persons with richer resources on which to draw, a disaster threatens the disruption of established relationships and the fulfillment of their cherished life aims. Young adults may be less seriously affected in a flood than those of middle age, who may lose the economic security they have worked so hard to attain. These issues may be less important for elderly persons, but such persons often suffer from cognitive impairment that reduces their coping ability.

Environmental factors also affect adjustment. Supportive families may help child victims of a flood recover quickly, whereas children from irritable or violent families are more impaired.[4] The surviving relatives of disaster victims who have supportive networks and receive bereavement counseling tend to experience fewer postbereavement problems. Additionally, those who view the victim's body are better able to come to terms with the death and adjust to their loss than those who do not have this opportunity.[7]

The victims of disasters are not limited to those who suffer personal losses; rescue workers may also be victims. In the third article, Beverly Raphael, Bruce Singh, and Lesley Bradbury describe helpers' reactions to disasters. The immediate psychological response usually is shock and disbelief. Helpers tend to feel better when they have specific tasks to perform. In fact, they may experience a sense of elation as they become involved in the disaster work. This "high" can drive helpers to work without relief and push them to their physical limits.

Rescue workers and other helpers may experience severe disaster-related stressors, such as helplessness associated with an unexpected disaster that results in large numbers of dead and injured people, the smell and sight of mutilated and decomposed bodies, and the suffering of injured victims and their relatives. These sights may "trigger" thoughts of their own mortality and of the chance of losing their loved ones. Helpers may be frightened by the life-threatening actions they must take to rescue the injured who are in pain and imminent danger of death. They may feel frustrated and inadequate when they are unable to execute their mission due to the danger of using certain equipment, or when they feel unprepared or lack the required knowledge. Raphael and her associates[6] found that workers who are frustrated in their efforts to carry out helping actions or who have diffuse roles are more likely to feel guilty and depressed. In contrast, rescue workers who have a clear purpose and are actively involved in helping are likely to feel that they have made a worthwhile contribution.

Paramedics, like disaster workers, are routinely exposed to death and dying. Palmer[5] found that paramedics are able to adapt to these stressors in part because their training desensitizes them to severe injury, blood, and death. They manage unpleasant and even gruesome tasks by using humor and by distancing themselves from the suffering and horror they see by using radio codes and special language. For example, a dead body is referred to as a "Signal 27" and fatally burned persons are dubbed "crispy critters." Paramedics also cope by controlling their emotional response to patients and by reminding themselves that their efforts usually improve the victim's chance to live.

In this chapter, Raphael and her associates note that workers react to their disaster experience in varied ways. For some, nightmares and recurring memories serve to release their emotions, whereas others may experience psychosomatic and stress symptoms. Some workers are helped by sharing their thoughts and feelings with family members. Others need to seek professional help to come to terms with their disaster experience. Psychological debriefing sessions give workers an opportunity to share feelings, release pent-up emotions, and integrate the horrors to which they have been exposed. Rescue workers then may empathize with the plight of disaster victims, form special bonds with them, and channel their anger at man-made disasters by taking up the victims' cause. Moreover, some workers come to value life more highly and to redirect their own lives as a result of their experiences.

References

1. Baum, A., Fleming, R., & Singer, J. Coping with victimization by technological disaster. *Journal of Social Issues*, 1983, *39*, 117–138.
2. Berren, M. R., Beigel, A., & Barker, G. A typology for the classification of disasters: Implications for intervention. *Community Mental Health Journal*, 1982, *18*, 120–134.

3. Gibbs, L. M. Community response to an emergency situation. Psychological destruction and the Love Canal. *American Journal of Community Psychology*, 1983, *11*, 116–125.
4. Gleser, G., Green, B., & Winget, C. *Prolonged psychosocial effects of disaster: A study of Buffalo Creek*. New York: Academic Press, 1981.
5. Palmer, C. E. A note about paramedics' strategies for dealing with death and dying. *Journal of Occupational Psychology*, 1983, *56*, 83–86.
6. Raphael, B., Singh, B., Bradbury, L., & Lambert, F. Who helps the helpers? The effects of disaster on the rescue workers. *Omega*, 1983–1984, *14*, 9–20.
7. Singh, B., & Raphael, B. Postdisaster morbidity of the bereaved: A possible role for preventive psychiatry? *Journal of Nervous and Mental Disease*, 1981, *169*, 203–212.
8. Valent, P. The Ash Wednesday bushfires in Victoria. *The Medical Journal of Australia*, 1984, *141*, 291–300.

21

A Typology for the Classification of Disasters

MICHAEL R. BERREN, ALLAN BEIGEL, and STUART
GHERTNER

Over the past 25 years, a wide spectrum of social psychological literature has been published concerning disasters. Articles have appeared that provide descriptions of the extent of the destruction,[6,7,16] assessments of the social and emotional consequences of disasters,[5,9,11,13,19,24] and analyses of those intervention services provided to minimize the potentially devastating social and emotional consequences.[4,8,10,20,21,25]

Types of disasters described include, among others, airline crashes,[4] earthquakes,[2,10] mass kidnappings,[21] tornadoes,[16,22,25] floods,[6,8,13,17,19,20] fires[1,14] and war-related events.[11,12,18]

Despite these many descriptive articles, very few investigators have focused on theoretical concepts that could provide cohesion to this important area of research. Although several authors have studied the psychological stages through which victims pass following a disaster,[5,9,24] their reports appear to make the erroneous assumption that all disasters are similar (disaster equivalency).

This chapter appears in abridged form from *Community Mental Health Journal*, Summer 1980, *16*, 103–111. Copyright 1980 by Human Sciences Press, Inc., 72 Fifth Avenue, New York, New York 10011. Reprinted by permission.

MICHAEL R. BERREN, ALLAN BEIGEL, and STUART GHERTNER • Southern Arizona Mental Health Center, Tucson, Arizona 85719.

In this chapter, we present the hypothesis, based on our own experiences in responding to disasters and a review of the existing literature, that to understand and predict psychological reactions to disasters one must first recognize the important characteristics that differentiate disasters from each other. It is our contention that these factors must be taken into account in planning strategies designed to reduce their emotional and social consequences.

A Five-Dimensional Disaster Typology

A study of the literature and a recent involvement with the aftermath of a disaster leads us to a formulation that describes five primary factors which can be used conceptually to distinguish one disaster from another. The five factors are (1) type of disaster (a natural event as compared to a disaster perpetuated by man); (2) duration of disaster; (3) degree of personal impact; (4) potential for occurrence (recurrence); and (5) control over future impact.

By using this typology to analyze different disasters more accurately, it is our hypothesis that it will be possible to predict (more definitively) the psychological impact of a specific disaster based on its classification. This should, in turn, lead to a better understanding of how to target interventions more specifically and effectively.

Type of Disaster

Much of the literature uses the terms *disaster* and *natural disaster* synonymously. Not all disasters, however, are natural disasters. Catastrophic events can range from natural disasters or acts of God to disasters that are purposefully perpetuated by man. An earthquake occurring in a remote, primitive area is an act of God. Man has no hand in creating or intensifying the disaster. At the other end of the spectrum, the holocaust against the Jews during World War II[12,13] and the mass kidnapping of children in Chowchilla, California,[23] are clearly man-made disasters.

Most disasters are the result of events that fall somewhere between the extremes cited. The disastrous flood that occurred at

Buffalo Creek has been described as a combination of natural forces and man's compromising of nature.[6,19] At Buffalo Creek, a dam collapsed and literally destroyed the town below. Reports following the dam's collapse confirmed many suspicions that negligence on the part of the company controlling the dam was in part responsible, although not necessarily intentional.

Airline crashes are often the result of a combination of natural events such as bad weather and human error. The worst airline disaster in history, the collision of two jumbo jets in the Canary Islands, was a function of fog and apparent miscommunication between the control tower and one of the planes.[15]

Duration of Disaster

Many disasters might last for only a few seconds or a few minutes. Others are preceded by years of impending doom. The major destruction caused by a severe fire, such as at the Coconut Grove or Beverly Hills occurred within less than an hour.[14] Prior to the fires, the victims were not suffering from precatastrophic problems or concerns.

The Buffalo Creek flood serves as an example of a disaster at the other end of the duration continuum. The area residents, for some time, had lived with the possibility that the dam could eventually collapse. "The flood had been part of the mental as well as the physical geography of Buffalo Creek, a feared event buried in the minds of people. The massive convulsion of the physical world that took place on February 26, 1972, was a mental imprint come true."[19] Another example of a disaster with a long precipitating history as well as duration is the famine in the Sahel region of Africa.[7] The preceding years of drought set the stage for the eventual and predictable disaster.

Degree of Personal Impact

Two earthquakes of equal magnitude will have a significantly different impact depending on where they occur. Similarly, a single earthquake, tornado, or flood will have a different impact upon the individuals who are classified as "victims." Some might suffer nothing more than the temporary inconvenience of living in a city piled with rubble, long supermarket lines, and poor telephone service. For others, the same disaster may result in the loss of family members or friends as well as loss of major material possessions such as a home.

This example points out that the term *victims* describes, in reality, a heterogeneous group who experience varying consequences as a result of the disaster. Furthermore, the personal impact of a disaster significantly affects both the victims' perceptions of the disaster as well as their lives after the disaster. This finding was demonstrated by Janney, Masuda, and Holmes,[10] who in 1977 found that victims' short- and long-term attitudes related to perception of life were changed significantly following an earthquake that devastated a town in Peru. Citizens of a similar town, only 2 miles away, that was not damaged severely by the earthquake did not have these changes in attitude.

Potential for Occurrence (Recurrence)

Some disasters have a greater probability for occurrence than do others. Regardless of how fearful of flying one might feel, the probability of being in an airplane crash is extremely low. Likewise, fires similar to that which occurred at the Coconut Grove Supper Club[14] are rare. Conversely, the possibility of having a major springtime flood in one of the states bordering the Mississippi River is fairly high. Although not a certainty, its occurrence is not totally unexpected. Also spring tornadoes in Texas and Oklahoma, summer hurricanes coming off the Carribean or Gulf of Mexico, and brush fires during the hot, dry summer in the Los Angeles area occur with some regularity. All have a relatively high potential for occurrence. Although a single community cannot be singled out ahead of time as a specific target for a disaster, the chances are good that certain types of disasters will regularly occur within specific geographic regions. Thus although no one could have predicted ahead of time that Wichita Falls would be devastated by a tornado in the spring of 1979, the fact that a major tornado touched down in north Texas in the spring of 1979 was not surprising.

Control over Future Impact

There are some disasters that man has the opportunity to prevent from occurring again or at least to reduce their potential devastating consequences. A recent example took place in Tucson, Arizona, following the crash of an Air Force jet 100 feet from a junior high school.[3] Soon after the crash occurred, citizens' groups began to exert pressure on the local Air Force base to put an end to flights over populated sections of the city. The community acted in an attempt to reduce the (potential) future impact of another air disaster and was successful. Most landings over populated areas of the city were eliminated. Thus even if another Air Force jet crashes while landing, the probability of disastrous consequences to those on the ground has been greatly reduced.

In contrast, the long, dry Southern California summer creates a high risk for fires breaking out in exclusive foothill housing areas. These fires occur on a regular basis and lead to extensive damage. Although certain precautions are taken, the community is unable to significantly reduce the probability of extensive damage. Nature is too powerful a foe and man's occasional carelessness makes fires almost inevitable.

Application of the Typological Classification

Jet Air Force Crash in Tucson, Arizona

On the afternoon of Friday, October 27, 1978, an Air Force 7-D Corsair II jet fighter crashed in the street approximately 100 feet from the fence surrounding Mansfeld Junior High School. Upon impact, the aircraft ignited into a wall of flame several stories high. Two individuals were burned to death in their car, and six others received mild to severe injuries. The crash and subsequent deaths and injuries were witnessed by over 100 students who were eating lunch on the school grounds. The noise and vibration created by the crash resulted in students and teachers running hysterically through the schoolyard and the school building. Within 2 hours, most major signs of the crash, such as ambulances, fire, smoke, and crowds had been eliminated. The Tucson crash can be classified as follows.

Type of Disaster.   The crash was more an act of God than a
disaster purposefully perpetrated by man. Apparently, part of the
plane's carburetor system failed, and a crash landing was inevitable. The pilot was perceived by some as a hero for staying with the
plane long enough to steer it clear of the junior high school.
Others felt that the location of the crash was a function of pilot
error since he should have ditched the plane over the desert surrounding the city.

Duration of the Disaster.   Within 2 hours after the crash,
most evidence that a disaster had taken place was gone. Only a
charred airplane and two burned parked cars remained in the
street. A meeting previously scheduled for that evening in the
school auditorium was held. By the next morning, the jet and two
cars had been removed, and the street was being repaved.

Although the crash and resultant fire lasted for only approximately 35 minutes, the panic of students wanting to call their
parents and the behavior of terrified parents attempting to get
through police lines to find their children continued for several
hours. Compared to natural disasters that have destroyed entire
communities and left hundreds homeless for long periods of
time, the major consequences of this disaster were relatively short
in duration.

Degree of Personal Impact.   For the students, the personal
impact of the crash was minimal. Although it is true that immediately after the crash, many students were traumatized and hys-
terical, only one student was injured. Even though the crash could
have resulted in numerous fatalities and massive property loss,
the students never faced any real danger nor did anyone have any
major material losses since the plane landed on a side street and
missed the school. In comparison to other airline crashes, the
Tucson crash would have to be classified as being of moderately
low personal impact.

Potential for Occurrence (Recurrence).   The probability of
any air disaster is extremely low, and the probability of a crash
occurring at a particular spot (i.e., next to Mansfeld Junior High
School in Tucson, Arizona) is infinitesimal. The occurrence was
highly unlikely, and the probability of these individuals being
victims a second time is extremely remote.

Control over Future Impact.   Parents of students at the school
and citizens in the community had the opportunity to reduce the

even minimal chance of an Air Force jet crashing again in the vicinity of the school or a populated area. Through the political process, numerous hearings, and a major investigation community pressure was placed on the local Air Force base to change their landing approach patterns over the city. Prior to the crash, the approach pattern ensured that virtually every plane landing at the Air Force base (approximately 175 a day) flew over the junior high school, the University of Arizona, and other densely populated areas of the city. Use of an alternate pattern resulted in a 75% reduction in the number of low-flying Air Force jets over the junior high school and other populated areas. Thus with this particular disaster considerable opportunity existed for exerting control and preventing similar disasters.

Mass Kidnapping of School Children in Chowchilla, California

On July 17, 1976, 26 students and a school bus driver were kidnapped by armed bandits wearing ski masks. The ordeal lasted over 27 hours during which time the children and bus driver were taken on an 11-hour bus ride and then buried alive in a large truck. After hours underground, the children and bus driver were able to dig a tunnel to the surface and escape. While they were captive, the children had no access to restrooms or food. Many of the children believed that death was imminent.[23]

Type of Disaster. The kidnapping was obviously a disaster perpetrated by man. The kidnapping was well planned and the ultimate goal of the kidnappers was apparently extortion.

Duration of Disaster. The kidnapping lasted just over 27 hours from the time of initial contact with the masked bandits to eventual escape. During their captivity, the victims could not escape from the reality of what was happening and that death was a distinct possibility. The intensity of the situation did not lessen during the 27 hours and, as time passed, the situation became more frightening.

After they escaped, the major part of the disaster was over. Although there was no long-term cleanup phase, as in a tornado or earthquake, the 27-hour ordeal should still be considered a fairly long-term event.

Degree of Personal Impact. The children experienced an extraordinary amount of emotional trauma during the kidnapping. Many thought they would either be shot or suffocate underground. Most expressed the concern that they would never see their families again. Physical suffering was less severe, and most physical problems (cuts, scrapes, bladder infections, cramps, etc.) were readily treated.

A second set of victims, the parents, also suffered mental anguish during the time of their child's captivity. They had no idea whether they would ever see their child alive again. Most parents reported dwelling on images of the last moment they had seen their child on the morning of the kidnapping. Even though there was no loss of life or loss of major possessions, the kidnapping was a disaster that had high personal impact for the victims.

Potential for Occurrence (Recurrence). Kidnappings, especially mass kidnappings, are rare events. The probability of these students or even this community being faced with a second kidnapping would have to be considered remote. The victims were not kidnapped because of their political views, their race, or religion. The children were not even from wealthy families. They had no characteristics that would have predicted their mass plight, and they had little in common except for living in the same town and being in the same school bus at the same time.

Control over Future Impact. Even though the chances of a second kidnapping are extremely low, many families modified their lives to reduce the probability even further. Some parents began driving their children to school. Others talked about moving from Chowchilla (which in reality would do nothing other than reduce the slight risk of being kidnapped in Chowchilla and increase the slight risk of being kidnapped somewhere else). Despite these actions, if someone wanted to kidnap any of the children again, they could probably do so. Consequently, there is relatively low control over future kidnappings.

Discussion

Recognition of the importance of providing crisis intervention and follow-up support after disasters is increasing. Newspaper and professional accounts testify to the community need for the intervention steps taken by local mental health associations, mental health centers, the Red Cross, and other human service providers.

This classification model can be utilized to identify crucial elements of a disaster and to assist human service providers in the planning of their intervention activities. A limited example of how the typology can lend itself to identifying specific appropriate courses of action, however, can be seen by comparing the classification of the Tucson air crash with that of the Chowchilla kidnapping. Based on the analysis that the classification typology yields, the two groups of children required different initial intervention activities.

The Tucson children, due to the low personal impact of the disaster, were accepting of group discussions (coordinated by the local mental health center) the day following the crash.[3] The classroom discussions, both didactic and experiential, were designed to clarify facts and feelings related to the crash.

It is unlikely that a similar course of action would have been wise in the case of the Chowchilla children. The intensity of the individual trauma suffered suggests that one-to-one intervention would be a more logical first step and that ongoing therapy would be required for some of the victims.

For some disasters, where prevention or reduction of future impact is feasible, mental health intervention services might be oriented toward consultation and education services that can assist others to take steps necessary to reduce the potential impact. For example, following the Air Force jet crash, the emphasis was on community effort to eliminate planes from flying at low altitudes over the city. The low need for mental health services to reduce the degree of personal impact allowed resources to be used for this purpose.

In other instances, priority for intervention services should not be oriented toward this type of activity. Fire survivors and their relatives will be less benefited by or interested in this kind of intervention and are more likely to require direct services to help them deal with their grief and other emotions arising from the disaster.

References

1. Abe, K. The behavior of survivors and victims in a Japanese nightclub fire. *Mass Emergencies,* 1976, *1,* 119–124.
2. Anderson, W. A. Disaster and organizational change: A study of the long-term consequences in Anchorage of the 1964 Alaska earthquake. *Disaster Research Center Monograph,* 1969 (Ohio State University).
3. Berren, M. R., Beigel, A., & Ghertner, S. *A case study of providing emergency mental health services immediately after an aircraft accident.* Paper presented at the Western Psychological Association Meeting, San Diego, Calif., 1979.
4. Duffy, J. C. Emergency mental health services during and after a major aircraft accident. *Aviation, Space and Environmental Medicine,* 1978, *49,* 1004–1008.
5. Edwards, J. G. Psychiatric aspects of civilian disasters. *British Medical Journal,* 1976, *1,* 944–947.
6. Erikson, K. T. *Everything in its path: Destruction of community in the Buffalo Creek flood.* New York: Simon & Schuster, 1976.
7. Glantz, M. H. *The politics of natural disaster: The case of the Sahel drought.* New York: Praeger, 1976.
8. Heffron, E. F. Project Outreach: Crisis intervention following natural disaster. *Journal of Community Psychology,* 1977, *5,* 103–111.
9. Hocking, F. Psychiatric aspects of extreme environmental stress. *Diseases of the Nervous System,* 1970, *31,* 542–545.
10. Janney, J. G., Masuda, M., & Holmes, T. H. Impact of a natural catastrophe on life events. *Journal of Human Stress,* 1977, *3,* 22–23, 25–34.
11. Klein, H. Delayed affects and after-effects of severe traumatisation. *Israel Annals of Psychiatry and Related Disciplines,* 1974, *12,* 293–303.
12. Klein, H., Zellermeyer, J., & Shanan, J. Former concentration camp inmates on a psychiatric ward. *Archives of General Psychiatry,* 1963, *8,* 334–342.
13. Lifton, R. J., & Olson, E. The human meaning of total disaster. The Buffalo Creek experience. *Psychiatry,* 1976, *39,* 1–18.
14. Lindemann, E. Symptomatology and management of acute grief. In H. J. Parado (Ed.), *Crisis intervention: Selected readings.* New York: Family Service Association of America, 1965.
15. Meisler, S. KLM takeoff not cleared, prober says. *Los Angeles Times,* March 29, 1977, p. 1.
16. Moore, H. E. *Tornadoes over Texas: A study of Waco and San Angelo in disaster.* Austin, Tex.: University of Texas Press, 1958.
17. Okura, K. Mobilizing in response to a major disaster. *Community Mental Health Journal,* 1975, *11,* 136–144.
18. Prince, S. H. *Catastrophe and social change.* New York: AMS Press, 1968.
19. Rangell, L. Discussion of the Buffalo Creek disaster: The course of psychic trauma. *American Journal of Psychiatry,* 1976, *133,* 313–316.
20. Richard, W. Crisis intervention services following natural disasters: The Pennsylvania Flood Recovery Project. *Journal of Community Psychology,* 1974, *2,* 211–219.

21. Sank, L. J. Psychology in action: Community disaster: Primary prevention and treatment in a health maintenance organization. *American Psychologist,* 1979, *34,* 334–338.
22. Taylor, J. B., Zurcher, L. A., & Key, W. H. *Tornado: A community responds to disaster.* Seattle: University of Washington Press, 1970.
23. Terr, L. Children of Chowchilla: A study of psychic trauma. In *Psychoanalytic study of the child.* New Haven: Yale University Press, 1979.
24. Tyhurst, J. S. Individual reactions to community disaster. *American Journal of Psychiatry,* 1951, *107,* 764–769.
25. Zarle, T., Hartsough, D., & Ottinger, D. Tornado recovery: The development of a professional–paraprofessional response to a disaster. *Journal of Community Psychology,* 1974, *2,* 311–321.

22

The Human Meaning of Total Disaster

The Buffalo Creek Experience

ROBERT JAY LIFTON and ERIC OLSON

In late 1972, we were asked by lawyers from the Washington, D.C., firm of Arnold and Porter to consult on the psychological effects of the Buffalo Creek, West Virginia, flood disaster. At that time a case claiming damages for "psychic impairment" was being prepared on behalf of more than 600 people who had survived the February 1972 flood. The flood resulted from massive corporate negligence in the form of dumping coal waste in a mountain stream in a manner that created an artificial dam, resulting in increasingly dangerous water pressure behind it. After several days of rain the dam gave way, and a massive, moving wall of "black water" (containing the coal waste), more than 30 feet high, roared through the narrow creek hollow, devastating the mining hamlets along the 17-mile valley. In less than an hour the water

This chapter appears in abridged form by special permission of The William Alanson White Psychiatric Foundation, Inc. from *Psychiatry*, 1976, *39*, 1–18. Copyright 1976 by The William Alanson White Psychiatric Foundation, Inc.

ROBERT JAY LIFTON • City University of New York, John Jay College, New York, New York 10019. **ERIC OLSON** • Sven Rinmansgaten, 3 TR/S-11237, Stockholm, Sweden.

reached the foot of the hollow at Man, West Virginia, and in that time 125 people were killed and nearly 5,000 made homeless.

The ensuing days and weeks after the flood constituted what Kai Erikson called a second trauma, the deepening awareness that the fabric of community life had been irreparably destroyed.[1] The claim of "psychic impairment" in the lawsuit against the Pittston Company, whose Buffalo Mining Company subsidiary had built the dam, was based on the effects on the survivors' psychological well-being of the flood experience itself as well as the destruction of the community. The lawsuit was settled out of court in August 1974 for 13.5 million dollars, approximately half of which was based on "psychic impairment."

In connection with our consultation in the case we made, together and individually, five trips to Buffalo Creek between April 1973 and August 1974 and have conducted a total of 43 interviews involving 22 Buffalo Creek survivors. In addition we have talked with several ministers and volunteer workers in the area and read through the extensive documentation of the disaster compiled by a variety of observers and professional consultants working with the survivors.

The psychological impact of the disaster has been so extensive that no one in Buffalo Creek has been unaffected. The overwhelming evidence is that everyone exposed to the Buffalo Creek disaster has experienced some or all of the following manifestations of the general constellation of the survivor.[2]

Death Imprint and Death Anxiety

The first category of these survivor patterns is that of the *death imprint* and related *death anxiety*. The death imprint consists of memories and images of the disaster, invariably associated with death, dying, and massive destruction. These memories were still extremely vivid during interviews conducted 30 months after the flood, so that one can speak of them as *indelible images*. The memories of destruction were all-encompassing, so that a sense very close to the feeling that "it was the end of time" was present in many survivors. As one man whom we interviewed in May 1974 put it: "Everything came to an end—just stopped. Everything was wiped out."

Over the period of our visits we could observe the extent to which the anxiety and fear associated with these images took on chronic form—fear so strong in many as to constitute permanent inner terror. The fear tends to be associated with flood and disaster, with nature and the elements, and especially with rain and water. As one man put it in May 1974:

> *When it rained hard last week it was like the past came out again. I took the family down to the cellar and [at times like this] I just know the whole flood is going to come back. . . . It's like you might step out of the trailer and get caught in something. Everytime it rains I get the feeling that it's a natural thing for the floods to come.*

In other words, what is ordinarily "unnatural" destruction has become, psychologically speaking, "natural"—what one expects to happen. The same man, like many others, is unable to sleep when it rains, because "I don't want to be caught in bed with the flood." He goes on to recognize that the fear is irrational: "Knowing that the water couldn't get to me now doesn't help." He feels compelled to "keep checking the river" and to "keep pacing the house." For water has become the enemy—"I used to love to swim, but I can't go back to water no more"—and "the weather more or less controls my thoughts."

And many others expressed similar feelings about the weather 27 months after the flood. One woman particularly troubled with insomnia stated: "When it starts raining I get afraid. I didn't use to be that way but now I am. I'm afraid of thunder and lightning." Another woman (interviewed at the same time): "I have a real scary feeling when it rains—even though there's no danger up there." And still another, greatly troubled by insomnia and general anxiety: "If it rains I get a very uneasy feeling. The clouding up now makes me feel uncomfortable."

A related symptom, also widespread, is a fear of crowds. Gatherings of large numbers of people become associated with the disaster. One man (in May 1974) told us that he avoids crowds because he imagines another disaster and "if there are 12 people in the crowd only some people would escape and some would be lost. If I was there by myself I could get away." He was expressing a characteristic feeling that his survival was a matter of luck, perhaps a fluke, and that in the grotesque competition for survival created by such a disaster he would be better off on his own. Involved here also is the shattering in the survivor of the illusion of invulnerability we carry with us in both ordinary and dangerous situations, and a related sense of having been rendered precariously vulnerable to the next threat. Another man said that he stays away from crowds because "I get nervous when I get with a crowd—all that feeling comes back," and added that "if you get around a crowd it seems like somebody will bring up the subject and I just don't like to hear it. I can't keep from crying like a baby."

Terrifying dreams, still recurring regularly 27 months after the disaster, are especially vivid expressions of death anxiety. Two such typical recurrent dreams we encountered were:

> I dream I'm in a car on a pier surrounded by muddy water—or else in a pool of muddy water. I feel like I've got to hold on to the side of the pool. If I do I'm all right. I know that I can't get out. I have to stay in it.
>
> I've never been to no funerals except the ones right after the flood. . . . In the dream there is a big crowd at the funeral—the whole family is watching. I'm being buried. I'm scared to death. I'm trying to tell them I'm alive, but they don't pay no attention. They act like I'm completely dead, but I'm trying to holler to them that I'm alive. They cover me up and lower me down, but I can see the dirt on me. I'm panicked and scared. I become violent trying to push my way through the dirt. . . . I think I'll suffocate if I don't fight my way out. I feel like I'm trying to shout that I'm alive.

In both cases the dreamer is threatened by a disaster-related form of death and must struggle desperately to remain alive. The first dream suggests being locked in a continuous struggle without being able to leave the lethal environment (the muddy pool). The second dream reflects the state of being "as-if dead"—both dead and alive—characteristic of the most severe kinds of survivor experience. Both dreams reflect the survivor's perpetually fearful anticipation. As one man put it, "Sometimes me and my wife don't go to bed at all. . . . It's hard to live under a dread all the time."

That dread, moreover, tends to become a collective family

experience in ways that further stimulate fear in each individual—as a father of four children told us in May 1974:

> *We all want to leave. . . . Me and my oldest son stayed in the house right after the flood. The boys [now ages 18 and 16] say, "I can't go to sleep in this bedroom." My youngest daughter [age 11] won't go upstairs by herself, even in the daytime. She seems afraid. The whole family seems afraid. They get most shook up when a storm comes up. Their nerves are already on edge. It don't take much to get everyone shook up. After a bad storm it's a couple days before they sleep. During the tornado warnings they were all shook up, and I wanted to go to the school [on higher ground and the place where survivors congregated after the flood].*

The tornado warnings (of April 1974) he mentions were especially traumatic to Buffalo Creek survivors, intensifying dread and reactivating the entire disaster experience. This phenomenon of reactivation contributes greatly to the survivor's sense of permanent vulnerability. As a Baptist minister explained in May 1974:

> *I told you [in a previous interview] people had quieted down a bit. But when they announced all those hurricanes people came to the church and stayed all night. . . . Just let something blow up and they flare up again.*

This diffuse, death-related anxiety comes to pervade the Buffalo Creek environment to the point of contagion. As in other overwhelming disasters (such as Hiroshima), outsiders coming in, such as mental health professionals and clergymen, describe experiencing some of the fear and dread described by people exposed to the disaster.

We may sum up this first category by saying that Buffalo Creek survivors remain haunted not just by death but by grotesque and unacceptable forms of death; feel ever vulnerable to these forms of death; and perceive their overall environment—including nature itself—as threatening and lethal rather than life-sustaining.

Death Guilt

The second category is that of *death guilt*—the survivor's sense of painful self-condemnation over having lived while others died. Survivors we spoke to 30 months after the disaster were still plagued by the feeling, however irrational, that they could or should have done something to save close relatives who perished. One of the plaintiffs, who made a series of desperate efforts to save his wife before she went under, has since experienced a mixture of preoccupation with memories of her and his failure to save her, and anger at the coal company because "they killed my wife." Psychologically the two emotions merge, and like other survivors of extreme situations, he inwardly experiences a certain amount of personal responsibility for having "killed her." Also involved is the survivor's characteristic feeling that his life was purchased at the cost of another's—that the other person's death permitted him to live, that had he died the other might have lived instead. These feelings, very widespread in Buffalo Creek, are inseparable from the death-related fears already described and are among the most painful emotions known to humankind.

Death guilt is reflected in the preoccupation of survivors with dead relatives—for example, one plaintiff's constant thoughts about his many dead cousins, and another's brooding over his dead mother, sister, and three brothers. The latter, Mr. T., in addition to his persistent feeling that he should have done something to save them, told us in May 1974 that he would still "sit and study and wonder" because "so much happened at one time," asking himself again and again: "Why didn't the family get out after they were warned?" He would conclude that "You can't ever get that answer . . . as if there's something left out, and maybe it's better that I can't figure it out." Contributing greatly to that sense is his continuous struggle to fend off a sense of guilt and responsibility for those unacceptable deaths.

Death guilt is perhaps most vivid in recurrent dreams. Some of these dreams include the reappearance of dead relatives, either in everyday situations or in uneasy reunions in which it is not clear whether they are or are not actually alive. Much more disturbing, and still frequent after 27 months, were dreams in which death guilt was more direct. The wife of Mr. T. had been unusually close to his dead mother:

I dreamed we knew the dam was going to break. In the dream Mrs. T. had a white dress on. She asked me to follow her out in the yard. She just kept

*going back into a hole that looked like a mine. I don't know why she wanted
me to come with her—she held out her hand, but I was afraid.*

The dream suggests the dreamer's sense that she should have
shared the disturbing fate—the death—of her mother-in-law.

Still more characteristic were recurrent dreams of actual disaster events or scenes resembling them in depicting grotesque
death, as described by a survivor in May 1974:

*I dreamt about the baby I found with half its face torn off and the truck full
of bodies. Sometimes in those dreams you're running, or trying to get hold of
someone to help them out of the mud. Just last week I had that dream. I woke
up pulling on my wife. After that you just can't go back to sleep. That was
about 3:00 A.M. last Friday night. There's nothing you can do at that time
of night until 7:00 or so in the morning when you see people out.*

In such dreams the survivor experiences an image of ultimate
horror—a single image that comes to exemplify his entire disaster
experience in the combination of fear, pity, and guilt that it
evokes in him. Such images are especially likely to include children or women whose grotesque death one witnessed or failed to
prevent—since in most cultures, ours included, those two groups
(especially children) are viewed as particularly helpless and vulnerable, as beings whose lives the physically stronger members of
society are particularly responsible for maintaining.

One survivor contrasted his capacity to absorb his World War
II combat experience with his total inability to deal with residual
guilt from the flood disaster, as expressed in an image of ultimate
horror involving a mother pleading with him, while herself
drowning, to save her baby:

*When I was on the battlefield in World War II I was expecting the worst,
and it didn't bother me at all like this. When my buddies got killed I knew I
was no part of their getting killed. But when the flood came I didn't have
time to help that lady and her baby who cried for help.*

He went on to explain that "feelings about not helping people
during the war went away after I came home," but those related to
the flood had stayed with him for 27 months, both in his waking
life and his dreams:

*In my dreams I never get caught in the water. What hurts is the people
calling for me to come and help them but I can't do it. The ending of the
dreams is always the same—hitting my back on the railroad cars where I hid
from the water.*

People who have gone through this kind of experience are
never quite able to forgive themselves for having survived. Another side of them, however, experiences relief and gratitude that
it was *they* who had the good fortune to survive in contrast to the
fate of those who died—a universal and all-too-human survivor
reaction that in turn intensifies their guilt. Since the emotion is so
painful, the sense of guilt may be suppressed and covered over by
other emotions or patterns, such as rage or apathy.

But whether or not suppressed, that guilt continues to create
in Buffalo Creek survivors a sense of a burden that will not lift.
They feel themselves still bound to the dead, living a half-life
devoid of pleasure and with limited vitality.

Psychic Numbing

The third category is that of *psychic numbing*—a diminished
capacity for feeling of all kinds—in the form of various manifestations of apathy, withdrawal, depression, and overall constriction
in living. Psychic numbing is perhaps the most universal response
to the disaster, and the essence of what has been called the "disaster syndrome." Partly it is an extension of the "stunned" state
experienced at the time of the flood. That state was a defense
against feeling the full impact of the overwhelming death immer-
sion. The numbing persists at Buffalo Creek because people still
need to defend themselves against the kinds of death anxiety and
death guilt discussed before. Numbing, then, is an aspect of persistent grief; of the "half-life" defined by loss, guilt, and close at
times to an almost literal identification with the dead. As one of
the plaintiffs put it: "I feel dead now. I have no energy. I sit down
and I feel numb." Survivors withdrew from groups, from activities of various kinds, from one another. They describe being
disinterested in seeing friends or in many cases in doing anything.
Even in intimate relationships their capacity for both emotional

and physical feeling—including sexual feeling—tends to be greatly diminished. Their withdrawal may be accompanied by a wide variety of psychosomatic symptoms, such as general fatigue, loss of appetite, gastrointestinal difficulties, and aches and pains and dysfunction that can involve just about any organ system. The pattern has been described in other disasters as a breakdown in the ordinary psychosomatic balance or equilibrium, resulting in what used to be called *neurasthenia*. At Buffalo Creek one can observe a vicious circle of withdrawal and abandonment—as one survivor made clear in an interview in May 1974: "I want to be left alone. Now you don't care so much about other people; it's like everything is destroyed. It's like you're left alone." That is, his sense of having been abandoned and his tendency to withdraw reinforce one another.

Very common aspects of numbing at Buffalo Creek have been such things as memory lapses, general sluggishness and unresponsiveness, and confusion about details of one's immediate surroundings and about the passage of time in general. Those lapses, as one survivor makes clear, tend to be specifically associated with the disaster: "I can remember things from 1932 to 1972 better than I can the past 2 years. This past 2 years I can't remember what I do—weeks and months just go by." Numbing or avoidance of feeling can also be expressed in overactivity. Thus one woman said of her very troubled husband: "He works all the time. He gets himself overtired. He says, 'If I just sit down I'd die.'"

Numbing is closely related to the psychological defense of denial, and people said again and again in a variety of ways: "It's hard to believe that all this happened" or "I still can't accept that it happened." Numbing and denial are sustained because of the survivor's inability to confront or work through the disaster experience. He is thus left psychologically imprisoned in death- and guilt-related conflicts that can neither be dealt with nor eliminated. Feeling stays muted; psychological pain remains silent; and life experience in general is drastically reduced.

In recent years, authorities on disaster have come to recognize that psychic numbing occurs not only in survivors but in observers and evaluators of disaster. Medical and psychological professionals have been known to experience strong tendencies to ward off anxieties of their own around death and guilt aroused by their contact with survivors, which has in turn led them to deny the existence of these emotions and ignore or underestimate the psychological cost of disaster.

Counterfeit Nurturing and Unfocused Rage

A fourth category is that of *impaired human relationships,* and consists especially of *conflict over need or nurturing as well as strong suspicion of the counterfeit.* So much of their lives having been so suddenly and totally destroyed, survivors feel themselves in great need of love and support but at the same time unable to accept as genuine whatever affection or nurturing may be offered to them. While some have been able to help one another, there have also been instances of breakdown of the closest human bonds. One such case is that of two of the plaintiffs, a young married couple. Both remember their relationship prior to the flood as "calm and peaceful and loving." Now, according to the wife, her husband is "touchy about everything. Things with me and him are at a kind of halt, a standstill. . . . Something is always bothering him—it's constant—it never seems to stop." They very rarely have sexual relations or even sleep in the same room. The husband's perception is that life in general, since he lost many relatives in the flood, has consisted of "one aggravation after another." He says that his wife "has no desire for me. She's hateful and doesn't want to turn toward me." Yet each realized that the other was suffering. The wife said of the husband that "he's still grieving—he cries out in his sleep. He still sees pictures of his relatives. He still says he'd like to kill Jim V. [the former manager of the Pittston mining operation at Buffalo Creek] because Jim said the dam wouldn't break." And then she added:

> *I still grieve too. It hurts me awful bad that you can't walk down the road and see them [she too was very close to her husband's relatives]. Sometimes I think I see one of them. It hurts when you suddenly realize that they're dead.*

And she could conclude: "A big part of my touchiness does seem to be related to my grieving." Both, in other words, were so enmeshed in unrelieved grief reactions—unresolved death anxiety and death guilt—that neither could reach out to or even trust the other. They would go through brief periods of slight improvement in their relationship only to find the postdisaster pattern of mutual estrangement and distrust reasserting itself and still predominating 27 months after the flood.

Survivors have special need for family closeness but also a particularly strong tendency to grate on one another in a way that intensifies each other's resentment and fear. As one man put it, "My kids seem to be doing all right, but when I go to pieces now they go to pieces too."

Over the period since the disaster, the problem of anger and unfocused or unexpressed rage has increased. One woman, talking about the problem, said: "It's like that all over—everybody is angry and touchy." Often the touchiness is expressed toward fellow survivors in the various forms of envy, jealousy, and resentment that have been frequently observed following disasters and are characteristic of people who feel themselves weakened and victimized. At public meetings or in casual conversations, even seemingly positive suggestions for better help and support are sometimes received with suspicion—either because they are reminders of weakness or because of a tendency among survivors, bound as they are to the dead, to view any sign of energy and vitality on the part of fellow survivors—any strong affirmation of life—as somehow inappropriate or immoral.

But the hostility tends to be very diffuse, and many survivors told us of the frequent experience since the flood of violent impulses toward anyone who irritated them, and of enormous intensification of whatever difficulty they had experienced in the past in controlling their tempers. One of the plaintiffs put the matter characteristically:

> It used to be I could control my temper. Now my temper just goes. I just can't control it. When some little thing happens that seems unfair I get touchy.

And he added a bit later in the interview: "Since I lost my wife I can't get what I want. Nothing satisfies me." Anger, that is, continues to cover over grief and loss. And another male survivor: "I'm 46 years old. I've never been in jail. But if I could have got to some of those officials I probably would have hurt somebody. . . . I still get angry at times. I get all blurry and it flares up real quick. Before the flood if anything came up it seems like I could sit down and think and work things out." The quotation suggests the difficulty survivors have in finding adequate targets for their anger. Many select the former manager but seem to sense even as they do so that he as an individual is not an adequate target. Nor is it easy to personify an alternative target—as another man makes clear: "I can't say I feel angry at the people who built the dam because I've never seen one of them. . . . And I've never seen Jim V., the general manager, since the flood." A good deal of anger is directed toward the mine company, but it, too, ends in frustration:

> *There's a lot of people that's angry. They just don't care because what they worked on for years was completely destroyed. Then Pittston offers you just a little for all that. It makes you angrier than hell. To think they could treat old people that way; it makes you want to go out and fight somebody.*

This inability to find a satisfying outlet or target tends to lead people either to suppress their anger or express instead their continuous grief—as another survivor explained in May 1974:

> *I feel angry at the coal company, but I don't feel like taking it out on someone. When the kids come in late I get upset, but the kids don't cause any trouble. If my wife gets upset she sits and cries. She doesn't get angry.*

Some come to recognize, as one woman did, that anger too can be a painful burden:

> *I don't like to feel so angry. I don't like to lose control. I don't even like to talk about the road [a new road being built that angers many people]. The anger, a lot of it, is still there.*

Later in the interview the same woman added: "Anger, if not vented in the right way, will only hurt yourself. . . . The Church of God has helped me to control my anger. I feel I can cope more. If I let myself get pressured then I get upset." Generally speaking, the fundamentalist religion that most of the survivors have some connection with tends to teach that anger is bad and is not a proper response.

Thirty months after the disaster, survivors are left with diffuse anger they themselves disapprove of, rage they cannot express, and an overall sense that everything (and everyone) is suspect and that life itself has been rendered counterfeit.

Inner Form: The Struggle for Significance

The fifth category has to do with the significance or meaning surrounding a disaster, the capacity of survivors *to give their death encounter significant inner form or formulation.* At issue here is the survivor's capacity to find sufficient explanation for his experience so as to be able to resolve the inner conflicts described under the other four categories. Only by coming to some such meaning and significance is he able to find meaning and significance in the rest of his life. In many disasters, survivors are able to find some comfort, or at least resignation, in the deep conviction that what happened was a matter of God's will or of some larger power that no mortal could influence. No such comfort or resignation can be found among the people of Buffalo Creek. Some of them have attempted to understand the experience within a religious context, and in a church service attended by one of us (E. O.), the minister (not a survivor himself) declared almost boastfully that he had predicted the flood as a punishment for sin in the valley. Survivors we interviewed did not express any such concept but could well be unconsciously affected by a related sense that their own evil or sinfulness had something to do with their miserable fate. That feeling would be consistent with one interpretation of their religion and with inner feelings about disaster and illness prevalent not only in Christian societies but in many non-Western cultures as well. Mostly, however, the Buffalo Creek survivors are left without any acceptable or consoling explanation for the disaster. Instead they expressed a bitter awareness that the disaster was man-made and a conviction that God had nothing to do with it. Those feelings have become increasingly intense and unshakeable. Some, for instance, make an angry point about terminology, in bitter response to public statements that God's will was involved—as the following quotations from three different people suggest:

I call this a disaster, not a flood. This wasn't a natural flood.

A few individuals in charge of the coal company are responsible for this. God didn't put the dam up there.

They call it a flood. I call it a dam that Pittston built up there that broke loose. . . . Governor Moore said it was an act of God but God wasn't up on that slate dump with a bulldozer.

Similar feelings were expressed to us by a Freewill Baptist minister: "I believe the dam was made by man, not by God, and it collapsed because it was not made right." The same man, able to observe large numbers of survivors closely, concluded that because of the disaster "people are much more suspicious of God's justice." That last statement is of considerable importance because it suggests the extent to which people can no longer trust even a deity to put the moral world back in order. Precisely such a sense of the disruption of the moral universe occurs characteristically in the most severe forms of disaster, and is evident in every single survivor interviewed in Buffalo Creek. That sense of moral inversion—of wrongdoing going unpunished and responsibility unacknowledged while innocent victims undergo pain and suffering—further prevents psychological resolution and leaves people embittered and confused. They remain locked in their death anxiety, survivor guilt, numbing, and impaired human relationships, bound to the disaster itself and to its destructive psychological influences.

Still, many in Buffalo Creek continue to struggle to overcome their despair. One woman put it simply (in May 1974): "I just want to start living again." And a number of survivors expressed related aspirations toward restored vitality and renewal—whether through moving away from Buffalo Creek, adopting a child, being helped by family members, or in a few cases through medical, psychiatric, or psychological assistance. But many of the survivors, because of their limited educational and social background and equally limited financial resources, lack the capacity to take any significant steps toward renewal. Moreover, there are very limited community and professional facilities in the Buffalo Creek area. Ideally, survivors should have extensive community rebuilding in which they could have an active voice.

Survivors' overall psychological health could also be somewhat improved by any outcome in the situation which recognized their suffering, recognized also the responsibility of those whose actions or inaction caused the disaster, gave people who wished to leave the opportunity to do so, gave those who wished to rebuild on their land the opportunity to do so, and in a general sense conveyed to survivors the sense that at least a step had been taken to put the moral world back in order. Also of great psychological importance would be the capacity of people to embark upon a collective "survivor mission," consisting of actions or policies that might provide something of a sense of meaning and "survivor wisdom" from a situation that was otherwise totally destructive. Survivors of Hiroshima, for instance, have been able to benefit somewhat from the sense that conveying the horrors of their experience to the outside world could enable man to learn something about the effects of nuclear weapons and possibly avoid using them again. And at an individual level, parents whose children die of leukemia can derive solace from a "survivor mission" of energetically supporting scientific research that might prevent such tragedies in the future. Buffalo Creek survivors could, in a parallel way, derive some benefit from contributing to policies and programs that would insure greater safety and protection for mining areas and miners and prevent such disasters from occurring again.

References

1. See Kai T. Erikson, *Loss of communality at Buffalo Creek*, and James L. Titchener and Frederic T. Kapp, *Family and character change in Buffalo Creek*, both presented at the American Psychiatric Association meetings, Anaheim, California, in May 1975, at a symposium, "Disaster at Buffalo Creek: Studies of 160 Families," jointly sponsored with the American Psychoanalytic Association. We worked closely with Erikson and Titchener throughout.
2. Lifton, R. J. *Death in life*. New York: Random House, 1968.

23

Disaster

The Helper's Perspective

BEVERLY RAPHAEL, BRUCE SINGH, and
LESLEY BRADBURY

At the time of major disaster, as at the time of personal crisis, attention is directed toward those who are most obviously and acutely affected by the tragic events. They are defined as "victims," and those who offer them assistance are seen as the "helpers." The psychological stress, trauma, and grief experienced by the victims are obvious, and morbidity is revealed in many studies.[1]

This chapter seeks to draw attention to the stresses experienced by the "helpers" and the needs they may have for psychological support and preventive services. The writers' conclusions are drawn from personal experience in disaster work; discussions and communications with disaster personnel from a wide range of services and disasters; and questionnaire and interview responses from workers involved in the Granville rail disaster.

BEVERLY RAPHAEL and BRUCE SINGH • Faculty of Medicine, University of Newcastle, New South Wales, 2308, Australia. **LESLEY BRADBURY** • Repatriation General Hospital, Sydney, Australia.

Roles of Helpers in a Disaster

Short, in a most useful paper, delineated very clearly the ways in which certain popular images produce a polarization of two clear kinds of roles: "victims" who are seen as resourceless, weak, helpless, and "helpers" who are seen as being resourceful, strong, powerful.[2]

"Helpers" may be involved in many different aspects of assistance. Typically there are (a) disaster control and direct rescue operations; (b) medical tasks—triage and treatment of dead and injured; (c) information and communications; and (d) support services for injured and relatives.

Persons who undertake such helping roles at the time of disaster may either have specific training gearing them to their tasks (for example, police, ambulance, rescue squads, and so on) or may be spontaneous or voluntary workers who offer their services in response to the crisis.

Our work in this field and contact with those who have worked in many different disaster situations leads us to believe that such disaster work has high psychological impact; that, for most workers, it is at least temporarily stressful; and that, for some, it may lead to long-term psychological difficulties. In fact, the "helpers" themselves may become the other, unrecognized victims at the time of disaster.

Immediate Psychological Reactions of Helpers

The first response of all those in whose community a disaster occurs is usually that of shock and disbelief, a sense of overwhelming unreality. The awfulness of the death, loss, and destruction rapidly mobilizes a response of "we must do something"—"what can we do to help?" Persons who have specific and purposeful tasks and who are able to carry these out feel reassured and positive. There may be a sense of heightened involvement, even elation. This "high" of involvement and activity appears to drive people to the limits of endurance, to strength, power and courage. It may lead disaster workers to stay at their posts or tasks well beyond the time of their normal functioning and sometimes beyond that of their optimal performance. They may refuse to hand over to others equally experienced, feeling they are the only ones who can see this through. The person so involved sometimes describes a sense of being "split"—one part carrying out the tasks with no exhaustion, the other taking in, but not responding to, the emotionally draining and distressing sights revealed by the rescue tasks.

When practical difficulties prevent the worker from carrying out roles and tasks for which he was trained, frustration and helplessness may become disturbing feelings. After the Granville disaster, many workers, particularly those involved in direct rescue operations, described the enormous sense of helplessness and frustration engendered by their inability to use certain equipment because of fear of fire; the impossibility of moving the giant concrete slab that crushed the carriages; and the despair of knowing that there were trapped persons who could not be reached. Frustration appears to be the overwhelming experience in such circumstances. The feeling of helplessness is distressing when those involved see the magnitude of what must be done and realize that it cannot be achieved.

If those involved believe themselves to be unprepared, inadequately trained, or possessing insufficient knowledge, helplessness is linked to a sense of personal inadequacy. This may lead to prolonged and guilty recrimination after the event and may even interfere with their capacity to carry out routine work. These feelings seem to be experienced by many different categories of helpers regardless of their degree of training.

A further group who experience difficulties are all those people who come with their desperate wish and longing to help in a variety of ways, for whom no helper role exists. These may offer holidays, blankets, toys, child care for the affected—yet their offers may be inappropriate for the needs of victims at the time. Such people are frequently left with futile, resentful feelings, and an unwillingness to offer help again.

Anger is another early response which is particularly prominent in man-made disasters. This anger, which is initially directed at the agencies seen as responsible for causing the disaster, may generalize into many areas of the helper's life, especially work and family, as he takes up the cause of the "victims" with whom he has been so closely involved.

Reactions to Encounters with Death and Destruction

Most major disasters are so classed because of the death and destruction they encompass. All helpers are likely to have some confrontation with these either at close quarters or through contact with bereaved families.

The majority of workers who are directly involved in contact with dead and injured bodies are distressed by the death and mutilation. This is especially so when young children are involved as in Aberfan, or when the bodies are decomposed or disintegrated so as to bear little resemblance to a whole person. From Aberfan to Mount Erebus, workers relate stories of plastic bags containing parts of bodies, impossible to identify—pieces of bones and teeth and charred disfigured remains. Workers at the Granville disaster site recalled the crushed bodies revealed after the slab was finally lifted looking like "sardines in a can . . . squashed like a pizza."

Many emotional experiences may be triggered by this, such as the awareness of one's own mortality—that one, too, could end like this; the pain of possible loss of one's own loved ones in this way; relief that one did not die or lose a loved one this time. Sometimes this may be associated both with survivor elation and with survivor guilt—pleasure at one's survival, yet guilt that one could even momentarily feel pleasure at such a time. Vicariously, too, one can see and come close to death yet not be "caught" by it, and a sense of personal invulnerability may arise.

There may be an even more direct threat to one's own life—for instance, rescue workers were in danger during their work at Granville when the concrete slab shifted as they struggled beneath it. This threat to life and awareness of such nearness to massive death may leave frightening residual anxieties which have to be worked through subsequently. On the other hand, many workers may reevaluate their lives, seeing more meaning and value in their relationships and experience. They see the whole of life as being more precious, valuing each person more, and material possessions less.

Sometimes the painful aspects of these encounters with death are locked away—to be released at another time or with some minor trigger. One worker spoke of how, on seeing some tomato sauce a week later, the memories of blood and destruction welled up again and could be dealt with. Another could release painful memories about the bodies when a crushed doll's head triggered memories of a body difficult to identify because of similar crushing injury.

It seems especially painful to recall the massive confrontation with death. One body or two can be encompassed, but, as workers in many different disaster situations have commented, a morgue full of cold, gray, dead people is not easily forgotten.

Empathy and Identification

Whatever tasks helpers may be involved in at the time of disaster, their empathy for, and identification with, the dead, the injured, and their families enable even those who might at other times be seen as "hardened" to become gentle, supportive, and caring. Most workers whose traditional roles give them unpopular public images (for example, police) may be distressed by a stereotyped view held of them suggesting that they do not feel for the families affected, when, in fact, their distress and concern is great. Often the empathy and identification lead to special bonds with the "victims," which may continue long after the disaster is over.

Grief

The end product of these immediate responses to the encounter with death, the empathy and identification, is inevitably some level of grief. The worker grieves for those who died, for his community, and for himself and the losses he will one day suffer. Nearly all workers experience this grief personally sooner or later—a time when they cry for their disaster. For many men this is a very private time, for the social expectations may make it difficult for them to acknowledge their emotion, whereas women workers may be more sanctioned in their release, although seen as vulnerable because of it. It is important that this need for emotional release is fully recognized by workers and their support systems, and seen as a positive step in adjustment to the human side of disasters.

Coming to Terms with the Experience

Most helpers come to terms with the experience in multiple and individual ways.

1. Initially, the traumatic memories and dreams about the disaster usually intrude a great deal. Gradually they lessen in frequency and emotional intensity, especially as the emotions they trigger are released and cleared. Some workers wake for many nights with terrifying dreams or experience scenes of the disaster in slow motion. For some, these experiences do not lessen in intensity with time and support, and they are left with a "traumatic neurosis" which interferes with longer term adjustment. In this type of disorder, dreams and memories persist, and other psychosomatic and stress symptoms may appear; there may be irritability, sleep disturbance, bouts of anxiety and depression, and a falloff in interpersonal relationships and work.

2. The disaster stress experience is shared with others, talked through, put outside oneself and reintegrated, and emotional release of the painful experiences is gradually attained. Many workers are supported to this end by the debriefing sessions held by their teams. Such debriefing may have a strictly practical orientation (for example, geared toward improving equipment and techniques, and report writing) but usually some psychological catharsis occurs. Many a wise team leader encourages this specifically, sometimes in a facilitatory group so that much of the experience can be dealt with and set aside. Teams who undertook active psychological debriefing after the Granville disaster found it, for the most part, helpful in their subsequent adjustment.

There is often a strong sense of really being able to share the experience only with those who also have gone through it, and hence there is a special facilitatory effect of the shared group experience.

Others find benefit from sharing and talking about the experience with members of their families. This, too, is important for families, for they need to be especially aware of the subtle disturbance caused by the disaster experience, and may feel cut off if none of it is shared with them. Many workers have suggested that, but for their spouses' special understanding, divorce might have resulted from being psychologically disturbed at such a time.

3. For some, there is need for professional help to talk about and to integrate into their own experience of the world the enormity of death and disaster. It is often difficult for workers to seek and accept this, as they are seen as the strong ones who must help and support others. So difficult has this been for some disaster workers that denial has persisted, with a sense of shame and failure. The help that has been so desperately needed has not been obtained, and long-term consequences of depression and decompensation have resulted. The levels of such morbidity are difficult to define, but our studies have suggested they are not insignificant. Most of those involved in a disaster, "victims" or "helpers," rise to great human heights, but they may also be stressed by this intense experience; in the days and weeks that follow, psychological understanding and support can facilitate the adjustment process.

ACKNOWLEDGMENT

Grateful acknowledgment is made to all those people and organizations from many disasters, who have shared their experiences to make this paper possible.

References

1. Kinston, W., & Rosser, R. Disaster: Effects on mental and physical state. *Journal of Psychosomatic Research*, 1974, *18*, 437.
2. Short, P. "Victims" and "helpers." In R. L. Heathcote & B. G. Thom (Eds.), *Proceedings of a symposium on natural hazards in Australia.* Canberra: Australian Academy of Science, 1979.

X

Coping With Unusual Crises
Violence and Terrorism

With rising crime rates and the worldwide spread of terrorism, growing numbers of people live in fear of victimization or actually become victims. The threat of violence or bodily assault typically arises suddenly and unpredictably. The abrupt fright and immediate danger of physical injury or death create an acute crisis. In their attempts to manage such an event and its aftermath, victims often progress through three stages of reactions.

In the first, or *impact*, stage, individuals feel helpless and chaotic and describe a sense of disrupted personal integrity. They often seek reassurance and direction in order to establish a provisional equilibrium. The second, or *recoil*, phase entails a long-term struggle to face the personal violation that was experienced and to overcome the vulnerability, guilt, anger, and other complex emotions that were aroused. Finally, there is the *reorganization phase* in which the survivor assimilates the painful experience and achieves a new psychological balance.[1] Victims whose body is penetrated (as occurs in rape or a stabbing), who believe they are going to be killed, are victimized by someone they know, or are attacked in a place they consider safe (as when an intruder attacks a victim in a bedroom), experience the most psychological distress and thus may have more difficulty coming to terms with their victimization.[2]

The victims' plight often is mirrored by members of their family who share similar feelings. Family members may find it

331

hard to comfort the victim because of their own reactions to the crisis. Strained family relationships and communication breakdowns often result. For instance, husbands and boyfriends of rape victims may encounter fear, jealousy, a sense of loss, and guilt for failing to protect their partner. Conflicts can arise when the man resolves his feelings more quickly than his partner and then resents her "dependency" and continued search for comfort and forgiveness. In turn, the woman may see her partner as insensitive. In other instances, distressed family members may blame the victim for not taking proper precautions, such as when parents hold their adolescent daughters responsible for being raped.

Family members of murder victims face unique problems in working through their grief. They may agonize over the pain and suffering the victim experienced before dying, feel responsible in some way for the murder, and be unable to find meaning in such a sudden, senseless death. Trials, parole hearings, and unsympathetic reactions from the community add to the family's stress and hinder accommodation to their loss.[3] Months after the murder of his wife and young son, one man made a special effort to read the autopsy and police reports. The detailed information about his wife and son's deaths helped him overcome his grief. Other families of murder victims obtain a renewed sense of purpose by becoming active in organizations such as Parents of Murdered Children.[3] (For a discussion of the reactions of children who witness a murder and their experiences with the legal system, see Pynoos & Eth.[5])

Unlike adults, children do not have the benefit of a lifetime of experience to help them cope with victimization, and so the traumatic effects may linger. In Chapter 3, we saw the lasting impact that the death of a parent can have on children. In the first article, Lenore C. Terr provides another example of the longterm adjustment that children may require following a life crisis. Terr discusses the lingering psychological consequences that the Chowchilla schoolchildren experienced after being kidnapped. The children reported cognitive disturbances and extreme fear during the event and continued to dread further trauma long afterward. They were afraid of mundane events—cars passing, the dark, the wind, and being left alone—and saw them as potential warnings of another kidnapping. Most of the children lost their aura of personal invulnerability and naive sense of trust in the world.

As with the Buffalo Creek disaster victims (see Chapter 22), the children's tensions were expressed in repetitive dreams of their own death. They also identified "predictive" omens, that is, they reinterpreted events that occurred just before the kidnapping as warning signs. In this way, the children tried to establish some retrospective control over the event and understand why it had happened, or how they might have avoided it. The children also reconstructed the kidnap experience in their play and re-enacted the fears, fantasies, or actual behavior that occurred just before or during it. Although they showed some aftereffects of the trauma 4 years later, the use of these active coping strategies probably helped many of the children to resolve their fears and maintain their good school performance. In general, children who initially were physically and emotionally healthier showed better long-term adaptation, as did those who were located in well-functioning and more socially integrated families.[8]

Although most adults are better equipped than children to handle the trauma of being victimized, they, too, may require a lengthy period of adjustment. In the second article, Ann Wolbert Burgess and Lynda Lytle Holmstrom discuss the effects of rape victims' adaptive and maladaptive responses on their recovery. Some rape victims consciously put thoughts of the rape out of their mind, whereas a contrasting strategy—dramatization—helped other victims to cope. By overexpressing their thoughts and feelings about the rape, some women were able to relieve their tension. Other victims handled their tension by finding a reason for the rape, such as blaming it on the fact that the rapist was sick or holding themselves responsible for being in a vulnerable situation such as hitchhiking. Dale Miller and Carol Porter[4] note that the victim gains a sense of control by identifying actions that may have led to the negative event (as with the "omens" noted by the Chowchilla children). Some women minimized the rape by comparing themselves to victims who had worse experiences or by believing they were lucky not to have been killed or forced into perverse acts.

In general, rape victims who assessed themselves positively, had high self-esteem, and coped by using active cognitive and behavioral strategies recovered most rapidly. Women moved or traveled to escape reminders of the place where the rape occurred. They also changed telephone numbers and thus acquired some measure of environmental control. Other women gained intellectual control by reading or writing about rape or assisting other victims at rape crisis centers. Supportive counseling may help women learn to manage rape-related fears and anxieties. (For a discussion of a stress inoculation program for rape victims, see Veronen & Kilpatrick.[9])

Victims can cope effectively in many ways. They may become more engaged in their work and other structured pursuits or involve themselves in activities related to the crime, such as phoning the police and following the progress of the investigation. Cognitively, victims may work through their feelings by remembering and dreaming about the details of the event, reliving it and reconstructing it in their mind, and repeatedly discussing it with a comforting friend. Victims also may release their pent-up anger through fantasies and dreams of revenge.[1] Burglary victims, like rape victims, try to regain control over their environment. They engage in "security behavior," such as buying increased insurance and installing new locks and alarm systems and being careful to use them. In general, individuals who assume some responsibility for being victimized or who feel that there is something they can do to prevent it from happening again tend to have fewer problems.

Terrorism is a particularly vexing crime because there is little an individual can do to escape seemingly random hostage taking, hijacking, and bombing. In the third article, Frank Ochberg describes the harrowing experience of Gerard Vaders, a newspaper editor, who was held hostage on a train for 13 days along with some of his fellow citizens. A group of South Moluccan terrorists captured the train in an attempt to win independence for their homeland. Vaders initially tried to keep his emotions under control, appraise the threat, and prepare physically and mentally for what might ensue. From the beginning he coped by assuming the role of journalist: he decided to risk taking notes during his captivity. In this familiar role he was able to focus his attention and maintain professional self-esteem.

By the second day, Vaders expected to be executed. He was

tied like a curtain in a doorway of the train for 7 hours and told, "Your time has come." So he prepared himself for death, reviewed his life, and asked that he be allowed to give a fellow hostage a final message for his family. The terrorists listened as he spoke openly about difficulties in his family and his feeling that he had failed as a human being. During this time the terrorists came to know Vaders as a person; this probably was the reason they spared his life. As the days passed, he began to experience the Stockholm syndrome in that he came to feel some sympathy for the terrorists.

After his release, Vaders lost weight, suffered from abdominal symptoms, and temporarily drank and smoked more. Relationships with his family underwent significant changes. Vaders's daughter found it hard to cope with the criticism to which her father was subjected as a result of stories he wrote chastising the government. But he strengthened his alliance with his estranged wife, and they considered reconciliation. One year after the incident, Vaders was functioning well in his job and had joined a national committee to help set policies for handling terrorism in his country. (For a personal account of the experiences of an Iranian hostage and his family, see Rosen & Rosen.[6])

A major psychological task of recovering hostages is to accept new information about themselves and the world. They may need to come to terms with resentment toward their government's policies and the positive feelings they develop for their captors. Survivors also need to resolve guilt feelings that stem from believing that they failed to live up to the expectations of their peers, and that they took cowardly actions or lost their nerve while in captivity. Hostages can face their feelings more easily if society sanctions their actions. Eric Shaw notes that the Iranian hostages' good adjustment can be attributed to the fact that the American people gave them much support and treated them as national heroes when they returned home.[7] When the healing sanction of society is absent, as was the case with the Vietnam veterans, adjustment can be painful and prolonged (see Chapter 27).

References

1. Bard, M., & Sangrey, D. Things fall apart: Victims in crisis. *Evaluation and Change,* Special issue, 1980, 28–35.

2. Everstein, D. S., & Everstein, L. *People in crisis: Strategic therapeutic interventions.* New York: Brunner/Mazel, 1983.
3. Magee, D. *What murder leaves behind: The victim's family.* New York: Dodd, Mead & Co., 1983.
4. Miller, D., & Porter, C. Self-blame in victims of violence. *Journal of Social Issues,* 1983, *39,* 139–152.
5. Pynoos, R. S., & Eth, S. The child as witness to homicide. *Journal of Social Issues,* 1984, *40,* 87–108.
6. Rosen, B., & Rosen, B., with Feifer, G. *The destined hour: The hostage crisis and one family's ordeal.* Garden City, N.Y.: Doubleday, 1982.
7. Shaw, E. Political hostages: Sanction and the recovery process. In L. Z. Freedman & Y. Alexander (Eds.), *Perspectives on terrorism.* Wilmington, Del.: Scholarly Resources, 1983.
8. Terr, L. Chowchilla revisited: The effects of psychic trauma four years after a school-bus kidnapping. *American Journal of Psychiatry,* 1983, *140,* 1543–1550.
9. Veronen, L. J., & Kilpatrick, D. G. Stress management for rape victims. In D. Meichenbaum & M. E. Jaremko (Eds.), *Stress reduction and prevention.* New York: Plenum Press, 1983.

24

Psychic Trauma in Children

Observations Following the Chowchilla School-Bus Kidnapping

LENORE C. TERR

The Chowchilla school-bus kidnapping commanded international attention. All 26 children (age range, 5–14 years) who enrolled in the Alview Dairyland summer school disappeared for 27 hours, and they eventually escaped from their captors. After their return the children disclosed that their school bus had been stopped by a van blocking the road, three masked men had taken over the bus at gunpoint, and they had been transferred to two blackened, boarded-over vans in which they were driven about for 11 hours. They were then transferred into a "hole" (actually a buried truck trailer), and the kidnappers covered the truck trailer with earth. The children were buried in the hole for 16 hours until 2 of the oldest and strongest boys (ages 10 and 14 years) dug them out. By then the kidnappers had left the vicinity.

Upon return to Chowchilla the children and their parents

This chapter appears in abridged form from *American Journal of Psychiatry*, 1981, *138*, 14–19. Copyright 1981, the American Psychiatric Association. Reprinted by permission.

LENORE C. TERR • 450 Sutter Street, San Francisco, California 94108.

were bombarded with questions and attention from the news media. Personnel from the local community mental health center talked with the superintendent of schools, but they did not interview the children individually. A meeting was arranged for the parents and some of the interested children, and at the meeting a mental health center physician told the parents that he predicted only 1 of the 26 children would be emotionally affected by the experience. Partly because no parent was willing to admit that his or her child was the 1 in 26, there was a lag period of 5 months before the parents asked for help for their children.

By November 1976, however, some parents had become intensely concerned about their children's emotional reactions, and they disclosed this concern in an article, "Chowchilla: The Bitterness Lingers" in the *Fresno Bee!* Dr. Romulo Gonzales, a Fresno child psychiatrist who knew of my interest in research on psychic trauma, forwarded the article to me, and I phoned one of the parents who had been quoted. She responded at once to my offer of limited crisis treatment and a research study.

I met initially with a small group of parents and eventually interviewed each of the 23 child victims who had remained in Chowchilla, as well as one or both parents. I did not interview the school-bus driver or the kidnappers because I wished to "see" this traumatic event from only the children's point of view. Verbal and signed consent was obtained from the parents, and each child was told of the research and treatment objectives of the interviews.

A detailed review of my Chowchilla findings and theoretical speculations has been published.[2] In this short summary I present and discuss the findings from the Chowchilla study that have not been noted or emphasized in earlier literature on psychic trauma. I discuss the children's initial signs of traumatic disruption, repetitive phenomena, and fears. For the purposes of this study I have used Freud's 1920 definition of *psychic trauma,* "an extensive breach being made in the protective shield against stimuli."[3]

Surprisingly little research has been done in the past 50 years on the psychodynamic effects of pure psychic trauma, particularly without the contamination of death or guilt. Perhaps one reason is that very few group situations like the Chowchilla kidnapping have arisen in which individuals were exposed to sudden extreme anxiety and returned entirely unharmed.

In this study each child was interviewed for at least 1 hour (many saw me for 2 to 3 hours), and one or both parents were interviewed 1 hour or more. Every child showed signs of the emotional effects of psychic trauma. The children's ages quoted in the examples were their ages at the time of the kidnapping; the children's names have been changed.

Initial Signs of Traumatic Disruption

Omens

During and shortly after the kidnapping several children thought back to a specific event before the kidnapping. This prior event together with the trauma of the kidnapping became a complex that often determined the children's personality changes, future fears, and reenactments.

For example, the morning of the kidnapping Sheila, who was 11 years old, had argued bitterly with her mother. She wanted to skip school that day, but her mother would not let her stay home. Sheila left her mother with the parting statement, "You're the meanest mother in the world!" Sheila did not consciously think about her "parting shot" during the kidnapping episode, yet it became indelibly associated with her perception of trauma. Her mother stated, "She slams into my bedroom pouting, saying, 'Mom makes me do everything. Mom doesn't care about me.'" Her mother overheard Sheila telling her 5-year-old sister, who was not kidnapped, "Mom is going to tear my ears off!" Sheila was unaware of a link between her accusations of her mother after the kidnapping and her remark to her mother the morning of the kidnapping. Her personality had changed from that of a sweet, slightly bossy child to an angry, obstinate individual.

Bob, age 14, was one of the boys who dug the children out. His mother drove him home each day from summer school. However, on the morning of the kidnapping Bob dawdled so much in getting ready for school that his mother ordered him to take the bus home. Thus, the kidnapping inadvertently became the "punishment." Bob now feels that he was placed on the bus by "chance" in order to help the children escape. He is acknowledged by almost all the children as the hero of the incident. He has mentally reversed the "punishment" into the "privilege" of heroism.

Bob indulged in a dangerously inappropriate episode of heroism 18 months after the kidnapping. One weekend day a strange vehicle parked near Bob's family home, and his parents asked him to check who was there. A few minutes later his parents heard shouts outside in an Oriental language. They rushed out and discovered that Bob had shot his BB gun at a Japanese tourist whose car had broken down just beyond their property. Bob had indelibly associated the privilege of heroism with the fear of strange vehicles (he recalled that the kidnapping had begun with a strange van, seemingly "in trouble," blocking the road). This time Bob was not going to wait to be kidnapped; instead he shot the tourist to protect his family. Luckily, the man was not seriously injured.

Johnny, 11, had taken part in a class play the day of the kidnapping. He played the part of Samuel Adams in a production entitled, ironically, "We Must Be Free." After mentioning the play in his interview Johnny followed with the joke, "A guy has a lucky ring; [he] looks at it and falls into a manhole." Johnny's association of the ironic play title to the trauma itself was one factor in the inappropriate clownishness he exhibited for at least 8 months after the kidnapping. During the traumatic event Johnny also thought back to a movie he had seen with his father, "Dirty Harry." His father had asked him during a scene in which a school bus is commandeered by an escaping criminal, "What would you do if that happened to you?" Johnny felt he had been given a warning he had failed to heed, and he spent much of the year after the kidnapping year building his strength so that he would be prepared for the next time.

Johnny's sister, Jackie, who was 9 years old, was also worried about an omen during the kidnapping. On the school bus Jackie usually sat with her own friends, not with Johnny. During the kidnapping she consciously and repeatedly thought about why they chose to sit apart. In her interview 6 months after the kidnapping Jackie contemplated,

Most of the kids went with their sisters, but Johnny was up front. I was bothered because I wasn't with Johnny. I think about it mostly at night before going to sleep. That day I decided to sit in back. Usually I sit in front near Johnny. Johnny doesn't like me. He doesn't like to sit with me. He picks on me. He always hits me. He's always mad at me.

In the year following the kidnapping Johnny and Jackie argued and fought more than they ever had before.

As seen in these examples, omens may have to do with causality (an angry mother forcing a child to go to school), ways a child could have been warned (the meaning of a play title or a father's innocent question), or ways the trauma could have been experienced more easily (sitting with a brother). A child whose defenses and coping mechanisms have been surprised and overwhelmed retrospectively struggles during and after a trauma to understand Why? How could I have been warned? or How could I have gotten through this better? When the child finds an answer, it is so permanently connected to the trauma itself that its influence can be discovered in the child's posttraumatic psychopathology. In my opinion the omens or portents in ancient or primitive societies were most likely formed in the same way during and after disasters.

To my knowledge there is no psychiatric literature that deals directly with the concept of omen formation as a mechanism by which the "breached ego" attempts retrospectively to regain control and mastery. There are, however, a few scientific papers that touch on parts of this idea. Chodoff and associates[4] discussed "the search for meaning" by parents whose child is dying. Cain and Fast[5] gave examples of children who look for "reasons" for their parents' suicide, usually guilt-laden superego-motivated reasons. Neubauer[6] made the psychoanalytic observation that there is a connection between the individual's initial conceptualization of a trauma and his later behaviors or character formation. Despite the paucity of psychiatric observation and theory on omen formation, the literary allusions to this phenomenon are diverse and insightful. In the *Iliad*, Shakespeare's *Julius Caesar*, *The Rime of the Ancient Mariner*, and especially in *The Scarlet Letter* there are numerous examples of omens and some insights into their nature.

Fear of Further Trauma

One striking sign that the ego has been breached is the immediate fear that develops of further trauma. Similar to Rado's concept[7] of traumatophobia, the fear of further trauma causes children to resist any change that could force them into further jeopardy. As a matter of fact, several children were terrified to escape from the "hole." In describing their fears, all the children mentioned either fear of losing their parents, fear of dying, or fear of worse things happening.

Any changes that occurred during the traumatic series of events were greeted with extreme fear. As the children were moved single file out of the school bus or the van, seven children believed they would be shot. Debbie, 10, recalled, "In the van, I thought they'd shoot the first two, the middle two, and the last two, so I went third to get out."

When the kidnappers filled the gas tanks of the vans with gasoline, Alison, 10, who is asthmatic, believed that she was being asphyxiated. "People cried, but I cried the most. I felt I couldn't breathe in there. . . . When they put gasoline in, it made everybody cough, and I felt I was suffocating." One year after the kidnapping Alison's mother related, "The new car makes her go crazy. She says in the back of the car it doesn't get cool enough. She huffs and puffs and says she can't breathe." Long after the kidnapping "fear of further trauma" continued to operate as a force behind the "fears of the mundane" from which 21 of the 23 children suffered.

Disturbances in Cognition

A third indicator of the ego damage that immediately occurs during a psychic trauma is disturbance in cognitive functions, such as perception, time sense, and thought. Eight children either misperceived their kidnappers or hallucinated during their ordeal. Youngsters mistakenly identified the kidnappers as a bald man, a lady, a black man, a man with a peg leg, a chubby man, a man in the front seat of the green van. Susan, 5, claimed she "saw the men take their masks off on top of us. They were lying down for a nap. I could see them on top of the hole. They didn't see us getting out." Bob, the hero who dug the children out of the hole, hallucinated several times as he dug. He firmly believed he had permanently "lost [his] mind" until he discussed and understood the hallucinations during his psychiatric interview several months later.

It is of interest to note that no child employed massive denial during the kidnapping. All details were remembered, though some were "seen" incorrectly or ordered in the wrong sequence.

Sense of time was confused in eight children. They believed that symptoms that had begun after the kidnapping had occurred before. (Parents confirmed that the onset dates were after the kidnapping.) The youngsters who experienced "time skew" became increasingly anxious because they believed that their symptoms may have been predictive. The autonomous ego functions[8] of time sense, perception, and thought are particularly vulnerable to psychic trauma.

Repetitive Phenomena

The literature on psychic trauma in adults is replete with examples of repeated traumatic dreams, repeated talking about the traumatic event, and repeated unbidden daytime visions of the traumatic event. Many of these findings were confirmed in the Chowchilla group. Further types of repetitive phenomena were discovered: dreams of the child's own death, posttraumatic play, and reenactment. (Reenactment has been mentioned previously in the psychiatric literature,[9-11] but I could not find any specific clinical examples.)

Repetitive phenomena are examples of the repetition compulsion described by Freud in 1914[12] and 1920.[3] In the Chowchilla children the repetitions were found to be very specific. They did not repeat an attitude or a general feeling; instead they repeated a specific event.

Traumatic Dreams

The children's dreams could be grouped into four types: (1) terror dreams with no morning remembrance of the dream content; (2) exact repetitions of the kidnapping events; (3) modified repetitions with different kidnappers, victims, outcomes, or settings; and (4) deeply disguised dreams. The children had more unremembered terror dreams early after the kidnapping than later after the event. There was also a tendency, however, for children who were nonverbal about their emotions to dream this type of terror dream exclusively. Unmodified dreams also tended to occur earlier in the posttraumatic period than modified or deeply disguised dreams. One very interesting finding was the dream in which the child allowed himself/herself to die.

Barbara, 9, dreamed that "three men stopped the kidnapped kids on the road, and they killed us and then they put us in a hole." During the kidnapping Barbara realized she had been buried underground. To Barbara, burial is a mental representation of death. In another of Barbara's dreams, "We [her family] were riding in a car. Men in a van got us, kidnapped us, killed us, and put us in a grave." She went on to associate, "We were at the cemetery where my grandma is buried. We don't go there much."

Jackie, 9, has repeatedly dreamed of being lined up, shot, and killed. She related, "I was the last one off the van. I was really scared. I thought they'd shoot the first and last person. I didn't expect to live when I got off the van." Jackie had imagined and accepted her own impending death; therefore she was able to dream about it.

Louis, 8, remembered two recent dreams in which he had died. "A dinosaur stabbed me, and a wolfman got me and ate me." Susan, 5, described a dream in which a "little big dog" bit her in her sleep and she died. During her actual stay in the hole she "tried to take a nap, but Louis got a little block [the stake holding up the roof] and he wouldn't put it back. Everybody woke up." (Many of the children said that the event of the ceiling collapsing was the most frightening aspect of being buried.) Susan's experience of taking a little nap in the hole and waking up with the ceiling collapsing was the same in her mind as being bitten by the dog while she was asleep and then dying.

These dreams of death appear to be dreams of the acceptance or knowledge of death as a past experience. They indicate that during the trauma, these children's egos gave up all disbelief in the reality of their own deaths, all sense of invulnerability, or, as Lifton calls it, "the sense of immortality."[13] The death dreams indicate that the trauma-shattered young mind believes in and unconsciously accepts its own death. Psychic trauma thus may provide an exception to Freud's 1915 statement, "In the unconscious, everyone of us is convinced of his own immortality."[14]

Posttraumatic Play

For the purposes of this study, I have defined "play" as an activity the child feels he or she enjoys either alone or in a group. I have included hobbies, artwork, and storytelling as types of play. Fourteen children repeatedly "played" the kidnapping experience. Even though their games lacked subtlety, only 1 of the 14 realized that the play was related to the kidnapping. Posttraumatic play was repeated monotonously with no relief of anxiety. I have described posttraumatic play in detail previously.[15] For this reason, I will give only two examples.

Mary, age 5, stated early in her interview, "I thought the hole was just down in the ground. I heard them put on dirt and I started crying. I wouldn't go to sleep or nothing. I thought they [the kidnappers] would come in there too. The hole was the scariest part." Later Mary confided, "There is a cement place at my grandma's which is like a hole. I put clothes in it and my Barbie dolls. I pretend they're stuck in the hole." Mary was unable to see a relationship between her play and her fear of the hole. The longer I discussed it with her the less she admitted she engaged in this kind of play.

Bob, 14, the children's hero, indulged in repetitious play during July 1977, exactly 1 year after the kidnapping. Bob's mother observed that every night during this time he took

the cushions off the couch and punches them until he's worn out. . . . We have barbells, but he wasn't using them. It was superaggressive, and he looked very intense. . . . He pounded the cushions so hard that he tripped the circuit breakers on the other side. I asked him to stop, but instead he moved the cushions to the other side [of the room]. I feel better with him gone for the summer.

This activity lasted about 2 hours every night for 2 weeks. It ended when his mother sent Bob away to spend the summer with relatives. Bob's physical fitness spree, an anniversary reaction, was, I think, a repetition of his digging effort, which had been originally traumatic for Bob as evidenced by the hallucinations he experienced as he dug.

Reenactment

Many of the child victims exhibited unusual behaviors, which included behaviors or fantasies that first occurred during the kidnapping. These postkidnapping behaviors were direct reenactments of attitudes, fears, or actions that had occurred before or during the kidnapping.

I might have used the term *repetition compulsion*, but this term has been more widely applied in recent years to the behavior and attitudes of individuals who have not necessarily been traumatized but who show evidence of an unresolved internal conflict. The behaviors of the kidnapped children were specific and almost exact repetitions of a fear, a fantasy, or an actual behavior that had occurred just before or during the kidnapping. The term *reenactment* will be applied to this specific type of repetition compulsion; in this sense it is a subset of repetition compulsions.

Sammy, 10, who is legally blind, reenacted at the schoolyard when, without any provocation, he pushed a much smaller girl and slapped her in the face. He bragged, "I gave them all a rough time. . . . I don't care. It doesn't bother me." During the kidnapping, Sammy, a previously unaggressive child, had been so frustrated when a kidnapper took his glasses that he had tried to hit him with his shoe.

Celeste, 9, underwent some repetitive reenactments that were mystifying to her and her family. She had argued with her mother the morning of the kidnapping and had later misperceived a kidnapper to be a "lady." On the bus when the kidnappers demanded that the children exit single file, Celeste hid behind a seat. She told me, "I didn't want the lady to see me." She then decided they might shoot her for failing to comply, so she left the bus. In the year following the kidnapping Celeste hid whenever she saw a woman or a girl she did not expect to see. For instance she squatted under a counter at the grocery store when her girlfriend came in, and she dove into the bushes when her school-teacher walked past her on the street.

Several other examples of reenactment have already been mentioned. Bob's shooting of the tourist, Alison's wheezing in the family car, Sheila's personality change based upon her prekidnapping argument with her mother, and Johnny's clownishness and physical fitness program all demonstrate the power and the unconscious linkage of reenactment to trauma. Repeated reenactments have accounted for personality changes, poor school performance, psychophysiological occurrences, and increasing anxiety in several of the kidnapped children.

Absence of "Flashbacks"

Although 6 older children (age 9–14 years) reported daytime visions of the episode, they used voluntary verbs when discussing how these thoughts came to their minds, such as *browse, think,* or *dwell.* There was no evidence of the type of sudden involuntary flashbacks previously reported in adults.[11] Furthermore, the children younger than 9 years did not complain of having visions or "seeing" the kidnapping at all. Perhaps the "voluntary" vision of the older children is a transition phase that occurs earlier than the involuntary flashback of adult posttraumatic states. Because no child employed massive denial during the kidnapping, perhaps intrusions could not occur. Furthermore, because there is a sequential development of the ability to daydream or fantasize,[8] the intrusive "flashback" may not develop until late adolescence.

Fears

Every child exhibited kidnap-related fears at the time of the psychiatric examination. Of the twenty-three, 20 children feared being kidnapped again, 12 were afraid of a "fourth kidnapper," 6 believed that the arrested kidnappers were coming back, and 10 believed there would be a second unrelated kidnapping.

Twenty-one childred feared common "mundane" experiences, 10 were afraid to be left alone, 15 feared vehicles, 9 feared the dark, 6 were afraid of strangers, 9 feared sounds, 3 feared confined spaces, and 3 were afraid of open spaces. Eight children experienced attacks of such acute anxiety that they screamed, ran, or called for help.

Rachel, age 12, noted

> *I don't like to turn off the lights. I'm afraid someone would come in and shoot and rob us. When I wake up I turn on the light. . . . I've been in Bakersfield helping my brother. . . . At night in Bakersfield it feels like someone broke in. Nothing is there. I hear footsteps again. I keep going to check. . . . I check where the sound is coming from. . . . I'm very frightened of the kitchen because no one's there at all. I completely avoid it. At home I kept feeling someone was looking in and watching me. I kept the light on. I was afraid they'd come in and kill us all or take us away again.*

Mary, 5, was interviewed on a windy day in early summer in one of her school's empty classrooms. She interrupted her interview several times saying, "What's that?"

"Just the wind," I reassured her.

Again, "What was that knocking? I thought it was a car, maybe kidnappers."

"Only the wind."

"I had nightmares and dreams about it. When I think they were in jail. And a van kept parking and stopping and the fan was on."

In Mary's case it appears the fan, a harmless sound associated with the horrors of the van ride, and the "hole" have now "contaminated" all wind. Again and again Mary asked, "What's that?" as the wind gusted outside the schoolroom. She accepted no reassurance.

The children's fear of another kidnapping has affected their attitudes about their ordinary environment: motor vehicles, the dark, the wind, "mouses and dogs," "hippies," the kitchen, and so forth. Many of these items are now believed to be signals or warnings of an impending kidnapping. The children have remained continuously on alert. They also fear reexperiencing the original traumatic anxiety. Certain sensory stimuli associated with the original psychic trauma are avoided by the group because they evoke the original overwhelming anxiety. These posttraumatic fears of the everyday environment have been designated "fear of the mundane."

Susan, 5, whose dreams indicated that she had accepted her own death[2] announced to her mother one morning, "Laverne [her toddler sister] is dead! She's not up yet." Mandy, 7, twice screamed that her little brother had been kidnapped, when he was actually playing next door or trying on clothes in a store dressing room. Exactly 1 year after the kidnapping, Johnny, 11, refused to sleep in his bedroom for many nights because he believed the ceiling was collapsing.

Sammy, 10, the legally blind child who is able to ride his bike (much to his mother's simultaneous pride and concern), experienced two panicky episodes, according to his mother.

Before Christmas during vacation he was biking with a friend [in the] sandhills. A station wagon, two guys, and a dog were there. He abandoned his bike and ran home. He said he didn't want to be kidnapped again. He cried a lot. I advised him not to panic and run. . . . Just before the fair in May there were strangers on the road, and he gave up biking there and refused to go further.

The vast majority of child victims believed they could be kidnapped again. Each of them in some way listened and watched for signs of danger in the dark, when alone, near cars or strangers, when confined, or when out in the open. They remained permanently on guard. No matter what anyone told them, they seemed unable to trust again. Bob, 14, summarized his feelings by saying "I'm much more cautious now. I know it can happen to me. Before I thought it only happens to other people." Lifton and Olson[16] referred to similar phenomena in adults as "shattering of the illusion of invulnerability." In children this effect is so marked it appears to be an interference with *basic trust* in the sense that Erikson[17] originally defined the term.

Many of the Chowchilla children had been well parented and well loved. Even so, after the kidnapping they could not fully trust the world. Ordinary routine became fraught with fears. No parental reassurance could be accepted. A Hawaiian professor of mathematics read a newspaper account of 8-year-old Tania's shattered trust and tried to help by sending her a calculation of the extremely low probability of future kidnapping. The latter barely touched the angry little girl, who depended upon a nightlight, feared vehicles, and jumped at the sound of the heater in her room. Tania's mother poignantly noted, "She had been very easy to get along with. Loving. When she first came back, she wouldn't kiss me. She wouldn't sit on our laps. My mother pointed out that now she's fearful of closeness because she might lose it."

Child versus Adult Response to Trauma

Although this report has described some similarities between child and adult response to trauma, several differences between adult and child reactions have been shown. (1) No period of amnesia or haziness about the experience took place in these children. (2) No denial that alternated with intrusive repetitive phenomena occurred in the children. (One wonders why denial is classified as a primitive defense when traumatized children do not use it but traumatized adults do.) (3) No true flashbacks were observed in these children. (4) The children "play" their trauma in a manner similar to the repetitive dreams and reenactments of both children and adults. (5) Major signs of ego dysfunction in these traumatized children were cognitive malfunctions, misperceptions, overgeneralizations, and time distortions. (6) Reenactment was an important finding in the children. Although there is some mention of adult traumatic reenactments in the literature,[10] the literal repetitiveness from actual traumatic fantasy or performance has not been emphasized in descriptions of traumatized adults; it may be a finding more characteristic of children.

Finally: despite the fact that the children in this group represented three developmental stages—oedipal, latency, and adolescence—the findings were surprisingly consistent and occurred across all of these phases. Further research into the effects of a single psychic trauma in infancy and in the preoedipal years may help to explain this finding.

References

1. Miller, G., & Tompkins, S. "Chowchilla: The bitterness lingers." *Fresno Bee,* Nov. 14, 1976.
2. Terr, L. Children of Chowchilla: A study of psychic trauma. *Psychoanalytic Study of the Child,* 1979, *34,* 552–623.
3. Freud, S. Beyond the pleasure principle (1920). In J. Strachey (Ed. & Trans.), *Complete psychological works,* standard ed., vol. 18. London: Hogarth Press, 1955.
4. Chodoff, P., Friedman, S., & Hamburg, D. Stress, defenses, and coping behavior: Observations in parents of children with malignant disease. *American Journal of Psychiatry,* 1964, *120,* 743–749.
5. Cain, A., & Fast, I. Children's disturbed reactions to parent suicide. In A. Cain & I. Fast (Eds.), *Survivors of Suicide.* Springfield, Ill.: Charles C. Thomas, 1972.
6. Neubauer, P. Trauma and psychopathology. In S. Furst (Ed.), *Psychic trauma.* New York: Basic Books, 1967.
7. Rado, S. Pathodynamics and treatment of traumatic war neurosis. *Psychosomatic Medicine,* 1942, *4,* 362–368.
8. Hartmann, H. *Essays on ego psychology: selected problems in psychoanalytic theory.* New York: International Universities Press, 1964.
9. Freud, A., & Burlingham, D. *War and children.* New York: International Universities Press, 1944.
10. Wangh, M. A psychogenic factor in the recurrence of war. *International Journal of Psychoanalysis,* 1968, *49,* 319–323.
11. Horowitz, M. *Stress response syndromes.* New York: Jason Aronson, 1976.
12. Freud, S. Remembering, repeating, and working through (1914). In J. Strachey (Ed. & Trans.), *Complete psychological works,* standard ed., vol. 12. London: Hogarth Press, 1958.
13. Lifton, R. The sense of immortality: On death and the continuity of life. *American Journal of Psychoanalysis,* 1973, *33,* 3–15.
14. Freud, S. Thoughts for the times on war and death (1915). In J. Strachey (Ed. & Trans), *Complete psychological works,* standard ed., vol. 14. London: Hogarth Press, 1957.
15. Terr, L. Forbidden games: Traumatic child's play. *Journal of the American Academy of Child Psychiatry,* 1981, *20,* 741–760.
16. Lifton, R., & Olson, E. The human meaning of total disaster. *Psychiatry,* 1976, *39,* 1–18.
17. Erikson, E. *Childhood and society.* New York: Norton, 1950.

25

Adaptive Strategies and Recovery from Rape

ANN WOLBERT BURGESS and
LYNDA LYTLE HOLMSTROM

Being raped generates an enormous amount of anxiety in the victim. This anxiety is the basis for an acute traumatic reaction called the *rape trauma syndrome*.[1] The nucleus of the anxiety is the impact of the life-threatening or highly stressful experience on the individual.

In an earlier paper[2] we looked at the coping behavior of the victim before, during, and immediately after the rape. The behavior was directed at coping with stress and consisted of avoidance, survival, and escape. In this chapter we will look at a wider spectrum of adaptive behaviors aimed at reorganization and the ways the victims dealt with their rape over 4 to 6 years.

This chapter appears in abridged form from *American Journal of Psychiatry*, 1979, *136*, 1278–1282. Copyright 1979, The American Psychiatric Association. Reprinted by permission.

ANN WOLBERT BURGESS • Boston City Hospital, Boston, Massachusetts 02118. **LYNDA LYTLE HOLMSTROM** • Department of Sociology, Boston College, Chestnut Hill, Massachusetts 02167.

Method

Sample

The original sample of adult rape victims consisted of 92 women seen during a counseling-research project based in the emergency department of Boston City Hospital in 1972–73. The crisis intervention model[3] and the research method[4] have been reported elsewhere. The data for this chapter were collected as part of a longitudinal follow-up study of all the sexual assault victims. The sample for this study consisted of 81 victims (88%) from the original sample, 78 who were reinterviewed, and 3 for whom there were good indirect data. Three of the 92 victims had died, and data on 8 additional victims were incomplete. The adult rape victim group was heterogeneous with regard to ethnicity, race, religion, social class, employment, education, marital status, and age.

Data Collection

We used a standard schedule of questions that were flexible and open ended.[5] Some of the questions had been asked during the initial interview at the hospital, and some were new. The combined sources of data provided the information on coping and adaptation and also served as a means to compare memory and recall of specific thoughts, feelings, and actions after the rape. The classification of length of recovery was developed by looking at the answers to two major questions: Do you feel back to normal, that is, the way you felt prior to the rape? and, Has the rape interfered in your life and, if so, in what areas? These data are victims' subjective reports of their own recovery over the intervening 4 to 6 years.

Data Analysis on Length of Recovery

The dependent variable in the analysis of recovery is the time required for the victim to feel recovered. Victims were divided into three groups: those who felt recovered within months (30, or 37%), those who felt it took years to recover (30, or 37%), and those who did not feel recovered by the time of follow-up 4 to 6 years after the rape (21, or 26%). Thus, when contacted 4 to 6 years after the rape, the majority of victims felt recovered (74%), while a minority did not feel recovered (26%).

Adaptive Responses to Rape

Research on adaptation to stress is still a relatively new field. One major problem appears to be the lack of a classification system to organize data on adaptive responses.[6] Given this constraint, the data on coping and adaptation by adult rape victims will be discussed under four major categories: self-esteem, defense mechanisms, actions, and maladaptive responses.

Self-Esteem

Self-esteem is the evaluative component of an individual's self-concept and implies a personal assessment of worth or competence. This evaluative process can apply to a specific role and to the totality of all roles assumed by an individual.[7] The application of this concept to a victim implies that the person could evaluate his or her specific role as a victim as well as the influence of the victim experience on various other roles in his or her life.

The spontaneous comments made by 45 of the victims were coded as positive or negative and categorized by length of recovery time. There was a clear association between self-esteem and length of recovery. Among the victims who gave a positive statement, 65% recovered in months, but among those with a negative statement none recovered this quickly. In contrast, among victims who gave a positive assessment none was still not recovered, but among those who gave a negative assessment, 50% were not yet recovered. Of course, such an association does not tell the direction of cause and effect. One possibility is that at the time of rape some victims have high self-esteem in general and others have low self-esteem, and the rape reinforces and confirms their existing evaluation of themselves. The other possibility is that the victims are not divided that way before rape and the way the victim handles the rape produces high self-esteem in some and low self-esteem in others.

Positive Self-Assessment. Victims who made a positive statement reflected acceptance and approval of either behavior or approach to situations and/or people. Examples of positive terms included *strong* ("I'm a strong person mentally"), *calm* ("I remain calm in difficult situations"), and *high tolerance for stress* ("I was glad I cooperated with the guys and didn't get hurt"). Some of the victims who gave a positive assessment were able to use words denoting humor to gain distance on the rape ("I can laugh about being robbed and maybe . . . I will be able to laugh about the other part").

Negative Self-Assessment. Victims who made a negative statement did not affirm or approve of their behavior. The negative terms included *doubt* ("gave me another self-doubt about myself"), *not functioning adequately* ("I have never been normal"), *regret* ("I regret not yelling . . . maybe I could have done more"), *guilt* ("I played along with them and that made me feel guilty"), *general life-style* ("one more mess in my life . . . the worst to date"), *bad luck* ("I was born with bad luck, something is always happening to me").

Defense Mechanisms

The tactics used by individuals to cope with anxiety may be unconscious, such as the ego mechanisms of defense[8]; may be conscious strategies used to deal with everyday stresses and strains[9]; or may be patterns of coping influenced by culture and society.[10] On follow-up, it seemed important to analyze the conscious cognitive strategies that victims used to master the anxiety generated by the rape. Four types of defense mechanisms were identified: explanation, minimization, suppression, and dramatization. Adult rape victims who use any or all of these mechanisms are more apt to recover in months or years than to be unrecovered 4 to 6 years after the rape. For example, out of 21 victims not yet recovered, only 5 used any type of conscious defense mechanism.

Explanation. The mechanism of explanation helps the victim cope with the anxiety by providing some reason for the rape.

Coming up with an explanation gives some understanding for the bizarreness of the acts and aids in returning some degree of control to the victim. The process by which a victim develops the explanation can be seen in the following victim's comments:

> *I was trying to think in my head of why it happened. Why it happened to me. Why it was necessary at that time and place. . . . I remember walking along the street and people "cat watching." It made me cross to the other side of the street . . . then the guys were on me. It's like being tricked. . . . I didn't have a chance.*

Explanations victims gave for the rape divide according to whom the victims assigned responsibility, the assailant or the victim. Victims who assigned responsibility to the assailant gave such reasons as sex ("He said he was horny"), revenge ("He enjoyed it in that he was getting back at me. He could get sex for a dime"), pathology ("He is sick . . . he needs help"), and exploitation of the victim's vulnerability ("He saw me drunk").

Victims also gave explanations focusing on themselves: their decisions ("If I hadn't gone, it wouldn't have happened"), self-reflection ("I was dumb," "I was idealistic," "I was conned," and "For 20¢ I was raped. I hitchhiked to save 20¢"), and being forewarned ("I went to a fortune-teller a long time ago who said a disaster was coming. When this happened, I said to myself, The disaster has happened").

Victims who use the mechanism of explanation may make themselves more vulnerable to judgmental reactions from others. Explanations often have a self-blaming quality to them. It is important to recognize that although victims may blame themselves for their decisions or behavior, they do not necessarily feel guilty about their actions. Their anxiety is decreased by providing a reason, which serves as a self-correcting mechanism. This contrasts with victims who feel guilty, which increases anxiety about the rape. This self-correcting mechanism may be seen in the following example: "I take experiences as they come as a stepping stone to learn from. The rape was a good learning situation . . . taught me to be more careful." A victim who uses explanation as a defense mechanism may have to contend with the reaction of the person to whom she is giving the explanation. Just the word *rape* conjures up many biases and prejudices in people.[11] The following comment from a victim puts the matter well:

> *I can talk about it calmly now. I do it in an explanatory way. When I tell people, I am really wary of their reaction. I don't want pity or want them to think of it as a weird thing . . . I want a human reaction.*

Minimization.   Minimization helps cope with the anxiety by reducing the anxiety to a smaller, more manageable context. Minimization decreases the terrifying aspects and allows the person to think of it in tolerable amounts. Victims who minimize rape do so in comparison to their perception of rape, their current situation, other victims, or to a prior experience.

Victims often have a perception or image of what it is like to be raped, and if the rape does not match the image they feel fortunate to have survived so well. Victims perceive rape as fatal ("I got off lucky . . . there could have been a bullet in the gun"), perverted ("Even though they had a knife, I kept thinking they were kids and they weren't going to use it . . . they didn't do anything perverse"), involving additional violence ("scared they were going to kill me . . . or take me out of the city or to a place with older men . . . all I had to do was lie there . . . didn't ask me to do anything unnatural").

Victims may have other conditions that they view as more upsetting than the rape. As one psychotic victim said, "The rape was nothing compared to the voices. I wish they would go away."

Victims may compare themselves to other victims and minimize their anxiety that way. Victims may focus on either the violence or the sexual component of the rape. One 62-year-old victim, who had been badly beaten, almost smothered by a pillow, and cut in the stomach with the assailant's knife, compared age and sexual experience:

> *I guess you see worse victims than me. I know it must be awful for some of these young girls. I know what sex is all about. I've been married and had kids. It would have been really awful if I was a virgin. Something like that would have really bothered me.*

Prior experience with upsetting events may give victims a clue to what must be done in terms of coping. Victims with this strategy talked of accepting the rape ("It's over . . . it must be accepted. There is nothing else I can do about it. It's better to be raped than die").

Suppression. Suppression provides cognitive control over thoughts of the rape. The person tries to put the memory of the rape completely out of her mind through a conscious effort. Victims using this mechanism do not like the subject of the rape to be brought up ("Don't refresh my mind to it") and talk in terms of being able to "block the thoughts" from their minds or actively keeping the thoughts from entering their minds. Victims using this mechanism often have had previous experience with such a mechanism ("It's better not to think of the rape so you don't get bummed out"). Cognitive control may be a way to neutralize the anxiety, as in the following case:

> It isn't my way to get upset. I don't dwell on things I can't change. I go in the other direction. Life is too short to go in the way of being upset and having your life ruined by such an event.

Dramatization. According to sociologist Zola, the defense mechanism of dramatization "seems to cope with anxiety by repeatedly overexpressing it and thereby dissipating it" (p. 627).[10] Victims using this mechanism usually have a small group of friends with whom they discuss the rape. One victim traveled to another country, talked with women, and helped establish a feminist clinic to deal with issues of sex and violence. Another victim who recovered within months said, "I don't cry much and when this happened I cried a lot. . . . I got everything out plus talked about it with so many people."

Action

In response to their rapes, victims exhibited three patterns of behavior: increased action, no change in action, or decreased action. Increased action was associated with faster recovery.

Of the victims who increased their action, 45% had recovered in months, but of those with decreased action, none recovered that fast. In contrast, with increased action, only 18% were not yet recovered, whereas 50% of those with decreased action were not yet recovered.

Increased Action. The most common action taken by victims was to change residence or to travel. Eight victims traveled outside the country within the first year after the rape. An important consideration in this type of action was the economic resources of the victim. Victims who had financial resources were able to travel and change residence. These victims moved from one apartment to another and often were able to completely change neighborhoods. Some victims moved to another state. As one victim said,

> *I think it was easier for me because I went to another city and wasn't reminded of it. I didn't have to see it every day. I could forget it. . . .*

Victims with less economic independence moved in temporarily with relatives and/or friends ("stayed with my aunt for a while . . . then lived with my mother . . . now have a place of my own"). Some victims had to delay their moving for such reasons as economics or work situations. When they did move, they commented on the positive component ("Didn't move till 1975 and feel so much better down here"). One victim who could not afford a move stayed with relatives and then rearranged her home. She had been raped in her bedroom and describes the change as follows,

> *Wouldn't sleep in my own bed. Stayed with friends for a while. Have changed my bedroom around and got a new bedroom set.*

There were other types of increased action that victims took. First, changing telephone numbers or getting an unlisted telephone number helped to provide some environmental control for the victim. Second, reading, watching television talk shows, or writing about rape helped victims gain intellectual control. Third, some victims became active in rape crisis centers to assist other victims. Of those victims who used this type of action, 70% recovered within months.

One-third of the victims reported no specific change in their actions. A minority of victims (17%) described a marked decrease in action. Victims talked of withdrawing from people ("I shut people out"), life events ("I hibernated"), or the world ("I disappeared and my family covered"). Victims talked of becoming substantially immobile ("I just lay on the couch for 2 weeks," or "I went to bed for a month").

Maladaptive Responses

Victims do not always cope with the anxiety of rape in adaptive ways. Some victims fail to cope with the stress of the rape and develop maladaptive responses. Eighteen (22%) of the victims reported either making a suicide attempt and/or seriously abusing alcohol or drugs after the rape.

The abuse of drugs or alcohol and/or acting on suicidal thoughts was associated with longer recovery. None of the victims who recovered in months coped by abusing drugs or alcohol or attempting to harm themselves, whereas nine victims (43%) who had not yet recovered did rely on one or all of these behaviors. Nine victims reported making some attempt at suicide. Sometimes the suicidal behavior is present before the rape ("When I was raped, I was very suicidal. I had attempted it several times"). Suicidal behavior may be part of a prior history of affective illness ("The rape made me manic, then depressed . . . then I attempted suicide"). Or the suicidal behavior may be a response to the failure to renegotiate a partner relationship after the rape.

The reliance on drugs and alcohol as a coping tactic after rape was used by 14 of the victims ("After the rape I stayed constantly drunk. I hit rock bottom. I drank to pass out . . . not to think of how bad things had gotten").

Not only do these figures on maladaptive response to rape indicate these victims to be a high-risk group, but the causes of death of the three women from the original sample who had died clearly indicate maladaptive responses. One victim committed suicide,[5] and two victims died from medical complications of alcoholism.

Quality of Life After Rape

An important dimension of the discussion on recovery from rape is some description of the quality of life for the victims in the three recovery-time categories. Although victims provided subjective data on their own recovery, additional indications of functional capacity in social task performance, partnership stability, and sexual functioning after rape should be reported.

Social Task Performance

Women in our society generally have one or more of three major social tasks: to be a housewife and/or parent, to be employed, and/or to be in school. On follow-up the majority of victims (81%) reported meeting at least one of these social tasks.

Recovery was most obvious in the resumption of social task functions. Of the 14 women (17%) who had completed some type of formal school program during the years after the rape, 10 completed an undergraduate college program, 4 completed high school, and 1 completed a vocational program. In addition, 5 women were in graduate school programs—law, social work, business administration, and education—and 6 women were completing undergraduate college programs. It was clear that women saw starting or completing an educational program as a positive aspect of their life ("Once I got some personal achievements . . . I was much better").

The majority of victims were working either part or full time. Of the 11 victims who were working for the same employer they had worked for at the time of the rape, most had received promotions. Other new positions included teacher, salesperson, freelance writer, grant investigator, health-related occupations, market analyst, bookkeeper, and administrative assistant.

It is important to differentiate between the several lengths of recovery of the victims who identified no specific task performance. Victims who felt recovered within months and who did not identify a social task ($N = 7$) were either under psychiatric aftercare supervision ($N = 2$), were retired or disabled and on pension funds ($N = 3$), or were in a social support network group ($N = 2$). In contrast, all victims who were not yet recovered and did not identify a social task ($N = 7$) had no strong social network ties and were socially drifting. In the years after the rape, they had been unsuccessful in gaining any personal achievements. The women were distressed at their life-style and, although they sought assistance, were unable to reorganize their lives in a meaningful way.

Partnership Stability

The stability of partnership relationships is associated with length of recovery. Fifty-one victims (63%) were in some type of partnership relationship at the time of the rape, including dating partners, dating and sexual partners, and marriage partners. Three patterns of partnership stability were noted after the rape. The most common pattern (30, or 59%) was disruption of the relationship, followed by no disruption of the relationship (14, or 27%), followed by semidisruption of the relationship (7, or 14%). Victims with partnership stability had a faster recovery than victims who did not have partnership stability. Of the 15 women who married within 4 to 6 years after the rape, only 4 married the partners they had at the time of the rape. Three who were married at the time of the rape were divorced by follow-up, and 2 who married within the 4 to 6 years had also divorced by the time of follow-up.

Sexual Functioning

The majority of victims who were sexually active at the time of the rape ($N = 63$) reported disruption in sexual functioning within the 6 months after the rape. Changes were reported in their frequency of sexual activity as follows: abstinence (38%), decreased activity (33%), increased activity (10%). Only 19% reported no change in sexual activity. Sexual symptoms included sexual aversion, flashbacks, vaginismus, and orgasmic dysfunction.[12]

Discussion

Recovery from rape is complex and influenced by many factors. These factors include prior life stress,[5] style of attack,[13] relationship of victim and offender (and whether it is an inter- or intraracial rape), number of assailants, language used by the assailant,[14] the amount of violence or the sexual acts demanded,[15] and postrape factors of institutional response to the victim,[4] social network response,[16] and subsequent victimization.[13] Clinicians should consider all of these factors in identifying victims who are at high risk for a slow recovery from rape and will remain vulnerable to many life stresses for a long time.

In this chapter we have reported the importance of high self-esteem and conscious coping and adaptive strageties in aiding recovery. Being raped sets into motion an evaluative process that affects the view victims have of themselves or their behavior during rape. The conscious defense mechanisms of explanation, minimization, suppression, and dramatization all help to neutralize the anxiety created by the rape, as do increased actions, such as moving, travel, or reading on the subject.

References

1. Burgess, A. W., & Holmstrom, L. L. Rape trauma syndrome. *American Journal of Psychiatry*, 1974, *131*, 981–986.
2. Burgess, A. W., & Holmstrom, L. L. Coping behavior of the rape victim. *American Journal of Psychiatry*, 1976, *133*, 413–418.
3. Burgess, A. W., & Holmstrom, L. L. *Rape: Victims of crisis.* Bowie, Md.: Robert J. Brady, 1974.
4. Holmstrom, L. L., & Burgess, A. W. *The victim of rape: Institutional reactions.* New York: Wiley, 1978.
5. Burgess, A. W., & Holmstrom, L. L. Recovery from rape and prior life stress. *Research in Nursing and Health*, 1978, *1*, 165–174.
6. Lazarus, R. S., Averill, J. R., & Opton, E. M. The psychology of coping: Issues of research and assessment. In G. V. Coelho, D. A. Hamburg, & J. E. Adams (Eds.), *Coping and adaptation.* New York: Basic Books, 1974.
7. Segre, J. M. *Self-concept and depression: Mothers returning to work or remaining at home.* Unpublished doctoral dissertation, Boston: Boston University Department of Education, 1978.
8. Freud, A. The ego and the mechanisms of defense. *The Writings of Anna Freud* (Vol. 2) New York: International Universities Press, 1936.
9. Kluckhohn, F. R. Dominant and variant value orientations. In C. Kluckhohn, H. A. Murray, & D. M. Schneider (Eds.), *Personality in nature, society, and culture* (2nd Ed.). New York: Knopf, 1956.
10. Zola, I. K. Culture and symptoms—an analysis of patients' presenting complaints. *American Sociological Review*, 1966, *31*, 615–630.
11. Feild, H. S. Attitudes toward rape: A comparative analysis of police, rapists, crisis counselors and citizens. *Journal of Personality and Social Psychology*, 1978, *36*, 156–179.

12. Burgess, A. W., & Holmstrom, L. L. Rape: Sexual disruption and recovery. *American Journal of Orthopsychiatry*, 1979, *49*, 648–657.
13. Burgess, A. W., & Holmstrom, L. L. *Rape: Crisis and recovery.* Bowie, Md.: Robert J. Brady, 1979.
14. Holmstrom, L. L., & Burgess, A. W. Rapists' talk: Linguistic strategies to control the victim. *Deviant Behavior*, 1979, *1*, 101–125.
15. Holmstrom, L. L., & Burgess, A. W. *Sexual behavior of assailant and victim during rape.* Paper presented at the 73rd annual meeting of the American Sociological Association, San Francisco, Calif., September 4–8, 1978.
16. Holmstrom, L. L., & Burgess, A. W. Rape: The husband's and boyfriend's initial reactions. *The Family Coordinator*, 1979, *28*, 321–330.

26

The Victim of Terrorism

FRANK OCHBERG

Victimization is nothing new. Coping with the stress of captivity has been studied in considerable detail during and after World War II. Since the victim of terrorism is often a symbol of the government under siege, and since hostages released by terrorists have an immense audience provided by the media in the aftermath of a dramatic incident, these victims have an impact on public opinion and public sentiment that may be profound. A public that overreacts in outrage against the victims' helplessness may precipitate harsh, simplistic counterterrorist measures. A public that joins the victim in identifying with the terrorist-aggressor may undermine the morale and confidence of the police. A public perplexed and alienated by the entire process may interfere with the bond of trust between government and governed that is necessary for the survival of democratic institutions. But, on the other hand, a public that is reasonably well aware of the repertoire of human responses that are effectively used by men and women under stress—even under the stress of terrorist threat and capitivity—such a public will be able to participate in

This chapter appears in abridged form from *Terrorism: An International Journal*, 1978, *1*, 147–168. Copyright 1978 Crane, Russak & Co., Inc. This article was originally entitled, "The Victim of Terrorism: Psychiatric Considerations." Reprinted by permission.

FRANK OCHBERG • 4383 Maumee, Okemos, Michigan 48864.

rational decision making about national policy on terrorism. There is another obvious reason to consider the victims of terrorism. They suffer. And their suffering may be misunderstood or neglected when the tumult and drama of the notorious event have subsided. There are medically sound approaches in the diagnosis and treatment of such suffering that can and should be brought to bear on these cases.

The clinical method of inquiry often begins with a close look at a single illustrative case, and we shall do so here. Although there are unfortunately many to choose from, none could be better than the experience of Mr. Gerard Vaders, a mature, sensitive, newspaper editor who was held for 13 days on that ill-fated train from Groningen, Netherlands, in December 1975. The point in presenting Mr. Vaders's story is to raise general issues about the hostage situation, about the role of the victim, about stress, coping, and psychological effects.

The Moluccan Train

The basic facts of the siege are well known. At 10:00 A.M. on December 2, 1975, the train from Groningen to Amsterdam was boarded and stopped by seven masked gunmen on a flat, dreary piece of land near Beilen. The engineer was shot, and during the ensuing period of negotiation under duress two hostages were executed. One terrorist and a hostage were injured when an automatic rifle discharged accidentally. The assaulting group was of the Free South Moluccan Youth Movement, and their cause was the separation and independence of their homeland from Indonesian rule. Their demands included release of political prisoners from Dutch and Indonesian jails, publicity of their cause, policy changes in the Netherlands regarding Moluccan independence, and safe passage out of the country. They held 72 hostages at the outset but allowed the number to dwindle to 23. Their weapons included pistols, automatic rifles, and sham explosives that were taped menacingly to all exit doors.

One year later the Moluccan terrorists were in prison beginning 17 year sentences, and Mr. Vaders was back in his bustling newsroom, telling me the story he would rather forget.

*How do I feel now? It is complicated. I know I need to get back to this life,
and to leave that other. But there are many who are still sitting on that
train, waiting. Waiting for Godot.*

*From the beginning it was different for me. I recognized the situation.
The moment the Moluccans came in, I felt back in the war. I was thinking,
"Keep your head cool. Face the crisis." I knew there would soon be choices.
Times to take risks. For instance, it was risky to sit there taking notes. That
destroys your anonymity. I made the choice and took notes.* [At this point I
asked if the feelings at the beginning of the siege were like any
others.]

*There was an early experience. I must have been 17. I was sleeping in
the room with my brother, and all of a sudden the SS were standing there
with machine pistols. They were on a reprisal raid because the Resistance
had murdered a Dutch collaborator. We were sent to a concentration camp
in Holland. Every morning we had hours of* appel—*lining up in freezing
weather. But I was young looking and had fair hair. I came to the attention
of the SS officer in charge. He asked my age and I lied, "16." I remember
him saying "My God, are we fighting children?" I was released the next day.*

*There was also a time of similar feeling during the Ardennes offensive,
when I came under fire. . . . And in 1948 in Indonesia two hand grenades
were thrown at me and I saw them at my feet. Neither one exploded.*

[Mr. Vaders resumed his narrative] *They threw the door open.
There were two or three of them wearing black woolen balaclavas. I knew
they were South Moluccans. The others thought PLO. But on their rifle
butts you could see the colors. I recognized it from Indonesia.*

Although the memories are vivid, it wasn't so much a memory as a
realization *that I would have to mobilize reflexes like in the war.*

*I still have guilt over the war. I did nothing bad, but not enough good.
Not enough for the Jews. My sister did more and was in Dachau. Then I
chose not to take too many risks.*

But on the train I did risk. I decided to write and to do it openly.

*For the first 10 minutes I felt cool. Cooler than usual. I was even
looking for humor in the situation. December 5 is our Santaklaus holiday
when we give poems as presents. I was thinking how I wouldn't have to write
poems this year.*

*The others on the train were either sitting still or following orders. The
Moluccans had us tape paper over the windows, and many were doing that.
One man seemed a little too aggressive. That was Mr. DeGroot.*

*I was taping windows, too. I asked them if anyone was hurt. They said
the driver wanted to be a hero and was shot. I asked if an ambulance should
be called. They said, "No. He's dead." But he wasn't dead yet, we later
found out. I sat down and took notes.*

They saw me writing and didn't say anything, but tied me up with my hands behind my back and they tied me by the arms to the doorway so that I was like a curtain. I faced away from the passengers and toward the pool of blood from the driver. People could walk past me, under my arms. I knew they were planning to execute hostages.

For a second I thought Mr. DeGroot was the minister for under-developed countries who had come to negotiate our release. But that was a mirage.

Then I thought that they executed DeGroot. We all did. One Moluccan was weeping and quoting the Bible and saying, "There is a time to kill. . . . I do not hate you but I have to do it." Actually, Mr. DeGroot escaped, but we never learned this until much later. At that time I was talking to them as much as possible.

One terrorist told me he couldn't hate the Dutch, that he was married to a Dutch girl. [That was a lie.] *They must have wanted us to like them.*

On the first day while I was hanging there they killed a soldier. [The first terrorist demand said hostages would be shot every 30 minutes until their request for a bus, a plane, and political recognition was granted.] *I could see one of them shooting and hear a howl like a dog.*

They let me down in the afternoon. Prins [a fellow hostage who had convinced everyone he was a doctor] *massaged my arms for an hour. This was my first contact with another hostage during the ordeal. I tried to keep up the contact.*

The first night I began shivering. They had used my coat to mop up the blood of the driver. Then one of the passengers finally gave me another coat. Afterward I learned it was the coat of the dead soldier.

The next morning I was full of fear. Sweating. Cramps in the stomach. Fighting away panic.

Now I took notes by stealth.

On the second night they tied me again to be a living shield and left me in that position for 7 hours. The one who was most psychopathic kept telling me, "Your time has come. Say your prayers." They had selected me for the third execution.

I had different impulses. One was to reason with them. But I suppressed that. I thought that would strengthen their resolve. The second impulse was to flee. I would have had to untie both hands, feet, and the door. I had one hand slightly free, but I would not have had time to do the rest.

I was preparing for execution. Making up a balance. My life philosophy is that there is some plus and some minus, and everyone ends up close to zero. Some say that is pessimistic. I think it is realistic. I was 50 years old. It had not been a bad life. I'm not happy with my life, but satisfied. I had everything that makes life human.

[But you weren't executed," I said. "How did you feel?"]

You won't believe this. Disappointed.

I had the impulse to say, "Let that man go and let me go in his place,"
but the words stuck.

I felt . . . I feel guilty. [He had a sad look then.]

In the morning, when I knew I was going to be executed I asked to talk
to Prins, to give him a message for my family. I wanted to explain my family
situation. My foster child—her parents had been killed—she did not get
along too well with my wife, and I had at that time a crisis in my marriage
just behind me. I hoped my wife would get a new purpose in her life by
concentrating on that child. There were other things, too. Somewhere I had
the feeling that I had failed as a human being. I explained all this and the
terrorists insisted on listening. Dr. Mulders and Dr. Bastiaans think that
saved my life. [I do also. He was no faceless symbol any more. He
certainly was no hero. All his human flaws were exposed, and the
Moluccans could not execute him.]

After that they didn't isolate me any more. They said, "We have others
to kill." I was sitting next to this woman and across from a young man
named Bierling (a 33-year-old father of two). They came and pointed to
Bierling and led him away and shot him.

[That must have been the point of maximum horror for Mr.
Vaders. Considering his feelings of guilt and shame from previous
"survivals," this one must have been excruciating.]

The days went by, and we somehow knew there would be no more
executions. Only Eli, the psychopathic one, wanted a fourth killing, but the
others talked him out of it. I was worried when Paul left. He was sensitive
and intelligent, and he seemed to balance out Eli. But Paul was wounded
when a gun went off and had to go to the hospital.

There was a growing sense that the authorities were mishandling the
situation. They sent us food but no utensils. The mayor of Beilen made a
stupid announcement.

And you had to fight a certain feeling of compassion for the Moluc-
cans. I know this is not natural, but in some way they come over human.
They gave us cigarettes. They gave us blankets. But we also realized that
they were killers. You try to suppress that in your consciousness. And I knew
I was suppressing that. I also knew that they were victims, too. In the long
run they would be as much victims as we. Even more. You saw their morale
crumbling. You experienced the disintegration of their personalities. The
growing of despair. Things dripping through their fingers. You couldn't
help but feel a certain pity. For people at the beginning with egos like gods—
impregnable, invincible—they end up small, desperate, feeling that all was
in vain.

I asked about aftereffects and learned that Mr. Vaders lost a great deal of weight and had a long illness that went undiagnosed from the summer of 1976 until a gallstone operation in November brought relief. His relationship with his wife improved dramatically. There was much discussion, reconciliation, and a decision to spend far more time together.

He wrote some stories that were critical of the government, and these aroused a great many threatening calls and letters. The government claimed he was sick, several colleagues spread rumors that he made a deal with the Moluccans to spare his life in return for a favorable press, and a police dossier emerged claiming that he had Communist connections. He drank more and smoked more, then cut it all out precipitously.

His daughter had a great deal of difficulty watching all the aggression leveled at him, dropped out of school, and needed some psychological support.

He had no dreams and no fantasies that he can remember during the siege, but beginning 1 week after release he had nightmares for 1 week in which he was threatened by guns. These have not recurred.

His negative feelings about the way the government handled the case have abated, and he is willing to help develop further policy. He sits on a national committee for this purpose. But he notes that the Ministry of Justice is very sensitive to criticism. "They think they do their best and that we should just express gratitude."

Significant Points in the Case

Gerard Vaders is a human being, alive today because he overcame the natural inhibitions that shroud intimate life details, and he displayed his true self to committed executioners. Ironically, this display of humanness could only occur after Mr. Vaders reconciled himself to death. Of course there can be no certainty in conjecture about precise reasons for the Moluccans' change of heart, nor can we know definitively why they chose him for execution in the first instance. As a notetaker and newsman (he told the Moluccans that much but never admitted editing the largest paper in North Holland), he stood out from the crowd. As a living curtain, suspended between compartments of the train, he was the nearest thing to an inanimate object. Disposing of curtains is easier than disposing of persons.

Mr. Vaders told me that he insisted on telling Mr. Prins all the details that should be conveyed to his wife and family, and he gave a great deal of background so that Mr. Prins could understand the message. The Moluccans tried to hurry this process at first, but Mr. Vaders was quite resolute and managed to overcome their objections. This is reminiscent of Judge DiGennaro, who was kidnapped by Italian terrorists and who told me, "I gave up all hope of life and I was free to be brave." Bravery did not mean attempting escape (he was bound and blindfolded throughout) but rather telling the captors exactly what was on his mind. Vaders showed a certain blend of courage and resignation that may have reminded the Moluccans of themselves.

His initial response to danger was classical. There was a period of arousal in which he felt cool, assessed the threat, and made physical and mental preparations. He was not particularly aware of bodily needs, visceral changes, or the falling temperature in the train during this beginning phase. However, he did suffer a collapse of sorts after the first night ended. There are phases in stress responses. Mr. Vaders may have entered what Hans Selye[2] calls the stage of exhaustion. Several other hostages in different settings have reported striking changes in their ability to function smoothly after dawn of the second day, or after the first period of sleep. The phenomenon is recognized; the mechanisms are not fully understood.

Mr. Vaders's response to danger was also idiosyncratic. Stress researchers have emphasized that both physiological and psychological patterns show striking individual differences, related to life history rather than the form or intensity of the threatening stressor. The other victims on the train were showing varied patterns of activity, emotion, and interaction throughout the siege.

To cope with captivity and the threat of death, Mr. Vaders employed several familiar coping strategies. First, Mr. Vaders assumed a familiar role. He became a journalist. In this role he could concentrate his attention, conserve his energy, and feel a certain amount of professional self-esteem. Preserving self-esteem is often more important to the individual than preserving life—a striking finding in the examination of these hostage inci-

dents. Furthermore, Mr. Vaders gathered information throughout his ordeal. Good copers do this. Others may constrict their
view of events in order to ward off threatening perceptions. Although denial of overwhelmingly negative input may be necessary
to preserve the ego, one's ability to scan the environment, to perceive quickly and accurately, and to gain further knowledge from
a peer group in a similar plight are all critical mechanisms for
coping with stress. Mr. Vaders employed these mechanisms.
Moreover, Mr. Vaders affiliated with his fellow captives. The ability to form and preserve affective bonds is necessary for normal
human development, is adaptive in negotiating the usual life
crises, and is critical in extreme situations such as captivity. Dr.
Leo Eitinger[1] and others who have studied concentration camp
survivors have documented and developed this point.

Mr. Vaders had a mild case of *Stockholm syndrome.* Named for
the dramatic and unexpected realignment of affections in the
Sveriges Kreditbank robbery, this syndrome consists of a positive
bond between hostage and captor, and feelings of distrust or hostility on the part of the victim toward the authorities. In Mr.
Vaders's case the negative display toward government was more
intense than the affection for the Moluccans. Both feelings began
in the early days of the siege, crested in the immediate aftermath,
and diminished over time. Some positive feeling toward the kind-
lier of the captors remains; negative feelings toward the government officials have abated. This is by now a recognized feature of
hostage situations. It does not occur in every instance but is frequent enough to be considered by police in the management of
protracted negotiations.

Finally, Mr. Vaders suffered a series of physical and emotional aftereffects that are characteristic of such situations. His
weight fell markedly, not only during the period of captivity and
restricted intake, but afterward. His protracted abdominal distress may or may not have been due to gallbladder disease. Gastrointestinal dysfunction after prolonged stress is not uncommon.
A variety of mechanisms and target organs may be involved.
Changes in eating, drinking, and smoking habits bridge the processes of physical and emotional reequilibration. For instance
emotion affects appetite, appetite affects nutrition, nutrition affects physical health, which in turn affects appetite and emotion.

Mr. Vaders did rather well psychologically, and as noted, his marriage emerged stronger than before the event. In several other cases victims have described feelings of "rebirth" and returned to family and friends with new resolve to place relationships on firmer ground. The fact that Mr. Vaders's daughter had difficult days is, sadly, a common occurrence. Loved ones do suffer by extension of the trauma into their lives, and they may not be protected by the mobilization of support that occurs within and around the victim. Mr. Vaders's nervous system was activated, his coping skills were employed, and his friends were rallied. This is not unlike the patient at death's door with a serious illness who ends up comforting his distraught relatives.

References

1. Eitinger, L. *Concentration camp survivors in Norway and Israel.* London: Allen & Unwin, 1964.
2. Selye, H. *The stress of life.* New York: McGraw-Hill, 1956.

XI

Coping with Unusual Crises
War and Imprisonment

Man's inhumanity to man reaches a pinnacle during wartime. The war that the United States fought in Vietnam was especially brutal. The guerrilla combat created different problems than those faced by soldiers during World War II. In Vietnam, the identity of the enemy was unknown. The Viet Cong shifted from combat to civilian roles, and so the Americans could not distinguish between friend and foe. Even when they were away from the front, servicemen always had to be alert because a friendly village might be the site of a surprise attack. Some soldiers reacted to the uncertain environment with rage and fear and outbursts of cruel violence. Americans tortured civilians and prisoners of war (POWs) and used ruthless tactics such as dropping napalm on an entire village in order to kill a few Viet Cong. Once the soldiers returned home, they faced a painful struggle to resolve feelings elicited by the havoc they inflicted during the war.

In the first chapter, Cindy Cook Williams describes how intrusive recollections such as flashbacks, nightmares, and recurring thoughts of wartime experiences can be healing processes that help Vietnam veterans come to grips with their war traumas and find meaning in them. Veterans faced the tasks of making sense of their participation in a war that was unpopular with the American people and reconciling the disparity between their actions in Vietnam and their personal value system. Veterans' preconceived visions of combat were destroyed by the realities of a war in which they struggled to survive, watched friends die in agony, and saw their values shattered. Many veterans who considered themselves decent people had to face the fact that they killed innocent civilians as well as soldiers.

Intrusive thoughts and images provide the content necessary to understand and work through alarming experiences, whereas denial helps gain temporary distance from disturbing memories. By shifting between painful recollections and periods of denial, veterans eventually can integrate their traumatic war experiences. However, some veterans act out violent behavior during flashbacks, whereas others cope with harrowing memories by becoming emotionally numb (much like survivors of a disaster; see Chapter 22). Still other veterans distance themselves from people, have problems forming lasting intimate relationships, or use drugs and alcohol to block out tension-producing memories.

Erwin Parson[5] notes that in order to make sense of their experiences in a war without victory, Vietnam veterans needed the American people's sanction and recognition of their efforts. Instead, the returning veterans experienced a "dysreception" that contributed to their postwar stress reaction. Herbert Hendin and Ann Pollinger Haas[3] have compiled compelling case material that vividly portrays veterans' posttraumatic stress disorders. They also studied a small group of veterans who adapted to combat without posttraumatic stress disorders. The veterans' personal resources aided their adaptation. These veterans maintained emotional and intellectual control in the face of combat and accepted rather than condemned fear in themselves and in others. They shunned excessive violence as a way of expressing their frustration at the Vietnamese. Moreover, they were able to impose their own structure on the chaos of the war and find a purpose in their combat experiences. They saw combat as a "dangerous challenge" rather than as a chance to prove their manhood or as a way of expressing anger and revenge.[3]

Despite its horrors, soldiers sometimes find that war creates positive changes. Israeli soldiers who fought in the Yom Kippur War found that it triggered a reevaluation of their personal values and priorities and made them more mature. Successful functioning under intense pressure increased the soldiers' self-esteem and self-confidence, as did the respect they received when they returned home. They were more tolerant of others and formed deeper relationships with them. Husbands felt closer to their wives and children. Finally, many soldiers appreciated life more fully after confronting life-and-death combat situations.[10] (For a study of the impact of military service on Vietnam and non-Vietnam veterans, and how these men's lives differed from non-veterans, see Card.[1])

Prisoners of war endure appalling adversity—inadequate food and shelter, torture, isolation and solitary confinement, and the uncertainty of not knowing when or if they will be freed. Immediately after capture, POWs typically are panic-stricken, fearful for their life, and plagued by thoughts of torture. Initial coping strategies involve regulating these emotions. Prisoners may block out fears by tunnel vision, paralysis, and dazed shock, and diminish their panic by focusing on details such as counting the number of captors. In the first minutes and hours, captives retain hope by telling themselves that their situation will improve and that they will be rescued soon. They may turn inward and focus on thoughts of loved ones, home, and freedom.[6]

Hypervigilance marks the next hours and days of captivity. Captives attend to all aspects of their captors' conduct and try to orient themselves by structuring their environment and keeping track of time as an aid to mental pacing. Communication with fellow captives is an essential source of support as prisoners engage in a cycle of resistance and compliance with their interrogators. Exercise and mental activities such as writing and learning a second language help to combat depression and the boredom of long-term captivity. Gradually, prisoners adapt, accept the fact that their captivity may be prolonged, and face 1 day at a time.[6]

Upon release, some Vietnam POWs worked through their feelings about captivity by talking about their experiences, giving lectures, and writing books. In the second article, David Jones discusses themes of effective coping he identified in books written by POWs. The underlying motif was that each man set an internal standard of behavior for himself that was reflected in loyalty to country. POWs remembered their heritage, believed that the American public supported and approved of them, and nurtured a heightened sense of duty to country. Prisoners also felt staunch devotion to their families. They idealized them and sought to survive and make their families proud. (For a remarkable personal account of a Navy captain who experienced 7 years of captivity and his wife's coping, see Stockdale & Stockdale.[8])

POWs' intense loyalty to each other was decisive in day-to-day survival and in facing isolation, interrogation, and torture. The men tried to resist their interrogators and used tactics such as playing dumb, providing trivial or garbled details, and writing confessions illegibly in order to avoid further torture, yet foil their captors' efforts to obtain useful information. Understanding and forgiveness were offered to those who were pushed beyond their limits and yielded under torture. The POWs helped the broken men regain their self-esteem and come to terms with their guilt. Finally, the POWs tried to remain loyal to their idealized self-image. POWs who have been found to cope best in captivity share some common traits—good physical health, a strong self-concept, a sense of purpose and satisfaction in life, and previous success and achievement. A rich and full life serves as a resource for the captive who must rely on memories of his past to combat boredom and isolation.

The families of POWs and men missing in action (MIAs) faced a prolonged, indefinite separation from their loved one and the uncertainty of not knowing if their husband or son was alive. Family members managed their plight by structuring their time, maintaining family routines, seeking support, and pursuing an active social life. Wives became more independent and learned to fulfill responsibilities that once belonged to their husband, such as making legal and financial decisions and disciplining the children.[4] (See Part V for a discussion of similar role changes experienced by divorced women.) Individuals and families who coped best with the stress of captivity were older, more mature, and better educated. They also had a sense of humor and were able to gain some control over their helplessness by becoming active in POW/MIA activities such as letter writing and making speeches.

Despite the extreme harshness of captivity, David Jones found that some POWs believed that the experience had enriched their lives. They were thankful for their blessings and more tolerant. Prisoners had time to review their past and to get to know themselves while in captivity; for some men this led to positive personality changes. Finally, many men considered the close personal relationships they developed with other prisoners as a lasting benefit. Likewise, some POW family members felt they matured from their ordeal. They experienced personal growth, became more self-confident, and learned how to relate to the public and stand up for their beliefs. POW couples found that their marital relationships deepened, and they communicated more openly, whereas their children saw themselves as more mature and responsible.[4] (For a general discussion of the benefits to children who grow up in a single-parent household, see Chapter 4.)

Perhaps no people in history endured more extreme conditions than the inmates of Nazi concentration camps. In the final article, Paul Chodoff describes the massive trauma of the Nazi camps and the common reactions of camp inmates. Holocaust victims experienced brutal and degrading living conditions, forced labor, torture, malnutrition, disease, the constant threat of death, and the agony of separation from family. Despite the unimaginable horrors of the camps, many inmates managed to survive.

Upon arrival at the camps, inmates experienced shock and terror, followed by apathy and then depression. Aapthy was adaptive in that it helped the prisoners blunt their initial fright and horror. Regression and denial were other common ways of trying to survive in the inhuman camp environment. The prisoners relied primarily on cognitive coping strategies because there was little opportunity to fight back and use problem-solving methods. Nonetheless, one of the most effective survival strategies was maintaining relationships with other inmates. In the desolate, bleak environment of the camps, inmates gained a semblance of control and took pleasure in little actions such as managing to get an extra food ration.

Some inmates were able to endure camp life by finding meaning in their survival. Inmates struggled to survive in order to bear witness to Nazi atrocities, to seek revenge, or because they hoped to be reunited with family members (for a dramatic account, see *Sophie's Choice*[9]). After their release, some survivors wrote books that informed the world of Nazi atrocities and eloquently recounted inmates' struggles to endure. Others hunted

Nazis in order to have justice affirmed. For many, the establishment of the state of Israel was seen as a way of making their horrific experiences meaningful.

After liberation, many survivors discovered that their homes had been destroyed and that members of their family were dead. They faced the burden of moving to a new country and establishing a new life. These new losses and the severe physical and psychological assaults of the camps left permanent emotional scars. Years later, some concentration camp survivors experienced "survivor guilt" for cheating death when so many others had died or for actions that they saw as endangering others' lives (see also Chapter 22). They were plagued by vague feelings that they had done something wrong. Many suffered from "concentration camp syndrome"—anxiety, depression, intense guilt, and a variety of enduring physical symptoms.

Some camp survivors married soon after their release. Marriage provided a way for them to recreate a family, overcome their grief, and make up for their losses. Yael Danieli[2] studied the families that resulted from these "marriages of despair" and found disturbed family relationships and a lack of normal parenting functions. But not all survivor families are mired in psychopathology. Maria Rosenbloom[7] notes that most children of survivors are leading productive lives. They see their family links to the Holocaust as having helped them form an identity, sensitizing them to others' suffering, and giving direction to their lives. The successes of the concentration camp survivors and their children are a glowing tribute to human resilience.

References

1. Card, J. J. *Lives after Vietnam: The personal impact of military service.* Lexington, Mass.: Heath, 1983.
2. Danieli, Y. Differing adaptational styles in families of survivors of the Nazi Holocaust. *Children Today*, 1981, *10*, 6–10, 34–35.
3. Hendin, H., & Haas, A. P. *Wounds of war: The psychological aftermath of combat in Vietnam.* New York: Basic Books, 1984.
4. Hunter, E. J. Captivity: The family in waiting. In C. R. Figley & H. I. McCubbin (Eds.), *Stress and the family: Coping with catastrophe* (Vol. 2). New York: Brunner/Mazel, 1983.

5. Parson, E. R. The reparation of the self: Clinical and theoretical dimensions in the treatment of Vietnam combat veterans. *Journal of Contemporary Psychotherapy*, 1984, *14*, 4–56.

6. Rahe, R. H., & Genender, E. Adaptation to and recovery from captivity stress. *Military Medicine*, 1983, *148*, 577–585.

7. Rosenbloom, M. Implications of the Holocaust for social work. *Social Casework*, 1983, *64*, 205–213.

8. Stockdale, J., & Stockdale, S. *In love and war: The story of a family's ordeal and sacrifice during the Vietnam years.* New York: Harper & Row, 1984.

9. Styron, W. *Sophie's choice.* New York: Random House, 1976.

10. Yarom, N. Facing death in war—An existential crisis. In S. Breznitz (Ed.), *Stress in Israel.* New York: Van Nostrand Reinhold, 1983.

27

The Mental Foxhole
The Vietnam Veteran's Search for Meaning

CINDY COOK WILLIAMS

Intrusive Thoughts and Images of War

Three types of intrusive and recurrent recollections about the war have been described by Vietnam veterans. These include (1) flashbacks or involuntary reenactments of a past event; (2) nightmares or night terrors; and (3) thoughts about the war that cannot be dispelled despite a desire to do so. Numerous anecdotal accounts of the occurrence of these recollections were found in the literature. One young Vietnam veteran's experiences with flashbacks and nightmares were described by Hogben and Cornfield[18] as:

> After entering the Marine Corps, he had eight months of combat in Vietnam. There he participated in much violence and frequently saw his buddies killed by mortar fire. . . . After discharge from the service, the patient noticed severe and frightening war-related nightmares for the first time. He was paralyzed on waking from the nightmares, but he was able to return to sleep. He also had intense, unprovoked day images of traumatic

This chapter appears in abridged form from the *American Journal of Orthopsychiatry*, 1983, *53*, 4–17. Copyright 1983, the American Orthopsychiatric Association, Inc. Reproduced by permission.

CINDY COOK WILLIAMS • Survey Research Center, Institute for Social Research, Social Environment and Health Program, University of Michigan, Ann Arbor, Michigan 48106.

war experiences and heard bullets and mortar shells whizzing by him. Loud fireworks provoked the visual reexperiencing of war scenes (p. 442).

In a study of 207 community college Vietnam veterans, De-Fazio, Rustin, and Diamond[5] found that over 50% of the respondents reported frequent nightmares. Frightening dreams and nightmares were found to occur more often among combat veterans as compared to noncombat veterans[9] and nonveterans.[23] Although in-depth investigation of the content of these dreams has not been reported, veterans often describe seeing themselves in helpless combat situations where their survival is at stake. In a typical dream, for example, the veteran may find that his rifle will not fire when he is faced with direct attack by the Viet Cong. Or he may dream of hiding in a foxhole surrounded by the enemy. It has also been reported that the onset of combat nightmares can follow environmental stimuli that remind the veteran of Vietnam.[5] Seeing a Vietnamese refugee on the street, experiencing a sudden downpour of rain in the summer, or merely having the heat in one's home exceed 80 degrees may be sufficient precipitators. Figley and Southerly[9] concluded in their study that these nightmares are characterized by (1) repeated occurrence; (2) dream content related to military service; (3) making veterans fight or fear sleep; and (4) waking them up.

Flashbacks or suddenly feeling and acting as if one were again in combat constitutes another type of intrusive phenomenon. For example, one veteran[23] experienced flashbacks to a Christmas Eve ambush "and the keening echo of the women and children dying in the road" (p. 91). Approximately 17% of the 549 Vietnam-era veterans studied by Kadushin, Boulanger, and Martin experienced flashbacks. Again, little in-depth research has been conducted on the content of flashbacks. However, anecdotal descriptions[1,14,15,24] cite environmental precipitators that resemble Vietnam. These stimuli can affect any sensory modality, such as the visual, auditory, and olfactory systems. Sometimes violent outbursts of behavior follow. One veteran saw some armed guards and thought he was again back in Vietnam. With no weapon to protect himself, he grabbed an innocent passerby for protection and forced this person into his home.[15] Kormos[24] described an ex-medic who hurled his brother down the stairs during a flashback; his behavior was so "automatic, that he didn't know how his brother had come to land in a heap on the floor—he was stunned by his own behavior" (p. 49).

The last type of recollection involves thoughts about the war that veterans are unable to dispel despite their desire to do so. Of the 2,453 Vietnam-era veterans sampled by Harris and Associates (cited in Fisher *et al.*[11]), 13% reported being frightened by memories of death and dying; 80% of these respondents indicated that their military service either caused or heavily contributed to these thoughts. One Vietnam veteran[15] described his experiences as follows:

> Sometimes my head starts to replay some of my experiences in Nam. Regardless of what I'd like to think about, it comes creeping in. It's so hard to push back out again. It's old friends, their faces, the ambush, the screams, their faces [tears]. . . . You know, everytime I hear a chopper [helicopter] or see a clear unobstructed green treeline, a chill goes down my back; I remember. (p. 2)

Again, it is the heavy-combat veteran of Vietnam who is more likely to report intrusive and recurrent memories of battle.[26] Similar to nightmares and flashback experiences, the onset can be precipitated by environmental stimuli resembling Vietnam and the combat situation itself.

What is the purpose of these reenactments that continue to recur despite the years separating these veterans from their combat experiences? Try as they may to leave the war behind, it appears that the past is still pursuing the Vietnam veteran.

The Search for Meaning

People who experience traumatic life events usually undergo a healing or restorative process. An integral part of this process is the search for the personal meaning of the tragedy or stressor.[6,12] Unsettling new experiences in one's life, such as death, war, and separation, often point out how incomplete or inadequate previous answers have been. Thus, a highly individualized and creative search for meaning often begins where previous explanations are found wanting.

What is it that Vietnam veterans must reformulate and rediscover? For one, these veterans are trying to make sense of an experience that many people in this country consider evil and pointless. A substantial proportion of the nation's people believe that the United States should have stayed out of the fighting in Vietnam. Although the public often believes that Vietnam-era veterans were drafted into the military, in reality the majority enlisted.[11] Interestingly, Laufer *et al.*[26] reported that Vietnam veterans were significantly more likely than noncombat veterans and nonveterans to have *supported* U.S. involvement in the war. Thus, expectations of serving this country as patriotic citizens, imitating the prototype of John Wayne, or stopping Communist infiltration were views often cast aside by these soldiers in the actual realities of war. Instead of meeting the usual challenges of adolescent and young adult development, many of these young men and women were faced with the sheer challenge of physical survival.[32] They watched as friends died. Boundaries of acting out one's violent impulses frequently became diffuse in this war and sometimes mixed with the pleasure of killing Vietnamese. It is easy to see how previous value systems and views about oneself often were blasted away in the face of the killing, fear, and fighting. Although not a Vietnam veteran, a World War II combat veteran[16] originally cited by Egendorf, Remez, and Farley[6] summarized it best:

> I am afraid to forget. . . . What protrudes and does not fit in our pasts rises to haunt us and make us spiritually unwell in the present. The deepest fear of my war years, one still with me, is that these happenings had no real purpose. . . . I strive to see at least my own life as a whole and to discover some purpose and direction in at least the major parts. Yet the effort to assimilate those intense war memories to the rest of my experience is difficult and even frightening. (p. 76)

It is evident that the Vietnam veteran's search for meaning involves issues on both a personal and societal level. And it may be that this search has only begun.

The Personal Search

Changing one's self-concept often involves a loss—a loss of previously held views about oneself. In his description of dissonance theory, Aronson[2] emphasized that "a person's tendency to change his attitude is motivated by an aversive state of arousal caused by the violation of the self-concept" (p. 152). Certainly war between nations and mankind has occurred since the beginning of time, and few would challenge that combat for many people is an aversive state of arousal. Laufer *et al.*[26] confirmed that the mere attempt to survive physically was one of the most important goals that men faced in Vietnam. But what is it that causes the Vietnam veteran such inner turmoil in his attempt to lessen the dissonance in his view of himself?

The Vietnam veteran who described himself as a "decent, good, reasonable, and fair" person before the war may now question the truth of these statements. For example, how would one fit into this self-concept the killing of other human beings—civilians and soldiers alike? One way people decrease the dissonance between their behavior and their self-concept is to deny that they *directly* harmed others. In some modern wars, the use of sophisticated weaponry and battle strategies often allowed physical distance between the "enemy" or opposing forces.[29] These soldiers frequently did not see the direct consequences of their actions. The nature of guerrilla warfare in Vietnam, however, did not easily provide combatants with this avenue of dealing with the killing. For those soldiers who faced the enemy during jungle maneuvers, the sudden personalization of the Viet Cong was a frequent reality. Hand-to-hand combat, sneak ambushes, civilian deaths, and body counts were inherent in this war.[4] Harris and associates (cited in Fisher *et al.*[11]) found that nearly 60% of their respondents acknowledged direct involvement in killing. In a study of Vietnam veterans seeking mental health treatment, Lund and Strachan[27] found that 35% reported killing civilians during their tour of duty. Although the psychological disturbance related to such actions was reported as being minimal while in the military, the veterans reported that it was a stressful and difficult issue to work through after leaving the service. Nearly half of those combat veterans in the Laufer *et al.* study[26] who had not sought help felt sad when they had seen Vietnamese killed or wounded. Thus, war may only suppress but not eradicate man's humaneness. It is this dichotomous behavior of mankind, however, that may be at the roots of the Vietnam veteran's search for meaning.

Intrusive Recollections as a Healthy Coping Strategy

Healthy or adaptive coping strategies require that the individuals actively search for the source of their own discomfort and distress. It requires *more* than superficial reflection, however. The process of searching requires an open and *honest* look at how one's life experiences fit into past views about oneself and the world.[6] It is the healthy personality, according to Jourard,[22] that is characterized by active growth, despite the pain this process can entail.

Catastrophic life experiences, such as war, natural disasters, and the Holocaust, cannot be undone. The memories and impact of these events live on among the survivors, and successful integration of these experiences requires healthy coping strategies. Horowitz and associates[20,21] found that an adaptive response to stressful events included the occurrence of intrusive and repetitive thoughts and images alternating with periods of ideational denial and emotional numbness. Within certain boundaries, it is the vacillation between these recollections and avoidance responses that provides a healthy coping response in eventually mastering these experiences. For example, the thoughts and visual images, whether intrusive or voluntary, provide the material upon which an individual can begin the process of understanding and working through these events. Yet the denial-numbing can also provide distance from the memories when the working-through process becomes too intense or threatening for the individual. It is within this context that recollections can be considered a healthy coping strategy. Interestingly enough, clinical outcome studies[3,7,30] designed to decrease intrusive cognitive ruminations generally report marginal treatment success. Although an initial decrease may occur in response to behavioral techniques, it is not uncommon for these thoughts to return. This raises the question of whether it may be counterproductive to attempt to "cure" such thoughts, since individuals who have gone through traumatic events may need these very thoughts and memories to integrate their experiences successfully.

Horowitz[19] emphasized that these "response tendencies among people are similar in nature in that they appear after a variety of stress events which differ in quantity and quality" (p. 81). Thus, it can be concluded that the Vietnam veteran's response to combat has similarities to the reactions of other "normal" people who have experienced stressful life events. Not only do many veterans search for an understanding of the deaths they have witnessed and sometimes caused, many also seek an understanding of the incongruity between their personal value system and their actions in Vietnam. Is such a search dysfunctional? In most instances, it is not. However, an imbalance in the recollection and denial-numbing continuum can lead to problems in everyday living.

Dysfunctional Consequences

Empirical evidence shows that the intrusive thoughts, flashbacks, and nightmares experienced by Vietnam veterans can be frightening, troubling and anxiety-provoking.[11,26] One way to buffer the pain is to become emotionally numb—to feel neither extreme pleasure nor pain. It is not uncommon for Vietnam veterans to describe themselves as being emotionally dead.[29,31] Goodwin[15] emphasized that

> some veterans I've interviewed actually believed that if they once again allow themselves to feel, they may never stop crying or may completely lose control of themselves; what they mean by this is unknown to them. (p. 14)

Although emotional numbing is adaptive in many instances, its excessive generalization to other domains of one's life can be dysfunctional.

It is not uncommon for the families (and particularly wives) of Vietnam veterans to complain that the men come across as cold and uncaring. Divorce and remarriage rates, for example, are higher among heavy-combat veterans compared to those who had experienced little combat.[8] Indeed, it appears that extreme emotional distancing could lead to failure in achieving the intimacy necessary to sustain some marriages. Thus, some Vietnam veterans may go through life with an impaired capacity to care or even love others—and suffer true estrangement and alienation.

Some Vietnam veterans may turn to alcohol and drug use to buffer the pain and anxiety associated with excessive recollections of the war. Alcohol use, for one, is a readily available form of self-medication. It can decrease anxiety, muscle tension, and agitation.

It also suppresses REM sleep—the phase of sleep associated with nightmares. Lacoursiere, Godfrey and Ruby,[25] however, pointed out that:

> What can begin as innocent self-medication for symptoms of traumatic neurosis can lead to a vicious circle. Repetitive symptom reduction by means of alcohol leads to tolerance and an increase in alcohol consumption to maintain symptom reduction, which leads to problems from the alcohol use itself (e.g., hangovers, gastritis, marital difficulties, and arrests for driving while intoxicated) and attempts to reduce or abstain from alcohol consumption. This leads to the alcohol withdrawal syndrome, with an exacerbation of many of the initial traumatic neurosis symptoms; this stimulates further drinking, closing the vicious circle. (p. 966)

Again, excessive use of chemical substances to mask the pain and anxiety of intrusive recollections can lead to dysfunctional consequences.

Recurring reenactments of the war through flashbacks and nightmares also can be maladaptive in some instances. During these experiences, the individual acts or feels like he is experiencing scenes from the war again. And, of course, the war involved violence. At times the violent behavior necessary for survival in Vietnam is acted out during flashbacks, nightmares, or night terrors. For example, wives report being choked or experiencing the strangling hold of their husbands' hands around their necks while sleeping in the middle of the night.[15,31] Again, research has not investigated the relationship between intrusive reenactments and violent acting out. This may be the greatest myth perpetuated by society about the Vietnam veteran, or it may be a common maladaptive response. Interestingly enough, in a laboratory experiment, Geen, Stonner, and Shope[13] found that acts of aggression tend to increase the probability of future aggression.

What characterizes the Vietnam veteran who suffers from dysfunctional responses related to his attempt to master his involvement in the war? One key factor may revolve around the issue of ventilation—not having the *opportunity* to talk about issues of concern, as well as not being *personally able* to discuss them. Many people find that ventilating or talking about traumatic events helps them master or integrate these issues into their self-concept and view of the world.

The antagonism between Vietnam veterans and the people of

the United States upon the homecoming of these soldiers is well documented.[11,26,28] During the time that the veterans returned home, Shatan[29] described their reception by the nation as:

> a welcome so equivocal that they may be treated both as trained killers and as those who "lost the war." This lack of moral acceptance, this defensive denial of their needs, further exacerbates their failure to mourn. They feel set aside from the rest of us by experiences whose horror they can barely convey. (p. 648)

In many instances, family members, friends, and other acquaintances did not want to hear about the war, specifically the experiences in combat. Many of the people who *did* listen did not understand. Thus, Vietnam veterans who tried to speak of their concerns often were met with overt or covert discomfort by the people at home.[10,17] In one of the few studies conducted on family relationships,[8] veterans who experienced heavy combat were less likely to have a family member they felt they could talk to ($r = -.25$, $p < .05$) or whom they felt understood them ($r = -.28$, $p < .05$). Similar experiences occurred among unmarried men who came home to girlfriends or who attempted to establish new relationships after the war. In a local Vietnam veteran organization, one veteran told the author:

> *Well, see, as a woman, you don't know what it's like to come back here after being in the jungle. I mean there were the "Sally Co-eds"—you know, the sorority types—they'd smile sweet and ask what the war was like. But their real worry was who was going to win the next football game or who was going to the dance. I mean, how can you relate to that? And it just wasn't them—it was most everyone. So you learned it wasn't worth it to talk—so you just kept it inside and let it brew.*

It may be that when unresolved issues continue to brew deep inside these veterans, the frequency of intrusive recollections increases. For some Vietnam veterans, the search for meaning may acquire maladaptive features in relation to society's inability to provide them with adequate opportunities to discuss and work through their combat experiences. And some may still be personally unable to talk about it, even in a supportive environment.

Summary and Conclusions

Many Vietnam veterans, particularly those involved in combat, continue to experience psychological distress nearly a decade after the war. The occurrence of intrusive and repetitive thoughts, nightmares, and visual images is frequently reported by Vietnam veterans still troubled by the war. These responses are not necessarily reflective of an illness, however; they can provide a healthy and adaptive pathway for the veteran to search for the personal meaning of his experiences in Vietnam. New explanations can be found—sometimes new values and beliefs about oneself and the world—when old meanings fail to provide needed answers. Without an open atmosphere in which to examine his war experience, the Vietnam veteran will continue to be assigned his fate—to hide and endure his pain alone in what one veteran has described as his "mental foxhole."[29]

References

1. Alarcon, R., Dickinson, W., & Dohn, H. Flashback phenomena: Clinical and diagnostic dilemmas. *Journal of Nervous and Mental Disease*, 1982, *170*, 217–223.
2. Aronson, E. *The social animal*. San Francisco: Freeman, 1980.
3. Blue, R. Ineffectiveness of an aversion therapy technique in treatment of obsessional thinking. *Psychological Reports*, 1978, *43*, 181–182.
4. Brende, J., & Benedict, B. The Vietnam combat delayed stress response syndrome: Hypnotherapy of dissociative symptoms. *American Journal of Clinical Hypnosis*, 1980, *23*, 34–40.
5. DeFazio, V., Rustin, S., & Diamond, A. Symptom development in Vietnam era veterans. *American Journal of Orthopsychiatry*, 1975, *45*, 158–163.
6. Egendorf, A., Remez, A., & Farley, J. Dealing with the war: A view based on the individual lives of Vietnam veterans. In A. Egendorf, Kadushin, C., Laufer, R. S., Rothbart, G., & Sloan, L. (Eds.), *Legacies of Vietnam: Comparative adjustment of veterans and their peers* (Vol. 5). Washington, D.C.: U.S. Government Printing office, 1981.
7. Emmelkamp, P., & Kwee, K. Obsessional ruminations: A comparison between thought stopping and prolonged exposure in imagination. *Behavioral Research and Therapy*, 1977, *15*, 441–444.
8. Faude, K., & Weston-Zarit, J. *Vietnam era veterans and family relationships*. Paper presented to the American Psychological Association, Los Angeles, 1981.
9. Figley, C., & Southerly, W. *Residue of war: The Vietnam veterans in mainstream America*. Paper presented to the American Psychological Association, San Francisco, 1977.
10. Figley, C., & Sprenkle, D. Delayed stress response syndrome: Family therapy indications. *Journal of Marriage and Family Counseling*, 1978, *4*, 53–60.
11. Fisher, V. *et al. Myths and realities: A study of attitudes toward Vietnam veterans*. Washington, D.C.: U.S. Government Printing Office, 1980.

12. Frankl, V. *Man's search for meaning*. New York: Simon & Schuster, 1959.
13. Geen, R., Stonner, D., & Shope, G. The facilitation of aggression: A study in response inhibition and disinhibition. *Journal of Personality and Social Psychology*, 1975, *31*, 721–726.
14. Goldman, P., & Fuller, T. Special report: What Vietnam did to us. *Newsweek*, Dec. 14, 1981, pp. 72–74, 76, 81–82, 84, 88, 91–92, 94, 96.
15. Goodwin, J. The etiology of combat-related post-traumatic stress disorders. In T. Williams (Ed.), *Post-traumatic stress disorders of the Vietnam veterans*. Cincinnati, Ohio: Disabled American Veterans National Headquarters, 1980.
16. Gray, J. *The warriors: Reflections on men in battle*. New York: Harper & Row, 1959.
17. Haley, S. Treatment implications of post-combat stress response syndromes for mental health professionals. In C. Figley (Ed.), *Stress disorders among Vietnam veterans*. New York: Brunner/Mazel, 1978.
18. Hogben, G., & Cornfield, R. Treatment of traumatic war neurosis with phenelzine. *Archives of General Psychiatry*, 1981, *38*, 440–445.
19. Horowitz, M. *Stress response syndromes*. New York: Aronson, 1976.
20. Horowitz, M., & Wilner, N. Life events, stress, and coping. In L. Poon (Ed.), *Aging in the 1980s: Psychological issues*. Washington, D.C.: American Psychological Association, 1980.
21. Horowitz, M., Wilner, N., Kaltreider, N., & Alvarez, W. Signs and symptoms of posttraumatic stress disorder. *Archives of General Psychiatry*, 1980, *37*, 85–92.
22. Jourard, S. *Personal adjustment: An approach through the study of healthy personality*. New York: Macmillan, 1967.
23. Kadushin, C., Boulanger, G., & Martin, J. Long term stress reactions: Some causes, consequences, and naturally occurring support systems. In A. Egendorf *et al.* (Eds.), *Legacies of Vietnam: Comparative adjustment of veterans and their peers* (Vol. 4). Washington, D.C.: U.S. Government Printing Office, 1981.
24. Kormos, H. The nature of combat stress. In C. Figley (Ed.), *Stress disorders among Vietnam veterans*. New York: Brunner/Mazel, 1978.
25. Lacoursiere, R., Godfrey, K., & Ruby, L. Traumatic neurosis in the etiology of alcoholism: Vietnam combat and other trauma. *American Journal of Psychiatry*, 1980, *137*, 966–968.
26. Laufer, R. *et al.* Post-war trauma: Social and psychological problems of Vietnam veterans in the aftermath of the Vietnam war. In A. Egendorf *et al.* (Eds.), *Legacies of Vietnam: Comparative adjustment of veterans and their peers* (Vol. 3). Washington, D.C.: U.S. Government Printing Office, 1981.
27. Lund, M., & Strachan, A. *The Vietnam combat exposure scale*. Paper presented to the American Psychological Association, Los Angeles, 1981.
28. Marin, P. Living in moral pain. *Psychology Today*, Nov. 1981, pp. 68, 71–72, 77, 79–80.
29. Shatan, C. The grief of soldiers: Vietnam combat veterans' self-help movement. *American Journal of Orthopsychiatry*, 1973, *43*, 640–653.
30. Stern, R., Lipsedge, M., & Marks, I. Obsessive ruminations: A controlled trial of thought-stopping technique. *Behavioral Research and Therapy*, 1973, *11*, 659–662.

31. Strickland, F. Personal communication. Ann Arbor, Mich.: VA Medical Center, 1982.
32. Wilson, J. Toward an understanding of posttraumatic stress disorders among Vietnam veterans. Testimony before the U.S. Senate Subcommittee on Veteran Affairs, Washington, D.C., 1980.

28

What Repatriated Prisoners of War Wrote about Themselves

DAVID R. JONES

The repatriation of the prisoners of war (POWs) held in North and South Vietnam took place in the spring of 1973. This group included 564 military men and 23 civilians; all except 71 of the military were officers, and most considered themselves career military men. The majority were Air Force and Navy fliers shot down between 1965 and 1968, with a second group shot down in 1972. Collectively, these men were older, better trained, and better educated than any group of POWs in history. As career military men, most had a fairly clear understanding of the strategic and political position of the United States in its support of the South Vietnamese government. As fliers, most were operating from fixed bases in South Vietnam or Thailand, or from aircraft carriers; in these locations, a great deal of attention had been paid to their health and welfare. Thus, their mental and physical health was generally excellent until their shootdown. Many were injured in the course of ejection and parachute landings, and their subse-

Reprinted with permission from *Aviation, Space, and Environmental Medicine*, 1980, *51*, 615–617. Copyright 1980 by Aerospace Medicine Association, Washington, D.C.

DAVID R. JONES • USAFSAM/NGN, Brooks Air Force Base, San Antonio, Texas 78235.

quent poor medical care, mistreatment, malnutrition, and outright torture are now widely known.

All of us can remember the national attention focused on the return of these POWs—the live television coverage, the joyful reunions, the interviews, the debriefings and medical examination, the speeches, and the gradual process of reassimilation into the military and the civilian communities. With the passage of time, national attention has turned elsewhere, and most of these men have returned to the privacy of their own careers. Some of us are still involved in their long-term follow-up at the USAF School of Aerospace Medicine. Medical processes, long-term demographic data, and their ultimate life stories are all of interest to us. In learning about them, we learn something about ourselves and about all humanity.

Some of these men have set themselves apart from the group as a whole. They chose to write books or to be interviewed at length for inclusion in books written by journalists, sharing an aspect of their memories and self-perceptions with the public. This active process is qualitatively different from answering questionnaires or being officially debriefed. People write books for a variety of reasons, but they share the desire to say something to other people, something they regard as important.

Was there a common message or theme? Did they manage to survive the years of captivity by using defenses familiar to us all? What ideas did they regard as crucial to their own survival?

I read six books in looking for answers to these questions: *The Passing of the Night* by Robinson Risner, *Five Years to Freedom* by James N. Rowe, *With God in a POW Camp* by Ralph Gaither, *They Wouldn't Let Us Die* by Stephen A. Rowan, *Survivors* by Zalin Grant, and *P.O.W.* by John C. Hubell.[1-6] The first three books were single-author accounts, and the last three were based on multiple interviews by the journalist-authors. In these accounts, I found that some 26 men clearly stated ideas that sustained them. These were expressed in different ways. Some men formulated them clearly and concretely early in captivity, while others developed them as they underwent their personal ordeals. Several commented that they had to keep these ideas simple and succinct so as to be able to adhere to them under heavy pressure from their captors.

There is a single theme common to all these accounts: a standard of behavior that each man set for himself. Although couched in different terms and at times projected onto outside—and perhaps idealized—figures, this standard was apparent in all accounts. Much of it was based on the *Code of Conduct for Members of the Armed Forces of the United States,* but this was refined and individualized as time went by and the realities of the POW environment in Vietnam became apparent. We will look at this theme as it was applied in the POW situation, tracing its application to the more concrete and immediate aspects of their lives.

Loyalty to Country

This loyalty was variously expressed as remembering their heritage, feeling that the U.S. public was behind them and would not let them down, and that their duty to their country did not end with their capture. As news of the increasing opposition to the war came to the POWs, some expressed their ambivalence about undergoing torture for refusing to endorse the statements of responsible public figures who opposed the war, even some who were presidential candidates. This ambivalence was frequently resolved by deciding that the right of Americans to express opposing opinions, the right of free speech, was precisely what they were sworn to defend as military men; to endorse an opinion opposing the war, no matter how respectable its source, would weaken their defense of this right, and they would not do it voluntarily.

Another form of loyalty to country was that given to the president of the United States. This loyalty was to the man as a symbol of the country, and not necessarily a personal or political loyalty to a particular president. The president symbolized the country and the national will.

Loyalty to Family

Some men expressed a strong sense of loyalty to their families. These men were sustained by a desire to be a credit to their families: not to disgrace them, not to betray them, and not to increase their suffering by being killed by their captors. One man clung to the last words his wife had said to him: "Don't make me a widow." As one might expect, during the years of captivity the men tended more and more to idealize their families and hoped to be able to return to them with a feeling of having been worthy of them.

Loyalty to Fellow POWs

Perhaps the most immediate and strongest loyalty, day by day, was to fellow prisoners. This took the form of mutual support and of continued opposition to their captors. It was necessary not only to establish personal standards of behavior but also to agree on group standards. The value of establishing one's membership in a supportive group in such dire circumstances cannot be overstated and is witnessed by the intense and dangerous efforts taken to establish communications with other POWs and especially with the new shootdowns, to help them avoid the terrible feeling of aloneness. The more experienced POWs knew the value of briefing new arrivals on the expected norms of conduct and of reassuring them when they felt they had disgraced themselves by giving up information under duress that went beyond the ideal of name, rank, service number, and date of birth.

This feeling was variously expressed as being responsible to each other, needing to be able to look the others in the eye, and knowing that the others were pulling for the one undergoing torture. In this regard, a great deal of support was derived from telling the other prisoners what one had said under duress, both as a catharsis, and—more practically—so that stories could be kept straight. With this, one experienced forgiveness and understanding, a sense of ongoing acceptance by the group. In transactional analysis terms, if the code of conduct represented the stern, inflexible ideal of the critical parent, then the day-to-day support of the other POWs represented the reassurance of the nurturing parent that one was doing one's best.

Opposition to the captors took a number of forms. It was expressed as "we're doing the right thing here," or "they only understand force." The North Vietnamese were "ignorant about democracy" and were despised as manifesting the teachings of communism. In a pragmatic way, one experienced POW communicated to new arrivals not to change their minds about the war on the basis of what their captors said. Another vowed to live to tell the tale of how his fellow prisoners died on a forced march from South to North Vietnam. I might add parenthetically that I heard one ex-POW say in a speech that he was sustained by the thought that, when it was all over, he would get to go back to the United States while his captors were stuck forever in North Vietnam. *They* were the captives, *he* was free!

With rare exceptions, the POWs placed a great deal of value on resisting interrogation. Much of the content of their books deal with this matter. They all agree that any of them could be "broken" by torture, and so they had to deal with two issues: how they could best resist and how to regain their self-esteem once they had broken under torture. Individually, they set various limits for themselves. Collectively, most of them accepted the interpretation of the code of conduct by the senior ranking officer in their camp. Most learned that simply answering the four questions allowed by the code and refusing to answer any others was too rigid a position to maintain, and so they prepared mental fallback positions. These included such tactics as playing dumb, giving a great deal of detailed but trivial information, giving information they knew their captors already possessed, giving garbled information, couching forced "confessions" in stilted or awkward phrases to destroy their credibility, and so on. Some were truly passive/aggressive in such situations, writing illegibly or finding other ways of annoying their captors but stopping just short of incurring further torture. Such small victories were important in maintaining morale. In spite of having decided to resist to their limits and to give nothing of value to their captors, many of these men were pushed past their limits. Once they broke under torture, they had to overcome their feelings of shame and guilt and bounce back, to reestablish a stance of resistance. As noted before, the communications network helped immensely to support them during this vulnerable period, and most were able to recover their self-esteem and their will to resist in a few days or weeks. The knowledge that it was possible to roll with the situation and to recover and that others had done so successfully in the past and would not condemn one for having to do so now was one of the most important sustaining factors in the camp.

Loyalty to Self-Image

In a sense, all of the previous aspects of the personal loyalties of the POWs had to do with their image of how an ideal citizen, family man, or military man would behave under the trying conditions of the POW camps. Each seems also to have had an idealized self-image that was important to maintain. For a few, articulation of this image approached magical thinking, a feeling of personal invulnerability. This may have represented an extension of the usual way that fliers use denial in order to perform dangerous missions. Some phrased it "I can get through today" or "I can hack it one day at a time." Others spoke in terms of "I *knew* I'd survive" or "I felt I'd make it." One put it more aggressively: "I'll be damned if you people are going to kill me!" Such phrases are convincing when written after the fact by survivors; one wonders if some of the prisoners who did *not* survive said the same thing.

Much was written in testimony of the personal sense of support from the religious convictions of the POWs. Not all the men felt that religion sustained them; in fact, some stated clearly that they had no particular religious conviction. As one put it, "God had not put me there, and God was not going to get me out of it." Nevertheless, many attest to the power of their faith, and several attribute miraculous occurrences in answer to their prayers: being able to get out of tortuously tightened handcuffs, ecstatic relief from severe and prolonged pain, or a feeling of a calm, complete inner certainty that they would survive. These men recounted their experiences as a testimony to the power of God and the strength of their faith. Some of the POWs described this personal, internal faith as being the most solid reality in their lives.

Some returnees felt that the POW experience had good aspects. None of the men initially regarded their captivity as a chance for personal growth or a potentially beneficial experience, but a number of them look back on it as having enhanced their lives. One phrased it as "I'm lucky to be alive." Others wrote of a new sense of tolerance, of being thankful for present blessings or of having had a chance to plan for the future. Some reviewed their past lives, their personalities, and their family relationships and seem to have performed what they regard as a self-analysis resulting in changes for the better. One spoke of deciding to sublimate his personal ambition and seek instead to serve his country by his contributions. Many mentioned their close personal ties with their fellow POWs as a lasting benefit of their captivity experience: this was a new experience for some of these action-oriented, nonintrospective men.

In this matter, Sledge, Boydstun, and Rahe[7] have a paper that indicates a positive relationship between the feeling of having benefitted or grown during the captivity experience and the amount of abuse or torture reported.[7] The men in charge of the prison camps apparently emphasized the personal degradation of their prisoners as a part of their effort to break their will and resistance. Filthy cells, rats and roaches, a bare subsistence diet, lack of protection from cold or heat, solitary confinement, being manacled and made to lie in their own waste, lack of medical care, attempts at humiliation, prolonged physical discomfort, and outright torture were all orchestrated in this attempt to degrade the POWs. Thus, the confrontation centered on the prisoners' self-esteem and sense of honor. Even though both sides knew that any given POW could be broken, could be forced to write letters against the war or to make tapes confessing his supposed guilt for war crimes, it was apparent that there was no lasting conversion to the North Vietnamese cause except in rare instances. Thus, the more pressure a man withstood, the more likely he seems to have had his self-esteem ratified by the experience, to feel that he had been tried and found true.

One factor was *not* apparent in the behavior of the successful resistors: overt identification with the aggressor. This behavior was evident in some of the young Army and Marine prisoners who were reported to have collaborated to some extent. But the fliers mainly report a contempt for their captors, and no admiration for them or imitation of them in the camp environment is apparent. There were only rare acts of kindness by individual guards, and only one report approaching an empathy between a flier and his interrogator. After the 1969 improvement in camp conditions, when torture was abandoned as a common policy, one of the chief torturers and interrogators asked a senior POW to meet with a delegation visiting from the United States. When he refused, the Vietnamese pleaded with him, appealing to him as a comrade in arms with whom he had shared many experiences in the previous 4.5 years. For a moment, the American thought that his former tormentor was going to put his arm around his shoulder in a gesture of comradeship. Do torturers identify with those who successfully resist them?

Conclusion

I have examined some of the factors that sustained the returned POWs, as reported in books by and about them. These factors range from more abstract and external sets of rules through more concrete, immediate loyalty to fellow POWs to an internal sense of honor and self-esteem. These men do not claim to speak for the entire group, but I suspect that they do speak for the majority of the "early shootdowns," the pre-1969 group whose captivity spanned 5 years or more. Had they not had mature coping skills, I suspect that today we would be more involved in discussing their loss of identity, their depression, their guilt or, indeed, their failure to survive. These skills have been pointed out in another context by Vaillant[8]: a healthy and continuing sense of humor, the sublimation of opportunities for personal comfort in the service of a greater cause, the ability to anticipate and tolerate extremes of stress in order to maintain a sense of self-esteem and integrity, and an awareness of continuing service to their country.

References

1. Risner, R. *The passing of the night.* New York: Random House, 1973.
2. Rowe, J. N. *Five years to freedom.* Boston: Little, Brown, 1971.
3. Gaither, R. *With God in a POW camp.* Nashville: Broadman Press, 1973.
4. Rowan, S. A. *They wouldn't let us die.* Middle Village, N.Y.: Jonathan David Publishers, 1973.
5. Grant, Z. *Survivors.* New York: Norton, 1975.

6. Hubbell, J. G. *P.O.W.* New York: Reader's Digest Press, 1976.
7. Sledge, W. H., Boydstun, J. A., & Rathe, A. J. Self-concept changes related to war captivity. *Archives of General Psychiatry*, 1980, *37*, 430–443.
8. Vaillant, George E. Theoretical hierarchy of adaptive ego mechanisms. *Archives of General Psychiatry*, 1971, *24*, 107–118.

29

Survivors of the Nazi Holocaust

PAUL CHODOFF

Homo homini lupus . . . man is wolf to man. The bloody chronicles of recorded history have, time and again, demonstrated the truth of this bitter adage but never more clearly than in the treatment of the Jews of Europe in the unrelenting grasp of the German Nazis of the Hitlerian Reich.

The guttering flames and the greasy smoke of Auschwitz have long since ceased to afflict our eyes and nostrils. The melancholy tale of the survivors has reached or is reaching its conclusion as the years pass. Only about 300,000 of them remain alive throughout the world. However, the lingering effects of the Holocaust are still a clinical issue for psychiatrists and mental health workers as the children of the survivors seek help and understanding of the influences which molded them and their families.

The Concentration Camps

The camps, first established by Heinrich Himmler in 1933 for the internment of "enemies of the Reich," including the Jews,

From *Children Today*, 1981, *10*, 2–5. Copyright 1981 by U.S. Government Printing Office.

PAUL CHODOFF • Department of Psychiatry, George Washington University, Washington, D.C. 20037.

followed the Nazi conquests and ultimately formed an extended network throughout the occupied territories, especially in eastern Europe. On January 20, 1942, at a meeting in Wannsee, a suburb of Berlin, and presided over by Himmler, the decision for the "final solution" of the "Jewish question" was reached. Some of the camps (Auschwitz, Treblinka) were designated as extermination camps and were equipped with disguised gas chambers and crematoria; in others (Dachau, Bergen-Belsen, Buchenwald), the killing was somewhat less systematic.

However, the differences among the various categories of camps was only relative. In all of them the conditions were, in the words of the Oxford historian, A. P. J. Taylor, "loathesome beyond belief." In addition to the out-and-out extermination measures, the physical stresses endured by the prisoners included malnutrition, crowding, sleeplessness, exposure, inadequate clothing, forced labor, beatings, injury, torture, exhaustion, various epidemic diseases, medical experimentation, and the effects of the long "death marches" from the camps in the closing days of the war.

The physically depleted state of the prisoners, the brutal and primitive conditions in which they lived, and the entirely inadequate medical facilities were responsible for an extremely high death rate, and they also had the effect of increasing the susceptibility of the inmates to the nonphysical stresses which they had to face. Chief among these latter was the danger to life, ever present and unavoidable. It is possible, to some degree, for a healthy personality to defend itself against a peril which, though very grave, is predictable, and is at least potentially limited in time, as in the case of soldiers in combat who can at least hope for relief and rotation out of the fighting zone. For the concentration camp inmate, however, as has been described by Viktor Frankl drawing on his own experiences in Auschwitz, the absolute uncertainty of his condition was a barrier to the erection of adequate psychological adaptive measures. In addition to the threat to life, the prisoners suffered the catastrophic trauma of separation from their families. To the agonizing fears about their own future were added equally agonizing doubts as to whether, even if they survived, they would ever see their relatives again. The very least price one had to pay to survive in the camps was to suffer the grossest kind of daily humiliation.

Regimented, imprisoned, without a moment of privacy during the 24 hours, the prisoner's human worth and even his sense of an individual human identity was under constant and savage assault. His entire environment was designed to impress upon him his utter, his protoplasmic worthlessness, a worthlessness which had no relationship to what he did, only to what he was. He was debased from individual human status by being identified not by the dignity of a name but only by a number and a badge of a particular color. His ineluctable inferiority was hammered into the prisoner by the SS jailers who needed to justify their own behavior by convincing themselves of the inferior, subhuman status of the Jews in their charge.

A former inmate of Auschwitz, who has also been a patient of mine, has described her experiences. The following excerpt will convey something of the physical and psychological stresses which confronted the concentration camp inmate, as well as a suggestion of the adaptive measures called forth by these stresses.

As I said we had selections every single day—some just slight—just picking people out as I mentioned before because of scars, because of pimples, because of being run-down, because of looking tired or because of having a crooked smile, or because someone just didn't like you. But then they were selected either to go to work or to the crematorium and in this case Dr. Mengele was involved in it.

Anyway, my turn came. I had a choice to make. Not only Mengele had a choice to make: I had. I had to make up my mind: Am I going to follow my mother, or is this it? Am I going to separate from her? The only way I was able to work out the problem was that I was not going to give myself a chance to decide. I will go ahead in front of my mother—that was unusual, she being my mother, out of courtesy I followed her all the time in any other circumstances—but in this case I was going first, and my mother followed me and I went. I think my heart was beating quite fast, not because I was afraid—I knew I would come through—but because I was doing something wrong. I was doing something terribly wrong. Anyway I passed Mengele. I didn't see him. I just passed, and I was sent into the room where I would be kept alive and I turned around and my mother was with me, so this was a very happy ending.

As I said, in the evenings if I had a chance I went over to talk to my

*friend . . . to the fence, to the electric fence, and at each end of the fence they
had the watchtowers where the Nazis were able to observe us . . . just for the
fun of it . . . the girl who was right next to me—I think they just wanted to
see if they could aim well because I don't know why—they shot her right in
the eye, and she lost her eye. Another time another girl was at the same place.
Her friend threw a package of food over to her and she ran towards the
fence to catch it and she touched the wire and there she hung. She looked like
Jesus Christ spread out with her two arms stuck to the wire.*

Adaptive Behavior in the Camps

What enabled a man or woman to survive such a hell? We
have no real answers to this question and must resort to such
generalizations as the almost miraculous and infinite adaptability
of the human species. Varieties of individual defensive and coping behavior which were more or less effective undoubtedly
played a role in whether a prisoner would live or die, but it cannot
be emphasized too strongly that such behavior was far less important than luck, accident and chance—where the prisoner happened to be when a selection for the gas chamber was taking
place, the quota of victims established for that day, the mood of
the selector at the time. However, accounts by survivors do agree
in describing a fairly consistent sequence of reactions to concentration camp life. This sequence was inaugurated by a universal response of shock and terror on arrest and arrival at the camp.
This fright reaction was generally followed by a period of apathy
and, in most cases, by a longer one of mourning and depression.
The apathy was often psychologically protective and may be
thought of as providing a kind of transitional emotional hiberna-
tion. In some cases, however, apathy took over to such an extent
that the prisoner became a "Musselman" and shortly slipped away
to death.

Among those prisoners who continued to struggle for life,
certain measures gradually came to be characteristic of long-term
adjustment. Regressive behavior of a greater or lesser degree was
almost universal, being induced in the prisoners by the overwhelming infantilizing pressures to which they were subjected
and by the need to stifle aggressive impulses.

It appears that the most important personality defenses among concentration camp inmates were denial and isolation of affect. Some form of companionship with others was indispensible, since a completely isolated individual could not have survived in the camps, but the depth of such companionship was usually limited by the overpowering egotistical demands of self-preservation except in certain political and religious groups.

The Postliberation Period

As soon after the end of the war and liberation as recovery of some measure of physical health permitted, most survivors of the concentration camps, as well as those individuals who had managed to evade capture during the war by an "on-the-run" existence, made their way back to their homes desperately eager for information about their relatives. More often than not their worst fears were confirmed; they found their homes destroyed or unavailable, and their communities substantially wiped out. Such frustrating aspects of postliberation reality were powerful factors in the inevitable disruption of the rosy fantasies about postwar life which had proliferated during imprisonment. A large number of the liberated prisoners, homeless, alone, bewildered and without resources, took refuge in the DP camps that were set up in various parts of Europe, and in some cases remained in them for years.

As the immediate postwar epoch drew to a close, the surviving remnant of concentration camp prisoners gradually settled themselves in more or less permanent abodes in their own countries of origin or in other lands, especially in the United States and Israel. For this latter group, to the multiple traumata they had endured was added the need to adjust to a new environment, new customs, and a different language.

Long-Term Effects

At this point one might expect the grisly story to come to an end for most of the survivors, with the passage of time allowing the gradual envelopment of their fears and memories in psychic scar tissue. This is not what happened.

In the late 1950s and early 1960s articles began to appear in the medical literature of many countries describing features of personality disorders and psychiatric illness still present many years later in a large number of these individuals, in some cases cropping up after latent periods of up to several years after the persecution. Even in those individuals who have not sought psychiatric treatment or evaluation and who appear on superficial examination to be well, a more careful scrutiny reveals evidence that very few of them were unaffected. For instance, in a Scandinavian report of 130 patients who were believed to have shown no aftereffects of the concentration camp experience, closer observation revealed that not a single person failed to show some psychopathology. Likewise, the life adjustment of 60 survivors in California who appeared to have made successful adaptations was found to have been attained at a considerable psychic cost.

Although it is not difficult to understand why people who have had this kind of experience would be chronically or episodically depressed, it remains unexplained why the depression of concentration camp survivors is so often tinged by feelings of guilt either openly verbalized or easily to be inferred from their behavior. Here we are dealing with a special case of the phenomenon of "survivor guilt" which also occurs in so many other settings. Its frequency among concentration camp survivors varies in different discussions of the subject; it has been put as high as 92% in one study. Survivor guilt, however, is not a unitary phenomenon. Concentration camp survivors may feel guilty because of specific actions on their part which endangered the lives and welfare of others or which they interpreted as having this effect. Mrs. S.'s behavior in getting into the selection line ahead of her mother is one example. Another is the guilty preoccupation of a survivor who berated herself for having appropriated the clothes of another woman who had died as her own were falling off.

There are other guilty feelings which are not related to particular misdeeds, fancied or real, but which are experienced as a nonspecific, vague, and pervasive conviction of having done something wrong and shameful even though this feeling cannot be attached to a remembered episode. Finally, there is that species of survivor guilt relating to the very fact that they remained alive when so many others died. This variety of survivor guilt is sometimes linked with expressions of wonderment and incredulity about the vastness of the human tragedy in which the individual had been engulfed and about the capacity of humans to behave toward other humans in so savage a manner.

Concentration Camp Syndrome

The essential features of the concentration camp syndrome include a core of anxiety complicated by various admixtures of symptomatic defenses against anxiety, an obsessive-ruminative state, psychosomatic symptoms, depression, and guilt. While the syndrome resembles in some respects the ordinary combat stress reaction, a more interesting analogy is the Japanese A-bomb disease or neurosis described by Robert J. Lifton in survivors of the Hiroshima bombing, who for many years afterward suffered from vague and chronic complaints of fatigue, nervousness, weakness and various physical ailments, along with characterological changes and feelings of "existential" guilt.

There is, of course, no question but that the primary cause of the psychiatric sequelae of the Nazi persecution, including the concentration camp syndrome, is the multiple, massive emotional and physical traumata to which the survivors were subjected. The survivors also encountered a whole series of environmental stresses even after their liberation, and these must be taken into account in attempting to understand the ultimate adaptive or symptomatic outcome in each case.

My encounters with more than 200 survivors of the Holocaust have left me not completely satisfied that their depression and guilt can be explained entirely by the usual combination of precipitating stress and morbid predisposition which psychiatrists invoke to explain such symptoms. Perhaps this is because the immense scale of the tragedy in which these survivors were enmeshed seems to render the ordinary language of psychopathology inadequate. The stubborn, even prideful refusal to forget displayed by certain survivors seems to involve something beyond masochistic personality mechanisms or a revival of past, incompletely resolved emotional conflicts. Instead, this refusal suggests a desperate attempt to preserve the memories of their murdered dead from the limbo of insignificance to which they have been consigned because of the bureaucratic, almost casual manner of their destruction. By remembering and continuing to remember, they cast a benison of meaningfulness on that destruction.

There is an ancient Talmudic legend of the Lamed-Vov, the 36 just men who take upon themselves the sufferings of the world. Perhaps those concentration camp survivors who ceaselessly lament the past are performing a similar function. Perhaps their sufferings can be thought of both as memorial to their dead and as an act of existential expiation for a species capable of such an outrage upon a common humanness.

Author Index

Subject Index

Retirement (*cont.*)
  marital problems and, 182–183, 216–219
"Role-cycling," 106

Self-esteem, 59–60, 141, 186, 192–193, 334, 355–356, 378, 401, 403
Self-concept, 12–13
  changes in the bereaved, 221
  changes in divorced women, 139, 141–142, 155–163
  of Prisoners of war, 402
  of Vietnam veterans, 389
Self-help groups, 16, 24–25, 291
Self-image. *See* Self-concept
Separation. *See* Divorce
"Separation distress," 140, 145
Single-parent families
  children's added responsibilities, 60–61, 66–71
  parent-child relationships, 60–61, 66–70, 156–157, 159
  low-income parents, 141, 155–163
  See also Divorce
Society of Compassionate Friends, 76, 242
Stepfamilies, 143, 165–166
  developmental phases and tasks, 167–175
  scapegoating within, 169–175
  See also Remarriage
Stepfamily Association of America, 143
Stockholm syndrome, 335, 371, 374
Survivor guilt, 290–291, 326, 382, 412–414. *See also* Death guilt

Terrorism, 334–335
  See also Hostages; Kidnapping

Thoughts, intrusive, 377–378, 385–387
Three Mile Island, 289, 291

"Uncoupled identity," 222

Veterans, Vietnam, 377–378
  dysfunctional responses, 391–393
  flashbacks and, 385–387
  intrusive thoughts, 377–378, 385–387, 390–394
  search for meaning, 387–394
  tasks of, 377–378
Victimization. *See* Victims
Victims, 331–335
  of burglary, 334
  coping, 332–334
  of disasters, 289–292, 297–298, 308–320
  families of, 331–332
  of incest, 258
  of kidnapping, 337–350
  of rape, 333–334, 353–364
  stages of reactions, 331
  of terrorism, 334–335, 367–375
Violence. *See* Kidnapping; Rape; Terrorism

War
  impact on soldiers, 377–381
  Vietnam, 377, 388–389
  See also Prisoners of war; Veterans
Widows
  a personal account by, 227–234
  tasks of, 221–222

DATE DUE